Research Methods
in Occupational Epidemiology

Monographs in Epidemiology and Biostatistics
edited by Brian MacMahon

Monographs in Epidemiology and Biostatistics

Volume 13

Research Methods in Occupational Epidemiology

Harvey Checkoway

University of Washington
School of Public Health and Community Medicine
Department of Environmental Health
Seattle, Washington

Neil Pearce

Wellington School of Medicine
Department of Community Health
Wellington, New Zealand

Douglas J. Crawford-Brown

University of North Carolina
School of Public Health
Department of Environmental Sciences and Engineering
Chapel Hill, North Carolina

New York   Oxford
OXFORD UNIVERSITY PRESS
1989

Oxford University Press

Oxford   New York   Toronto
Delhi   Bombay   Calcutta   Madras   Karachi
Petaling Jaya   Singapore   Hong Kong   Tokyo
Nairobi   Dar es Salaam   Cape Town
Melbourne   Auckland

and associated companies in
Berlin   Ibadan

Copyright © 1989 by Oxford University Press, Inc.

Published by Oxford University Press, Inc.,
200 Madison Avenue, New York, New York 10016

Oxford is a registered trademark of Oxford University Press

Library of Congress Cataloging-in-Publication Data

Checkoway, Harvey.
  Research methods in occupational epidemiology.

  (Monographs in epidemiology and biostatistics ; v. 13)
  Includes bibliographies and index.
  1. Occupational diseases—Epidemiology.   I. Pearce,
Neil E.   II. Crawford-Brown, Douglas J.   III. Title.
IV. Series. [DNLM: 1. Epidemiologic Methods.
2. Occupational Diseases—epidemiology.
W1 MO567LT v.13 / WA 400 C514r]
RC964.C42   1989   616.9′803′072   89-3255
ISBN 0-19-505224-2

9 8 7 6 5 4 3

Printed in the United States of America
on acid-free paper

To Anne, Lynette, and K. B.

Preface

Occupational epidemiology has emerged as a distinct subdiscipline within the general fields of epidemiology and occupational medicine during the past several decades. The impetus for this development has been an increasing awareness by practitioners of occupational epidemiology of the need to apply rigorous research methods to the study of the frequency and causes of work-related diseases and injuries. Moreover, the emergence of occupational epidemiology has been accompanied by a broadened scope of injury. Observations by workers and physicians of the occurrence of illness characteristic to certain occupational groups, such as debilitating lung diseases among underground miners, historically have motivated efforts by epidemiologists to estimate the extent of the problem and to identify causative factors. Such efforts continue to be important and necessary. Increasingly, occupational epidemiologists are addressing fundamental public health and scientific questions relating to the specification of exposure–response relationships, assessment of the adequacy of occupational exposure guidelines and extrapolation of hazardous effects to other occupational and nonoccupational settings. Fortunately, methodological advances in epidemiology and in the related sciences of toxicology, industrial hygiene, health physics, and biostatistics can facilitate research into these complex issues.

Our intent in writing this book is to synthesize the principles and methods that are used in occupational epidemiology. The principles and methods that are described and illustrated in the book are derived from general epidemiology and from the aforementioned ancillary disciplines; it is the synthesis of methods from these fields, as much as the substantive focus on health consequences of workplace exposures, that makes occupational epidemiology distinctive among other branches of epidemiology.

The book is divided into two main sections. The first section (Chapters 1–7) contains material on the historical development of occupational epidemiology, approaches for characterizing workplace exposures, and methods for designing and implementing epidemiologic studies. We describe the types and sources of health and exposure data required for epidemiologic studies and illustrate the features of the various study designs and suitable methods for statistical data analysis. The relative advantages and limitations of the different study design options, as they pertain to the investigation of particular health outcomes, are important, and often debatable, issues in occupational epidemiology. Accordingly, we emphasize this topic in the discussion throughout the book. We consider the first section of the book as a practical handbook for the design, implementation, and interpretation of research. Thus, this material should be suitable for epidemiologists, industrial hygienists, industrial medical officers, and others engaged in the practice of occupational health. Chapters 1–7 also contain theoretical discussions regarding study design, research validity, and data analysis; therefore, they should be useful teaching materials for introductory and intermediate courses in occupational epidemiology.

The second section of the book (Chapters 8–10) is devoted to more advanced topics. Here we elaborate on statistical techniques that can be applied to complex data configurations that arise in many occupational studies. Also contained in this section of the book are approaches for estimating doses to biological targets, where the methods described incorporate pharmacokinetic and metabolic models of exposure and effect. Chapters 8 and 9 were written to assist the epidemiologist who is confronted with the task of estimating dose–response relationships for exposures that may occur in complex temporal patterns. Chapter 10 presents some special applications of data derived from occupational epidemiology research. The discussion focuses on disease modeling (e.g., multistage models of carcinogenesis) and methods used in risk assessment. Risk assessment is gaining popularity in epidemiology because regulatory agencies increasingly are relying on data from occupational epidemiology studies as bases for environmental protection. We attempt to indicate the most desirable situations for successful risk assessment while highlighting the uncertainties that are inherent in this type of exercise. The second section of the book will likely be most appreciated by readers who already are familiar with occupational epidemiology methods and can therefore be used in advanced courses or seminars.

We should also point out what this book is not. We have not attempted to compile a systematic review of occupational diseases and associated risk factors. Readers are encouraged to consult available texts and scientific journal publications on occupational medicine and toxicology that are devoted to summarizing knowledge in these areas. We do, however, illustrate epidemiologic principles and methods with many real examples taken from the published literature, with the content spanning a range from acute toxicity resulting from chemical exposures to models of carcinogenesis. Likewise, our presentation of statistical and biomathematical modeling techniques is not intended to be a comprehensive review. Instead, we have focused on methods that we judge to be most informative and practical for common use.

Our interest in writing a textbook on occupational epidemiology developed as the scientific and practical problems encountered in our own research stimulated efforts to master existing methods and derive new and modified approaches. We hope that this book provides similar impetus to other researchers.

Acknowledgments

We are appreciative to the following colleagues who reviewed earlier drafts of this book and provided many helpful comments that improved the final product: Pier Bertazzi, Steve Blum, Chantal Brisson, Elizabeth Delzell, John Dement, Sander Greenland, Robert Harris, John Hickey, Stephan Lanes, Enzo Merler, Charles Poole, Carol Rice, James Robins, Kenneth Rothman, David Savitz, Carl Shy, Leslie Stayner, Walter Stewart, Duncan Thomas, Michel Vanhoorne, David Wegman, Noel Weiss, and Tim Wilcosky. Special thanks are extended to Sander Greenland, David Savitz, and David Wegman for reviewing the entire book and providing detailed, critical, and constructive comments.

We are grateful to John Dement for permitting access to data from his cohort study of workers in the asbestos textile industry and to David Brown from the U.S. National Institute for Occupational Safety and Health for providing these data to us.

Melinda Fujiwara's expert manuscript preparation and patience are greatly appreciated.

Seattle   H. C.
Wellington   N. P.
Chapel Hill   D.J.C-B.

Contents

4. Issues of Study Design and Analysis, 72

5. Cohort Studies, 103

6. Case–Control Studies, 170

Research Methods
in Occupational Epidemiology

1 Introduction

1. OVERVIEW

Epidemiology can be subdivided on two axes; subdisciplines, such as cardiovascular or infectious disease epidemiology, are oriented toward the disease outcomes, whereas others are oriented toward the study of causative exposures. Occupational epidemiology is the study of the effects of workplace exposures on the frequency and distribution of diseases and injuries in the population, and thus falls into the latter category of exposure-oriented subdisciplines. However, there is considerable overlap between the substantive concerns of various subdisciplines. For example, life-style and behavioral risk factors are important determinants of some diseases that also have occupational etiologies and therefore require consideration in occupational epidemiology research. Moreover, the methods used in occupational epidemiology are conceptually identical to those used in the study of diseases unrelated to occupational factors. For example, an epidemiologist studying the occurrence of respiratory disease symptoms among factory workers following an acute accidental exposure to an industrial chemical adopts investigative techniques familiar to the epidemiologist studying a food-borne epidemic of enteric illness. Similar parallels can be drawn for research methods used in studies of delayed effects of chronic exposures. In fact, some of the epidemiologic, statistical, and toxicologic techniques that have become standard methods in their respective fields were initially motivated by research needs in occupational health.

There are specific features of occupational epidemiology that differ from other areas of general epidemiology. Some diseases and their associated risk factors rarely, if ever, occur in nonoccupational settings. The pneumoconioses, such as silicosis or asbestosis, for example, are seen only among workers exposed to the causative dusts. Also, the study of the health of worker populations requires an appreciation of the peculiarities of occupational groups, such as generally favorable health profiles of workers relative to those of the

3

population at large, and an awareness of the data sources and their limitations for estimating occupational exposure levels.

2. HISTORICAL BACKGROUND

2.1. Recognition of Occupational Diseases

Concerns about adverse health consequences of hazardous occupational exposures date back to Hippocrates' warnings to physicians to explore patients' environmental, life-style, and vocational backgrounds as determinants of etiology and treatment (Lilienfeld and Lilienfeld, 1980). The Italian physician Bernardino Ramazzini is often acknowledged as the father of occupational medicine. Ramazzini described a number of occupational diseases and their causes in his book *De Morbis Artificum,* which was published in 1700 (Wright, 1964). Included among his presentations are descriptions of ocular disorders among glassblowers and neurologic toxicity among tradesmen exposed to lead and mercury.

The recognition of occupational hazards quite often has been prompted by anecdotal reports of debilitating and fatal conditions occurring preferentially among workers in certain types of jobs. A few historical examples, out of literally hundreds, serve to illustrate the development of occupational epidemiology.

Pneumoconiosis among miners of gold and silver in Joachimsthal and Schneeberg in the Erz Mountains at the border of Germany and Czechoslovakia is a good place to start. Premature mortality among these miners was reported by Agricola in the sixteenth century. The prevailing view at the time was that the miners' disease was a form of consumptive lung disease (Rom, 1983). In 1879 Hessing and Hartung recognized that underground metal miners were experiencing seemingly excessive rates of respiratory cancers (Hunter, 1978). In the 1930s mortality surveys revealed that nearly half of the miners' deaths were due to lung cancer and roughly 25 percent were due· to nonmalignant respiratory diseases (Pirchan and Sikl, 1932; Peller, 1939). The causative agent for lung cancer was subsequently identified as ionizing radiation (radon daughters) emanating from uranium and radium deposits in these mines (Lorenz, 1944). Since then numerous epidemiologic studies of underground metal miners in Europe and North America have documented dose–response relationships for radiation and lung cancer (Radford and Renard, 1984).

Percival Pott (1775), who identified soot as the cause of scrotal cancer in London chimney sweeps, is credited with providing the first clearcut evidence of chemical carcinogenesis from an occupational exposure. Pott's detailed descriptions of the abysmal working conditions of these young boys, who frequently climbed in the nude up narrow, sharp-angled chimneys that at times were still hot, stimulated social concerns. Reports of fires in chimneys delayed until 1840 passage of legislation prohibiting young boys from climbing up chimneys (Waldron, 1983). The carcinogenic potential of coal tar products was noted in diverse industries by the end of the nineteenth century, and an experimental model of soot carcinogenesis was first demonstrated in the 1920s (Decoufle, 1982).

The recognition of asbestos-related disease occupies an important place in the history of occupational epidemiology. Asbestos had been used for various artistic and ritualistic purposes for centuries before it was exploited on a broad industrial scale. Pottery containing asbestos dating from 2500 B.C. found in Finland and Herodotus' descriptions from 456 B.C. of the use of asbestos cloth to preserve ashes of the dead during cremation attest to its long history (Lee and Selikoff, 1979). Major industrial use of asbestos began following the discovery of large deposits in Canada, South Africa, and Italy during the last half of the nineteenth century. In 1907 Murray described a case of pulmonary fibrosis, detected at autopsy, in a British textile worker (Murray, 1907). The term *asbestosis* was first used by Cooke in 1927. Intensive investigations of the magnitude of asbestosis prevalence among exposed workers followed in the 1930s in the United Kingdom (Merewether and Price, 1930) and the United States (Dreesen et al., 1938). Fatal and nonfatal forms of asbestosis have subsequently been recognized in many exposed worker populations (Becklake, 1982). Seemingly excessive prevalences of lung cancer among asbestotics suggested a possible carcinogenic effect of asbestos fibers (Lee and Selikoff, 1979); these suspicions have received ample confirmation since the 1950s.

Studies of the mortality patterns of asbestos insulation workers by Selikoff and his colleagues during the 1960s and 1970s contributed greatly to the recognition of diseases related to asbestos exposure (Selikoff et al., 1964; 1979). Malignant mesothelioma of the pleura or peritoneum, first identified in 1960 (Wagner et al., 1960), has not been associated consistently with any other environmental agent (Craighead and Mossman, 1982). In fact, the association of malignant mesothelioma with occupational asbestos exposure is often cited as one of the most persuasive epidemiologic examples of an unambiguous demonstration of causality.

Alice Hamilton's 1925 book *Industrial Poisons in the United States* depicted a variety of occupational diseases, ranging from solvent-induced narcosis to "phossy jaw" among matchmakers exposed to phosphorus. Her work stimulated other physicians' concerns about health hazards in uncontrolled workplaces. The following excerpt from Adelaide Ross Smith's 1928 account of the work conditions encountered by women workers exposed to benzene in a small sanitary tin can factory in New York State is a vivid example:

> There was no direct ventilation of coated can covers. They emerged from the machine immediately after coating without having been heated and smelling directly of benzol. . . . The eight coating machines consumed 45 to 50 gallons daily of a compound containing 75 percent of benzol. Adjoining the coating room and connected with it by a wide-open doorway was another room where paper gaskets were made . . . [A twenty-six-year-old woman] was employed for some months in the room adjoining the coating machines. She had always been well and was not bothered by the work until she became pregnant. Then she suffered from severe nausea and vomiting. . . . Severe and prolonged nosebleeds were followed by bleeding from the gums and rectum and into the skin. She stopped work and improved. . . . A premature child was born at seven months and three hours after delivery the mother died following severe uterine hemorrhage.

This example is pertinent to contemporary occupational epidemiology for several reasons. The workplaces studied were small factories, where excessive exposures and adverse health sequelae continue to be underrecognized. Moreover, risks to women workers, especially those related to reproduction, increasingly have occupied the attention of epidemiologists.

2.2. Development of Systematic Epidemiologic Methods

Investigations of characteristic occupationally related diseases that are rare in the general population provided the impetus for epidemiologic research into workplace hazards. In the 1950s several important studies contributed to the methodology for studying less rare conditions. Studies such as those of lung cancer among gas workers (Doll, 1952) and bladder cancer among dyestuff factory workers (Case et al., 1954; Mancuso and Coulter, 1959) laid the groundwork for the historical cohort design that has since become a standard approach in occupational epidemiology (Gardner, 1986).

The history of occupationally related bladder cancer illustrates the development of the field. A specific occupational etiology for bladder cancer was first suggested by 1895 by the German surgeon Ludwig Rehn, who observed three cases among workers from a fuchsin dye factory. Bladder cancer was a recognized clinical entity at the time, but the occurrence of these three cases in a small worker population later proved to be excessive (Cole and Goldman, 1975). The misnomer *aniline cancers* was applied to these tumors for some years until the specific etiologic aromatic amine compounds were identified. Experimental research in the 1930s on industrial aromatic amines established beta-naphthylamine as a potent carcinogen (Hueper, 1938). In the 1950s Case and associates (1954) investigated the risk for bladder cancer among workers from 21 chemical factories in England and Wales. They observed bladder cancer rates 30 times higher among workers exposed to beta-naphthylamine, alpha-naphthylamine, benzidine, or a mixture of these chemicals. Case's findings indicated that beta-naphthylamine was the most potent human carcinogen. As a direct consequence of Case's report, and abetted by advances in diagnostic techniques, a bladder cancer cytodiagnosis and screening program was established in 1957 to serve the rubber industry in Birmingham (Parkes, 1969). Case's study also revealed that bladder cancers occurred, on average, 15–20 years after first exposure to these carcinogens. A prolonged period of induction and latency for occupational carcinogenesis is now a widely appreciated phenomenon (Armenian and Lilienfeld, 1974; Whittemore, 1977).

Numerous subsequent epidemiologic studies have confirmed Case's reports of aromatic amine carcinogenicity (Hueper, 1969). Some noteworthy and dramatic examples are reports of bladder cancer incidence risks ranging from 10 to 50 percent among workers exposed to beta-naphthylamine or benzidine (Goldwater et al., 1965; Veys, 1969; Wendel et al., 1974). Since the identification and, in some instances, prohibition of production and use of various industrial aromatic amine carcinogens, there have been vigorous efforts directed toward medical surveillance of workers with known current or past exposures (Schulte, 1986; Meigs et al., 1986).

3. SCOPE OF OCCUPATIONAL EPIDEMIOLOGY

The emergence of occupational epidemiology has followed the same course as that of other epidemiology subdisciplines; clinical observations of the occurrence of rare diseases among small groups have motivated methodological advancements that can accommodate investigations of both rare and more common health effects in large populations. Research has generally proceeded from small-scale investigations to studies of large populations of workers, often numbering in the thousands and tens of thousands of workers. Cohort studies of the mortality patterns among U.S. steelworkers (Lloyd and Ciocco, 1969; Redmond et al., 1975) and rubber industry workers in the United States (McMichael et al., 1976; Monson and Nakano, 1976) and England (Baxter and Werner, 1980) are important examples of epidemiologic studies of large industrial populations.

Despite the shift in emphasis from the study of characteristic occupational diseases to investigations of broader worker health profiles, the underlying objectives have remained constant. The first objectives are to determine the health consequences of workplace exposures and to make or recommend remedial efforts when indicated. Secondarily, occupational epidemiology provides data useful for making future projections of risks to other workers and, more generally, to members of the population at large who typically experience lower-intensity exposures than occur in the workplace. Future projection and risk extrapolation are usually termed *risk assessment*. Thus, there are both public health and scientific motivations for conducting research in occupational epidemiology. The immediate public concerns obviously focus on the protection of worker health. The identification of occupational causes of diseases provides the necessary information for setting occupational (and in some cases, nonoccupational) exposure standards so as to reduce risks to "acceptable levels." Problems of a more scientific nature, such as elucidating mechanisms of toxicity and dose–response relationships, can also be addressed in occupational epidemiology. The public health and scientific domains are by no means mutually exclusive, however, as both require observations of human health effects and measurements of exposures, and in some instances, both involve extrapolation of findings to other environments and populations. Furthermore, public health measures can be adopted with more confidence when there is a clear understanding of etiologic processes.

Exposure standard setting is a good example of the application of occupational epidemiology research findings to address both public health and scientific questions. Such findings are frequently used to set exposure limits below which adverse health effects are predicted to be minimal or nonexistent. Estimation of exposure standards involves assumptions about disease induction mechanisms and predictions of dose–response relationships that are best inferred from observations made on exposed human populations.

3.1. Identifying Occupational Hazards and Populations at Risk

Occupational epidemiology involves investigating the frequency of occurrence and causal factors for health effects that have nonoccupational as well as potential occupational etiologies. Lung cancer, for example, can be induced by occupational and nonoccupational exposures; in fact, in all industrialized countries the predominant risk factor for lung cancer is cigarette smoking, not occupational exposures. The practice of occupational epidemiology becomes increasingly complex when the diseases of interest are delayed effects of exposure that become manifest many years after first exposure, or when the health outcomes are subtle physiologic responses rather than overt diseases.

Several decision-making routes can determine which occupational health problems are studied. As the foregoing historical examples illustrate, a recognition of disease clusters among workers from particular occupations or industries can instigate epidemiologic research to identify causal factors. The investigations that ensue may be tightly circumscribed to the particular health problem at hand or may, depending on available resources and interest, burgeon into broader surveys of worker health. For example, the occurrence of aplastic anemia and other less severe forms of hematologic dysfunction among workers exposed to organic solvents at a factory might trigger a clinical and industrial hygiene survey to estimate the magnitude of the problem in relation to measured environmental concentrations of solvents. Knowledge of other consequences of exposures to solvents, such as neurotoxicity and leukemia, indicates the value of enlarging the scope of the study to include an assessment of risks for these conditions.

Findings from other disciplines can also provide direction to research in occupational epidemiology. A typical situation arises when a substance is shown to be carcinogenic in animals or mutagenic in cell culture assays. The logical next question is whether the substance displays similar effects in humans. Occupational groups exposed to the substance in question then become useful target populations for study because workplace exposures are generally greater than those occurring elsewhere. Governmental agencies often adopt this strategy for deciding which research areas to pursue. The principal limiting factor is the identification of an exposed worker population that is suitable for study. Research efforts often are complicated when the substance of concern is ubiquitous in the ambient environment and high-intensity workplace exposures occur only intermittently among small groups of workers who may also encounter other toxic substances. These difficulties have hindered epidemiologic studies of the possible carcinogenic effects of formaldehyde (Hernberg et al., 1983; Hayes et al., 1986), which were motivated by reports of cancer induction in laboratory animals (Swenberg et al., 1980).

Alternatively, one may choose to study workers exposed to a substance(s) that has never received attention as a potential toxin in either human or animal studies. Studies initiated on this basis are uncommon, regrettably, because funding agencies tend to discourage proposed research where no prior evidence of health significance exists.

Prior epidemiologic research can be a reasonable guide for directing planned investigations. Excessive disease rates among workers exposed to high intensities of certain substances can suggest the utility of investigating similar effects among workers who encounter low-level exposures. This approach to research planning is especially justifiable when the investigators purport to characterize exposure thresholds and other components of dose–response relationships. For example, reports of benzene-induced leukemia among workers in Turkish shoe factories (Aksoy et al., 1962) have provided the impetus for numerous epidemiologic studies of other industries where benzene occurs at lower intensities (Thorpe, 1974; Infante et al., 1977; Arp et al., 1983; Rinsky et al., 1987).

Investigative leads sometimes emerge from epidemiologic studies in which occupational risk factors are not the primary focus. Geographical patterns of disease rates and their correlations with the locations of various industries can sometimes indicate occupational hazards. "Ecologic" correlation surveys of this type prove to be most informative when the disease(s) is specifically related to a clearly identifiable occupational exposure, such as malignant mesothelioma and asbestos. Epidemiologic studies in which information concerning occupational exposures is obtained, even when these data are secondary to the main research questions, can also guide research. Efforts to screen hypotheses about occupational risk factors as contributors to the disease burden in the general population are enhanced when the collection of occupational data becomes routinely incorporated into population-based epidemiologic studies. Case–control studies of cancer conducted among patients from hospitals or disease registers are well suited to this approach (Siemiatycki et al., 1986). However, the need to avoid false positive associations resulting from a large number of factors studied without a priori evidence may complicate the analysis and interpretation of such studies (Thomas et al., 1985).

In some situations an epidemiologic study is undertaken as a means of assessing the health of workers with common exposures, such as trade union members or workers at the same company. Medical surveillance may be initiated in response to perceived health hazards or as a way of alerting workers and management to possible risks. Generally, surveillance studies encompass a wide range of health outcomes and tend to provide more descriptive data on baseline health characteristics than are obtained from studies focused on the etiologies of specific diseases. An efficient strategy for conducting worker health surveillance is to combine the program with ongoing environmental and biological monitoring surveys, such as those performed routinely to assure compliance with governmentally imposed exposure standards. Medical surveillance is most effectively conducted prospectively, although retrospective designs wherein past health events are linked to occupational exposures can also be used. Research into occupational causes of pregnancy loss among female workers is one area where prospective surveillance is particularly valuable (Wilcox, 1983).

In every case, no matter how pressing a scientific or public health issue may appear, the success of an occupational epidemiology study will depend on access to worker populations, and hence on the availability of data. The forces that dictate data access are frequently out of the investigator's control. Studies may be initiated at the request of companies or unions that can provide access to data, thus simplifying the epidemiologist's task. However, one may be forced to forgo genuinely interesting research projects when access to data is denied. This dilemma is by no means unique to occupational epidemiology.

3.2. Estimation of Effects

Occupational epidemiology, like all research sciences, involves estimating the magnitude of effect in the affected population. This effect estimate may then be extrapolated to predicted magnitudes of effects in other populations (i.e., risk assessment). A second use of the effect estimate is to evaluate (or "test") previously developed etiologic hypotheses. Some ("hypothesis testing") studies concentrate on one or, at most, several hypotheses for which prior evidence of causation is relatively strong. Other ("hypothesis screening") studies may evaluate a large number of hypotheses for which prior evidence is relatively weak, in order to identify hypotheses that merit further investigation.

For example, relative risks for some 30–50 different diseases may be estimated in one cohort study. Some of these may agree or disagree with prior expectations; others may lead to unprecedented findings. The hypothesis testing purist would be concerned only with those findings for which prior data and theory provide insight and would ignore all other findings. The epidemiologist with more liberal hypothesis screening tendencies would accept all findings as potentially valid, citing the importance of the current results as guideposts for further inquiry.

It is important to realize that hypotheses can seldom be tested definitively in an epidemiologic study because the research settings cannot be replicated closely. (Arguments about the observational versus experimental nature of epidemiology are moot here because occupational epidemiology nearly always requires observational research.) However, this is not to say that hypotheses cannot be formulated and evaluated against observations. Both the populations to be studied and the end points chosen for consideration are directly determined by prior expectations, hunches, and implicit predictions (i.e., hypotheses). Moreover, all hypotheses and their theoretical underpinnings are ultimately derived from and modified by observations.

In practice, then, the investigator, armed with a working knowledge of prior findings from epidemiologic and experimental research, is naturally attentive to the most relevant findings from his own study and draws conclusions in light of prior expectation. In addition, it is worthwhile to examine the data for other associations and to report the results accordingly. A balanced presentation of the findings includes a clear delineation of the results that relate to prior evidence and those that are unanticipated or lack corroboration.

A related issue concerns the role of statistical significance testing and the presentation of probability statements (p-values) denoting the likelihood of chance vis-à-vis reporting the estimates of the likely ranges of results, as exemplified by confidence intervals. Even when a specific hypothesis is under consideration, a decision about causality usually cannot be reached on the basis of a single study. Rather, a hypothesis can only be assessed in light of all available data from the relevant disciplines and theoretical predictions. Some investigators have created considerable confusion by attempting to decide the truth or falsity of a hypothesis with evidence obtained from a single study. This problem is exacerbated when decisions are made mechanically, as occurs when p-values are invoked as bench marks of causality. Both p-values and confidence intervals offer some useful information, although, given the long history in epidemiology of misinterpretation of p-values as distinguishing "significant" from "nonsignificant" findings, it is probably wisest to present confidence intervals if one or the other is to be selected. A refinement of this approach is the use of p-value functions to provide a more comprehensive assessment of the stability of study findings (Poole, 1986).

3.3. Causal Inference

Ultimately, the data derived from occupational epidemiology research are used for decision making. Regulatory agencies rely heavily on epidemiologic data when proposing occupational and nonoccupational exposure limits. Other common uses for these data include predictions about the future occurrence of disease in exposed workers and attribution of risk in cases of litigation.

These decisions require evaluations of the composite of evidence from epidemiologic and other research. An evaluation of scientific evidence can, in a most elemental way, be reduced to a simple question: "Does the exposure(s) cause the disease(s)?" Although this question can seldom be answered conclusively, a tentative answer is usually required for decision making. The issue of causal inference is one that has received considerable attention by epidemiologists. Criteria for causal inference in epidemiology have been developed (Hill, 1965), qualified (Evans, 1978; Weiss, 1981), and discussed in the context of inductive and deductive logic (Maclure, 1985).

Judgments about the value of an occupational epidemiology study are influenced by such factors as the adequacy of study design, the size of the study, the amount and precision of health and exposure data, and the appropriateness of the data analysis. These judgments are necessarily subjective, although research principles do exist that serve as guides. In fact, we devote the greater part of this book to an elaboration of such principles.

Attempts to codify guidelines for assessing research quality are invariably detrimental to the practice and application of epidemiologic methods. To illustrate, consider two studies of cancer among workers exposed to a suspected carcinogen. The first study consists of a case report of two workers with the same type of very rare cancer who both had been employed for 20 years in jobs routinely involving intense exposures to the agent in question. The second study uses a cohort design where 20,000 workers were each followed for 10 or more years. In the second study all that is known about workers' exposures is that the agent had been in the environment at various times, but there is no way to estimate exposure levels or to distinguish heavily exposed workers from those with less exposure. Comparisons with national and regional rates reveal slight excesses of some types of cancer but depressed rates for other cancers among the cohort. Using standard criteria for assessing the adequacy of research design, one would probably conclude that the second study is superior to the first. In fact, the first study does not even satisfy the rudiments of a research design; it can be viewed best as an anecdotal report. By contrast, the second study is large, relative to most epidemiology studies, and uses a well-recognized design. If, in deciding whether the particular agent is a human carcinogen, we rely solely on the evidence from the methodologically more sound second study, we would be forced to conclude that the evidence is equivocal, if not altogether negative. Nevertheless, the first study gives some apparently compelling evidence in support of a carcinogenic effect; there is a specificity of response that follows a prolonged, high level of exposure.

The preceding hypothetical example illustrates the type of ambiguity that can, and often does, arise in occupational epidemiology. Both studies provide incomplete answers to the research question. The best way to mitigate uncertainty in this case would be to seek more information, either by enlarging the first study to include more subjects or by obtaining more exposure data in the second study. It may be necessary to conduct a new study in a third setting if neither study can be improved satisfactorily.

References

Aksoy M, Dincol K, Erdem S, and Dincol G (1962): Acute leukemia due to chronic exposure to benzene. *Am J Med* 52:160–166.

Armenian HK, and Lilienfeld AM (1974): The distribution of incubation periods of neoplastic diseases. *Am J Epidemiol* 99:92–100.

Arp EW, Wolf PH, and Checkoway H (1983): Lymphocytic leukemia and exposures to benzene and other solvents in the rubber industry. *J Occup Med* 25:598–602.

Baxter PJ, and Werner JB (1980): *Mortality in the British Rubber Industries*. London: Her Majesty's Stationery Office.

Becklake MR (1982): Asbestos-related diseases of the lungs and pleura. *Am Rev Respir Dis* 126:187–194.

Case RAM, Hosker ME, McDonald DB, and Pearson JT (1954): Tumours of the urinary bladder in workmen engaged in the manufacture and use of certain dyestuff intermediates in the British chemical industry. Part I. *Br J Ind Med* 11:75–104.

Cole P, and Goldman MB (1975): Occupation. In: Fraumeni JF (ed). *Persons at High Risk of Cancer: An Approach to Cancer Etiology and Control*. New York: Academic Press, pp. 167–184.

Cooke WE, McDonald S, and Oliver T (1927): Pulmonary asbestosis. *Br Med J* 2:1024–1027.

Craighead JE, and Mossman BT (1982): The pathogenesis of asbestos-associated diseases. *N Engl J Med* 306:1446–1455.

Decoufle P (1982): Occupation. In: Schottenfeld D, and Fraumeni JF (eds). *Cancer Epidemiology and Prevention*. Philadelphia: W.B. Saunders, pp. 318–335.

Doll R (1952): The causes of death among gas-workers with special reference to cancer of the lung. *Br J Ind Med* 9:180–185.

Dreesen WC, Dalla Valla JM, and Edwards TI (1938): A study of asbestosis in the asbestos textile industry. *Public Health Bull* No. 241; Washington, D.C.

Evans AS (1978): Causation and disease: a chronological journey. *Am J Epidemiol* 108:249–258.

Gardner MJ (1986): Considerations in the choice of expected numbers for appropriate comparisons in occupational cohort studies. *Med Lav* 77:23–47.

Goldwater LJ, Rosso AJ, and Kleinfeld M (1965): Bladder tumors in a coal tar dye plant. *Arch Environ Health* 11:814–817.

Hamilton A (1925): *Industrial Poisons in the United States*. New York: Macmillan.

Hayes RB, Raatgever JW, deBruyn A, and Gerin M (1986): Cancer of the nasal cavity and paranasal sinuses and formaldehyde exposure. *Int J Cancer* 37:487–492.

Hernberg S, Westerholm, P, Schultz-Larsen K, et al. (1983): Nasal and sinonasal cancers: connections with occupational exposures in Denmark, Finland and Sweden. *Scand J Work Environ Health* 9:315–326.

Hill AB (1965): The environment and disease: association or causation? *Proc R Soc Med* 58:295–300.

Hueper WC (1938): "Aniline tumors" of the bladder. *Arch Pathol* 25:858–899.

Hueper WC (1969): *Occupational and Environmental Cancers of the Urinary System*. New Haven, CT: Yale University Press.

Hunter D (1978): *Diseases of Occupations*, 6th ed. London: Hodder and Stoughton.

Infante PF, Rinsky RA, Wagoner JK, and Young RJ (1977): Leukaemia among workers exposed to benzene. *Lancet* 2:76–78.

Lee DHK, and Selikoff IJ (1979): Historical background to the asbestos problem. *Environ Res* 18:300–314.

Lilienfeld AM, and Lilienfeld DE (1980): *Foundations of Epidemiology*. New York: Oxford University Press.

Lloyd JW, and Ciocco A (1969): Long-term mortality study of steelworkers. I. Methodology. *J Occup Med* 11:299–310.

Lorenz E (1944): Radioactivity and lung cancer: a critical review of lung cancer in the miners of Schneeberg and Joachimsthal. *J Nat Cancer Inst* 5:1–15.

Maclure M (1985): Popperian refutation in epidemiology. *Am J Epidemiol* 121:343–350.

Mancuso TF, and Coulter EJ (1959): Methods of studying the relation of employment and long-term illness in cohort analysis. *Am J Public Health* 49:1525–1536.

McMichael AJ, Andjelkovich DA, and Tyroler HA (1976): Cancer mortality among rubber workers. *Ann NY Acad Sci* 271:125–137.

Meigs JW, Marrett LD, Ulrich FU, and Flannery JT (1986): Bladder tumor incidence among workers exposed to benzidine: a thirty-year follow-up. *J Natl Cancer Inst* 76:1–8.

Merewether ERA, and Price CV (1930): *Report of Effects of Asbestos Dust on the Lungs and Dust Suppression in the Asbestos Industry.* London: Her Majesty's Stationery Office.

Monson RR, and Nakano KK (1976): Mortality among rubber workers. *Am J Epidemiol* 103:284–296.

Murray M (1907): *Report, Department, Commission on Compensation of Industrial Disease.* London: Her Majesty's Stationery Office.

Parkes HG (1969): Epidemiology and etiology of human bladder cancer: occupational bladder cancer in the British rubber industry. *J Natl Cancer Inst* 43:249–252.

Peller S (1939): Lung cancer among miners in Joachmisthal. *Hum Biol* 11:130–143.

Pirchan A, and Sikl H (1932): Cancer of the lung in the miners of Jachymov (Joachmisthal). *Am J Cancer* 15:681–722.

Poole C (1986): Beyond the confidence interval. *Am J Public Health* 77:195–199.

Pott P (1775): *Chirurgical Observations.* London: Hawes, Clarke and Collins.

Radford EP, and Renard KG (1984): Lung cancer in Swedish iron miners exposed to low doses of radon daughters. *N Engl J Med* 310:1485–1494.

Redmond CK, Gustin J, and Kamon E (1975): Long-term mortality experience of steelworkers. VIII. Mortality patterns of open hearth steelworkers (a preliminary report). *J Occup Med* 17:40–43.

Rehn L (1895): Blasengeschwulste bei Fuchsin-Arbeitern. *Arch Klin Chir* 50:588–600.

Rinsky RA, Smith AB, Hornung R, et al. (1987): Benzene and leukemia: an epidemiologic risk assessment. *N Engl J Med* 316:1044–1050.

Rom WN (1983): The discipline of environmental and occupational medicine. In: Rom WN (ed). *Environmental and Occupational Medicine.* Boston: Little, Brown & Co., pp. 3–6.

Schulte PA (1986): Problems in notification and screening of workers at high risk of disease. *J Occup Med* 28:951–957.

Selikoff IJ, Churg J, and Hammond EC (1964): Asbestos exposure and neoplasia. *JAMA* 188:22–26.

Selikoff IJ, Hammond EC, and Seidman H (1979): Mortality experience of insulation workers in the U.S. and Canada. *Ann NY Acad Sci* 330:91–116.

Siemiatycki J, Richardson L, Gerin M, et al. (1986): Associations between several sites of cancer and nine organic dusts: results from an hypothesis-generating case-control study in Montreal, 1979–83. *Am J Epidemiol* 123:235–249.

Smith AR (1928): Chronic benzol poisoning among women industrial workers: A study of women exposed to benzol fumes in six factories. *J Ind Hyg* 10:73–93.

Swenberg JA, Kerns WD, Mitchell RE, et al. (1980): Induction of squamous cell carcinomas of the rat nasal cavity by inhalation exposure to formaldehyde vapor. *Cancer Res* 40:3398–3402.

Thomas DC, Siemiatycki J, Dewar R, et al. (1985): The problem of multiple inference in studies designed to generate hypotheses. *Am J Epidemiol* 122:1080–1095.

Thorpe JJ (1974): Epidemiologic survey of leukemia in persons potentially exposed to benzene. *J Occup Med* 16:375–382.

Veys CA (1969): Two epidemiological inquiries into the incidence of bladder tumors in industrial workers. *J Natl Cancer Inst* 43:219–226.

Wagner JC, Sleggs CA, and Marchand P (1960): Diffuse pleural mesothelioma and asbestos exposure in the North Western Cape Province. *Br J Ind Med* 17:260–271.

Waldron HA (1983): A brief history of scrotal cancer. *Br J Ind Med* 40:390–401.

Weiss NS (1981): Inferring causal relationships: elaboration of the criterion of "dose–response." *Am J Epidemiol* 113:487–490.

Wendel RG, Hoegg UR, and Zavon MR (1974): Benzidine: a bladder carcinogen. *J Urol* 111:607–610.

Whittemore AS (1977): The age distribution of human cancer for carcinogenic exposures of varying intensity. *Am J Epidemiol* 106:418–432.

Wilcox AJ (1983): Surveillance of pregnancy loss in human populations. *Am J Ind Med* 4:285–291.

Wright WC (1964): Translation of: Ramazzini B. *De Morbis Artificum (Diseases of Workers)*. New York: Hafner.

2 Characterizing the Workplace Environment

1. OVERVIEW

The informativeness of an occupational epidemiology study depends in large measure on the amount, specificity, and precision of exposure data. Ideally we would like to be able to measure disease frequency in relation to quantitatively determined levels of exposure that are specific for individual workers. This would allow for estimation of dose–response relationships that can be generalized to other exposure settings. In practice, however, exposure measurement data often are either not available or do not exist because of technological constraints (e.g., assays for particular substances have not been devised) or because of limited resources. Instead, exposure levels usually have to be inferred indirectly from other data. This chapter summarizes some techniques for characterizing occupational exposures. Most emphasis is placed on estimating workers' exposure intensities and durations in an industrial setting. We also discuss procedures for evaluating occupational exposures for community- or registry-based studies, such as a case–control study of a particular disease conducted among hospitalized patients.

2. GENERAL CONCEPTS OF EXPOSURE AND DOSE

Data availability invariably determines the extent to which an occupational environment can be characterized. Before discussing the approaches to exposure assessment, it is worthwhile to review some of the basic concepts of *exposure, burden,* and *dose.* These terms have a wide range of meanings in various fields (pharmacology, epidemiology, risk analysis); therefore, we have chosen definitions that we feel are most useful in epidemiologic research. In this way we can establish a common terminology and place the methods of estimating exposure in context with the ultimate goal of occupational epidemiology—to elucidate the specific circumstances of exposure that result in disease. These topics will be taken up again in Chapter 9, where a more mathematical treatment of these topics is presented.

2.1. Definitions of Exposure and Dose Variables

A useful working definition of *exposure* is the "presence of a substance in the environment external to the worker." Exposure levels are assessed in reference to the intensity of the substance in the workplace environment and the duration of time during which the substance is encountered. Another term for *intensity* is *concentration,* which refers to the amount of the substance per unit of environmental medium (e.g., milligrams of dust per cubic meter of air). Concentration is a dynamic variable because it can change over time, although frequently in occupational epidemiology a single measure, such as the average concentration, is used to depict intensity. To illustrate, consider a worker in a paint manufacturing plant who works in an environment containing 50 parts per million (ppm) of toluene in air at some point in time. We can say that he is exposed to toluene at a concentration of 50 ppm at the time when the measurement is made. If, however, we had no information on the air concentration of toluene at this worker's location, we would still be correct in saying that he is exposed to toluene (assuming, of course, that toluene is present in air in at least detectable concentrations throughout the plant), but our assessment of exposure would only be qualitative.

Insofar as exposure is characterized by concentration and duration, it is possible to construct a time-integrated measure of exposure, known as *cumulative exposure,* which is the summation of the concentrations over time.

Exposure intensity and cumulative exposure both pertain to the environment external to the body. We can define two other terms, *burden* and *dose,* that refer to the amount of a substance that reaches susceptible targets within the body. Burden is the amount of a substance that exists in the body, or more specifically, the target organ or tissues, at a point in time. Burden can be expressed for the entire body or for some particular target, such as an organ.

Like exposure concentration, *burden* is a dynamic measure that changes over time. It is determined by prior cumulative exposure and by the persistence of the substance in the body. *Retention* is the general term used for persistence and is related to the body's ability to absorb, metabolize, and clear environmental agents. As a result, burden is a function of both the temporal pattern of exposure and retention. Burden is usually thought of in the context of exposure to substances, such as dusts or fibers, that remain in solid form for some time and that can lodge in body tissues. The concept also applies to other agents, including volatile chemicals (e.g., vinyl chloride monomer), which have shorter retention times. With many chemicals the notion of clearance encompasses actual physical removal from organs [sometimes resulting in sequestration into storage depots (e.g., adipose tissue in the case of fat-soluble compounds)], detoxification, and normal chemical degradation to other forms. Burden is an important factor in its own right in studies of effects of substances that have relatively long retention times (on the order of years), that remain biologically active in the body, and that, if sequestered, can be mobilized to reach target sites for activity.

The term *dose* has been used to denote various meanings in epidemiologic research, ranging from the amount of material taken into the body to the amount of biologically active material remaining at a critical organ or tissue. We shall define *dose* as the "amount of a substance that remains at the biological target during some specified time interval." Dose thus has two components: the burden and the interval of time that the material is present at the target. The *dose rate* is the analogue of exposure concentration and can change over time. Thus, it is often convenient to consider some summary indicator of dose rate, such as the average or peak, in an epidemiologic analysis.

Dose and dose rate are the variables of greatest scientific value in epidemiologic research; however, in most instances direct measurements of doses or dose rates cannot be made. In some cases it is useful to distinguish dose from the concept of *biologically active dose,* where the latter arises when only some fraction of the burden can produce an effect. Although it is possible to measure tissue levels of some toxins at the sites of biological activity, it is generally impossible to determine the amount that is or has been biologically active. For example, asbestos fibers can be quantified in lung tissue and related to the severity of pulmonary fibrosis (Whitwell et al., 1977; Roggli et al., 1986). These measurements are actually measures of organ burdens, rather than biologically active doses, because of the uncertainty about which fibers were active at the times when the disease process was initiated and, in some cases, exacerbated.

Because of the difficulties in obtaining reliable estimates of burden and dose, occupational epidemiologists often must rely on surrogates: exposure concentration, duration, and cumulative exposure. These variables are useful surrogates for dose, provided that assumptions about their relationships with dose are justifiable. In the simplest case, a linear relationship between cumulative exposure and dose would provide confidence that the former is, in fact, a useful surrogate measure. On the other hand, if the relationship is non-linear, because of complex patterns of absorption, retention, and detoxification, then metabolic models for environmental substances may assist in approximating doses. These topics are discussed further in Chapter 9.

3. TYPES AND SOURCES OF EXPOSURE DATA

Exposure data for occupational studies are obtained from a variety of sources and can be of varying degrees of completeness and accuracy. The following section describes the types and sources of these data, considering first data that are used in an industry-based study and second those obtained from community-based studies, where occupational exposure data are ordinarily less detailed.

3.1. Industry-Based Studies

Identifying Potentially Toxic Substances

The first step in characterizing the environment is to identify the agents that are likely to be toxic. This can be a relatively simple process when the study is motivated by concerns about a limited set of substances of proven toxicity (e.g., asbestos in an asbestos products plant). However, such an identification is complicated in industries where exposures vary greatly by type and intensity and where exposure may be to varying mixtures in which the pertinent chemical forms associated with toxicity are only poorly understood (Ballantyne, 1985). In the latter case, some judgment needs to be exercised in restricting the set of agents for study to those that, based on prior research, are likely to be toxic; that can be measured, or at least localized to various parts of the industrial process; and that occur in measurable concentrations. Such judgments typically require information and opinions from industrial hygienists, health physicists, safety officers, and toxicologists.

At times, symptoms or illness reported to plant medical officers by workers can give direction to the process of toxin identification. For example, reports of chest tightness or phlegm production suggest the importance of identifying pulmonary irritants, whereas reported skin rashes or dermatitis indicate the need to identify irritating or sensitizing chemicals that are handled. However, many substances, including some carcinogens, may not induce symptoms of early disease in either the ultimate target organs or other organs. Ionizing radiation is one such agent. Thus, complaints of illness should not serve as the only guide for environmental characterization.

The second step in characterizing the environment is to establish the most relevant routes of exposure for the agents of concern. Here again input from the previously mentioned ancillary disciplines is valuable. All the important routes of exposure should be identified. At a minimum, the routes considered should theoretically yield an exposure estimate that is proportional to the sum of all exposure routes for a given substance.

Specifying Available Data Sources and Needs

The types of exposure data needed in an industry-based study depend on the diseases of interest and the study design to be used. For example, a study of acute respiratory symptoms among actively employed workers exposed to formaldehyde might require only air measurements obtained concurrently with the health survey to establish an exposure gradient. However, a study of stomach cancer mortality among coal miners would require exposure data that span years or decades of employment because of the typically long induction time of the disease.

A list of the types of data that are useful for epidemiologic analysis is shown in Table 2–1. The entries are rank-ordered according to how well the data could be used to estimate true doses. The best situation occurs when we have quantified, personal exposure estimates for the agents of interest; the least informative case occurs when we have only knowledge of the fact of employment in a plant, industry, or trade where exposure probability is high. Exposure

Table 2–1. Types of exposure data in occupational epidemiology studies

Type of data	Approximation to dose
1. Quantified personal measurements	Best
2. Quantified area- or job-specific data	↑
3. Ordinally ranked jobs or tasks	
4. Duration of employment in the industry at large	↓
5. Ever employed in the industry	Poorest

information for most industry-based studies falls somewhere between these two extremes. In fact, the best case, quantitative personal exposure estimates, is uncommon in occupational studies. Studies of radiation-exposed workers monitored with personal dosimeters are an exception, but even these studies frequently suffer from incomplete monitoring (Checkoway et al., 1985b; Fraser et al., 1985). There is reason to question the value of a study in which exposure information is limited to the mere fact of employment at some time in the industry. A study of this type would be justifiable if it were known in advance that the characteristic agents were quite likely to be toxic and that a sizable proportion of workers actually had been exposed.

The next step in exposure characterization is to compile an inventory of existing data and to determine which data are most complete and usable for an epidemiologic analysis. In so doing we need to identify the agents that can be assessed quantitatively and those that must be evaluated qualitatively and ultimately what proportion of the work force can be included in the analysis of health effects in relation to exposure (i.e., how many workers will have "missing" data). It is convenient to distinguish two general facets of environmental characterization: historical exposure reconstruction and concurrent and prospective exposure estimation. These activities are discussed in turn, although it should be appreciated that an epidemiologic study may require one or both. The activities involved in historical or concurrent–prospective exposure estimation are conceptually identical, but differ in logistics.

Historical Exposure Reconstruction

In those unusual instances where past data on quantified, personal exposures exist, the principal concerns are the completeness of data and the ability to combine data obtained from different time periods when measurement techniques may have differed. Data completeness is of concern both for individual workers and for the study population as a whole.

For example, if in a study of nuclear workers, radiation film badges had been used only at certain times for some workers (i.e., when they were assumed to be at risk for significant exposures), then there will be periods for which the data will be absent. Such gaps in the data must be evaluated individually. Some workers may never have been monitored because they were considered "non-exposed" by plant management, or alternatively, they may have begun and terminated employment before a routine monitoring program was introduced. In the former case, it might be reasonable to assign unmonitored exposure values of zero or to classify these workers in a non-exposed category. Workers who were not monitored because of employment before monitoring should be included in an overall analysis of disease rates in the workforce but should be deleted from an analysis of exposure–response relationships (see Chapter 5).

In many studies personal monitoring data either do not exist or are sparse. As a result, environmental characterization involves developing an exposure classification scheme for the various work areas, jobs, and tasks in the industry.

A matrix of jobs and exposure levels can be created for both quantitative and qualitative exposure schemes (Gamble and Spirtas, 1976). A time dimension can be added if exposure concentrations have changed over time. Thus, for example, a certain job may be rated as having relatively high exposure levels in the earliest years of plant operation but may be assigned a low exposure rating for years after engineering controls were implemented.

The data sources useful for generating a job–exposure matrix are listed in Table 2–2. Process descriptions, flow charts, and plant layouts assist in the identification and localization of potential toxins. Historical archives containing such information are more likely to be maintained by large companies than in small industries. Walk-through surveys of plant sites are recommended as a means of gaining a firsthand view of current processes, work practices, use of protective equipment, and general environmental conditions.

Industrial hygiene or health physics sampling and monitoring data offer the most detail for characterizing the workplace environment. Superficially, it may seem that direct measurement data are the most useful for estimating workers' average exposures. However, the use of sampling data in this manner is not without pitfalls. There are some obvious shortcomings associated with measurement uncertainty, such as sample timing, location, and equipment cali-

Table 2–2. Data sources useful for developing a job–exposure matrix

1. Industrial hygiene or health physics sampling data
2. Process descriptions and flow charts
3. Plant production records
4. Inspection and accident reports
5. Engineering control and protective equipment documentation
6. Biological monitoring results

bration. Issues pertaining to measurement techniques are addressed suitably in industrial hygiene and health physics texts (Cralley and Cralley, 1982; Shapiro, 1981) and will not be discussed here.

The epidemiologist must be concerned with reasons why sampling was performed. Industrial hygienists and health physicists ordinarily devote their resources (often limited) to measuring exposures in plant areas where they believe the concentrations are likely to be highest. Similarly, the workers assumed to be most heavily exposed within a job category tend to be included preferentially in sampling surveys. Keeping in compliance with exposure limits (e.g., Permissible Exposure Limits) is one primary reason for this approach to sampling.

One result of compliance sampling is that assignment of exposure concentrations to unmonitored work areas, jobs, or workers becomes highly unreliable, if not impossible. The inability to confirm low-level concentrations is a weakness of many occupational epidemiology studies. Also, if compliance sampling is not recognized as such, average exposure concentrations will be overestimated. Thus, mean values will be skewed to levels more representative of times when exposures were elevated rather than reflecting true averages. The bias resulting from the overestimation of exposure concentrations will be slight in an epidemiologic study when the apparent mean values are directly proportional to the true means and where the proportionality is constant across exposure groups. (Proportionality is difficult to verify, however.) On the other hand, if the data from the study ultimately will be used for extrapolation to other settings, then the results will be an underestimation of the actual "risk per unit of exposure."

A feature that can lead to inaccurate estimation of exposure concentrations is the physical location of area measurement devices. Some devices are cumbersome and may impede normal work activities. As a result, they may be placed in locations removed from work stations. Miniaturization of measurement devices has made it possible to monitor exposures of individual workers, thus partially obviating concerns about improper location, although for some agents (e.g., cotton dust) area monitoring is the only available method.

In principle, personal monitoring should yield more precise exposure estimates than area monitoring, although personal monitoring is not without drawbacks. Wearing a monitoring device may cause some workers to alter their work practices, either becoming more careful to avoid unnecessary exposures or being less cautious than usual, depending on their perceptions of the reasons for monitoring. Furthermore, personal monitoring is often limited to workers considered to have the highest exposure potential; thus, results can be skewed upward.

Records of plant production, schedules, and materials purchased indicate when new materials are handled and produced at a plant and can assist in determining times during the year or day when exposures are likely to be highest. Ideally, industrial hygiene and health physics sampling reports should contain information on the specific dates and times during the day when sampling occurred. In practice, however, the data generally are too limited to permit distinctions between annual or daily exposure patterns.

Inspection and accident reports are especially valuable for documenting unusual exposure circumstances and for identifying special subgroups of workers that warrant further, more intensive follow-up (Moses et al., 1984). Furthermore, it is important to distinguish routine exposure monitoring from monitoring motivated by an episode of excessive exposure, such as a spill, leak, or radiation accident. For example, following an accident, industrial hygiene and biological monitoring efforts may be increased, so that the time between personal samples is reduced from the normal schedule. If the accident causes some workers to receive large intakes of a substance, then closely spaced biological monitoring of these workers will yield a higher average exposure estimate than would be seen if the ordinary monitoring schedule had been in effect. Unless there is some documentation that these particular measurements were made in response to an unusual exposure situation, the average exposure estimate would be elevated spuriously. Inspection of the dates of monitoring records may provide indications about the likelihood of unusual circumstances when specific documentation is lacking.

If they are properly applied and maintained, engineering controls can reduce exposures profoundly. Thus, changes in agent concentrations should be reflected in area and personal monitoring data. On the other hand, knowledge of the types and dates of engineering controls is very influential in estimating quantitative or qualitative exposure levels when industrial hygiene or health physics monitoring data are limited. When used properly, personal protective equipment, such as respirators, gloves, and hearing protection devices, can also affect doses significantly. Thus, some work areas may involve potentially intense exposures to specific substances, but workers in those areas may receive substantially reduced doses if protective equipment is used routinely or during special circumstances when exposures are greatest (e.g., cleaning of machinery). Therefore, use of protective equipment may invalidate an assumption of proportionality between exposure and dose.

Scaling exposure concentrations downward to reflect the use of protective equipment is one means of maintaining quantitative exposure estimates. In fact, some personal monitoring devices collect samples only when protective equipment (e.g., respirators) is not in use, thus permitting more accurate exposure determinations than are obtained from studies relying on area monitoring (Smith et al., 1977). However, unless there are reliable models for reducing exposure estimates when more typical monitoring devices are used, numerical scaling of exposure concentrations may compromise the accuracy of the data. It is generally better to incorporate information on protective equipment use into an ordinal exposure ranking scheme than to risk introducing more error into the data by applying "correction factors" to quantitative exposure estimates.

Biological monitoring has become more frequently used and reliable in occupational epidemiology in recent years (Lauwerys, 1983). Results of blood, urine, breath, and other types of biological monitoring can provide estimates of body burden, and by inference, organ doses. Also, biological monitoring data may be used to estimate environmental concentrations when the latter cannot be measured directly. Here again, workers selected for biological monitoring frequently are individuals suspected of being most heavily exposed. Consequently, care should be taken in applying biological monitoring results to compute average exposure levels for the worker population.

Example 2.1

Takahashi and co-workers (1983) compared mean levels of urinary arsenic in workers exposed to arsenic-based wood preservatives with those of a group of volunteers without known arsenic exposures. The exposed workers were classified according to the probable intensity of exposure, as inferred from job assignments. Their findings (Table 2–3) suggest that urinary arsenic levels discriminate well between the most highly exposed workers and the comparison group but are poorer predictors of lower exposure concentrations.

The interpretation of biological sampling for toxic substances depends on the properties of the agent in question, including its half-life in the body, metabolic fate (e.g., conjugation and elimination patterns), and transport to the tissues sampled. Biological

Table 2-3. Mean urinary arsenic levels among workers exposed to arsenic-based wood preservatives and a non-exposed comparison group

Group	No. of subjects	Urinary arsenic (μg As/L) Mean	(SD)[a]
Non-exposed	232	74	(73)
Possibly exposed	15	44	(36)
Low exposure	22	98	(76)
Moderate exposure	42	117	(158)
High exposure	10	148	(112)

Source: Takahashi et al. (1983).

[a]Standard deviation.

assays of radioactivity have proved to be a valuable method for estimating radiation doses from long-lived radionuclides (ICRP, 1972), for example. For substances with short half-lives in the body, biological monitoring is most useful for studies of acute health effects (e.g., carboxyhemoglobin or expired carbon monoxide and transient neurological deficits).

The mere fact that a worker has undergone biological monitoring sometimes can be used to assign him to an exposure category, even when the monitoring data cannot be expressed quantitatively. Thus, for example, if only workers who come into contact with lead undergo blood analysis, then a list of such workers could be isolated as a special "lead-exposed" group to be compared with workers presumed to be non-exposed. Also, some industrial toxicology programs sample workers more frequently if they are believed to be most heavily exposed. As a result, sampling frequency may serve as a crude index for exposure intensity.

Another type of biological monitoring involves assays of biological responses to toxins, rather than assays of the concentrations of the substances in body tissues. Cytogenetic assays, such as sister chromatid exchange (Vainio, 1985), fall into this category. The underlying assumption of this approach to biological monitoring is that the exposure concentration and/or duration (or dose) is proportional to the observed response. Care needs to be taken in inferring exposure levels from the results of biological response monitoring because individual susceptibility (and, hence, reactiveness) can influence the findings, as can confounding effects from other exposures, such as dietary factors and smoking.

Exposure ratings for particular jobs or tasks frequently rely on rankings provided by industrial hygienists, safety engineers, or

health physicists. The final ratings used for the analysis can be con-
sensus or average rankings provided by such personnel. Additionally, workers' ratings of the levels of their own exposures can offer
valuable insight (Jarvholm and Sanden, 1987).

Linking Exposure Data to Individual Workers

The problem of assigning exposure values to workers in situations
where personal monitoring data are not available is common in
occupational epidemiology. Worker personnel records constitute
the principal link between exposure data and individual workers.
These records typically contain the names of jobs held in a plant and
their associated dates of employment. The availability of detailed
work history records is virtually essential to the conduct of epidemiologic research in industries where job mobility occurs frequently. Figure 2–1 shows a sample work history record from a
cohort mortality study of phosphate industry workers (Checkoway
et al., 1985a). Each line entry denotes a job and/or pay change. In
this example, the worker began as "laborer" on May 29, 1962, and,
after several job changes, was assigned to "track helper" on Septem-
ber 6, 1963.

Large-scale epidemiology studies can generate tremendous volumes of work history data, sometimes hundreds of thousands of
lines of information. Summarizing the data involves reducing the
number of unique job or task codes to a manageable number,
thereby facilitating data editing for logic and transcription errors.
Care should be taken to avoid sacrificing information when coding
work history data; thus, obviously synonymous job descriptions
(e.g., "chemical operator" and "chem. oper.") can be combined,
but ambiguous job titles (e.g., "operator") should be kept distinct
from well-defined titles. Coding and editing work history information can be quite time-consuming, but this work is essential to study
validity.

Classification of jobs and work areas according to exposure levels
is often complex. The final classification scheme can be devised
either on a quantitative or qualitative scale, or it may consist of
groupings of jobs that are relatively homogeneous in duties and
materials encountered (Wilkins and Reiches, 1983). The last scheme
requires no explicit assumptions about exposure gradients,
although environmental concentration differences may be inferred
(Gamble and Spirtas, 1976). The following examples illustrate these
approaches.

EMPLOYMENT RECORD				HEALTH AND SAFETY
SERVICE FROM	POSITION	RATE	DEPARTMENT	REMARKS:
5-29-62	Laborer	1.75	Shipping	E
6-1-62	Temp. Rake Class. Feedman	1.90	B/L-Processing	TT
6-11-62	Temp. Table Operator	2.06	B/L-Processing	TT
6-16-62	Temp. Helper & Carleader	1.97	" "	TT
6-20-62	Laborer	1.75	T/S Oper.	T
7-25-62	Temp. Lineman Helper	1.90	M.Mtce.-Elect Shop	TT
8-1-62	Temp. Lineman Helper	1.90	Elec.Mtce.-Elec Shop T Dept. Change	T
10-22-62	Laborer	1.75	Den Triple	T
10-11-62	Laborer	1.75	Chem. Oper.	T
11-8-62	"	1.75	Shipping	T
11-14-63	Temp. Painter	2.39	Ch. Mtce	TT
11/21/62	Laboror	1.75	T/S Oper.	T
	5/21-63	1.80	CONTRACT RATE	MISCELLANEOUS REMARKS:
9/6/63	Card Helper	1.95	240/week	r-50

CODE –
CC – CLASSIFICATION CHANGE
D – DISCHARGED
E – EMPLOYED
EA – EVALUATION ADJUSTMENT
GI – GENERAL INCREASE

LO – LAID OFF
M – MILITARY SERVICE
MI – MERIT INCREASE
MP – MERIT PROMOTION
Q – QUIT

R – RESIGNED
RA – RATE ADJUSTMENT
RE – RE-EMPLOYED
RI – REINSTATED
T – TRANSFER
TT – TEMP. TRANSFER

Figure 2–1. Sample work history from a personnel file for a worker in the Florida phosphate industry. (Source: Checkoway et al., 1985a.)

Table 2–4. Asbestos concentrations in carding operation job categories at an asbestos textile plant

Job category	Mean fiber concentration (fibers/cc)			
	1930–35	1936–45	1946–65	1966–75
General area personnel	10.8	5.3	2.4	4.3
Card operators	13.3	6.5	2.9	5.3
Clean-up personnel	18.1	8.8	4.0	7.2
Raw fiber handling	22.8	11.0	5.0	9.0

Source: Dement et al. (1983).

Example 2.2

In their study of the mortality experience of asbestos textile plant workers, Dement et al. (1983) combined industrial hygiene sampling data with records of engineering control changes to estimate quantitative historical asbestos concentrations. Summarizing the air-sampling data offered a particular challenge because the results were expressed in million particles per cubic foot (mppcf) for the earliest years and in fibers per cubic centimeter (f/cc) for the later years of the study. Fortunately, there had been a "side-by-side" sampling survey using the two methods that permitted conversion factors to be derived expressing mppcf in units of f/cc (on which the current occupational and nonoccupational standards are based). The investigators next summarized the data according to Uniform Job Categories, an approach suggested by Esmen (1979), and computed average exposure concentrations for the component job categories of nine plant operations. The results for one operation, Carding, are summarized in Table 2–4.

Example 2.3

Pifer et al. (1986) conducted a historical cohort mortality study of workers in a chemical manufacturing plant where there are exposures to numerous chemicals and fibers. Because of the complexity of the workplace environment and the lack of adequate measurement data to support a quantitative exposure reconstruction, the investigators classifed workers into categories defined by chemical production divisions. The production divisions and the predominant environmental agents, indicating those that workers are most likely to encounter, are listed in Table 2–5. The analysis of the mortality patterns of these workers ultimately did not reveal any associations with process divisions or specific chemicals.

Example 2.2 illustrates the approach to reconstructing historical exposures on a quantitative basis. Dement and colleagues (1983) had the luxury of a relatively thorough set of measurement data spanning several decades. Had they been less confident in the numerical reliability of the data, they might have developed an ordinal exposure classification scheme, as has been used in other studies of asbestos-exposed workers (Acheson et al., 1984; Newhouse et al.,

Table 2–5. Exposure characterization of divisions at a chemical plant

Division	Major chemicals	Primary employee exposure
1. Research laboratories	Multiple components	—
2. Acetate yarn	Cellulose acetate, acetone, yarn lubricants, dyes	Acetone and lubricants
3. Acid	Organic acids, aldehydes, anhydrides, solvents, alcohols, plasticizers, diketene products, terephthalic acid, dimethylterephthalate, acetic acid	Limited (i.e., closed systems)
4. Cellulose esters	Cellulose acetate, cellulose acetate propionate, cellulose acetate butyrate, acetic, propionic, and butyric acids and anhydrides	Acetic acid and cellulose dust
5. Filter products	Cellulose acetate, acetone, yarn lubricants	Acetone and lubricants
6. Kodel fibers	Polyesters, modified polyacrylates, yarn lubricants	Lubricants
7. Organic chemicals	Multiple organic chemicals, aniline, sulfuric acid, dyes, manganese oxide, hydroquinine, aromatic chemicals	Hydroquinine
8. Polymers	Dimethyl terephthalate, ethylene glycol, cyclohexane dimethanol, butylene glycol, methanol	Limited (closed system)
9. Tenite plastics	Cellulose esters, polyethylene, polyesters, plasticizers, pigments, dyes	Cellulose esters and plasticizers

Source: Pifer et al. (1986).

1985). In Example 2.3 the lack of environmental measurement data necessitated a cruder classification scheme whereby exposure potentials can only be inferred qualitatively.

Exposure classification systems often require the compilation and synthesis of information from numerous sources. Lack of agreement among sources can pose a dilemma for the epidemiologist hoping to obtain a clearcut picture of the environment. To illustrate, Stewart et al. (1986) developed a formaldehyde exposure profile for ten facilities using data from job descriptions, historical and concurrently obtained air-sampling data, and ratings provided by industrial hygienists. This work was in support of a study of cancer risks in relation to formaldehyde exposure levels (Blair et al., 1986). Specific jobs were ranked according to ordinally assigned categories of intensity. The rating scheme incorporated historical air-sampling data. In addition, a current air-sampling survey was conducted at the facilities included in the study. The investigators found a poor correlation between the exposure ratings and the air-sampling results; roughly 35 percent of the original exposure estimates required changing. The lack of correspondence among the various sources of data in this study demonstrates how even seemingly unbiased data sources, such as industrial hygiene monitoring and rankings, can result in exposure misclassification unless special efforts are made to establish reliability.

The job–exposure matrix that is generated and ultimately used in the epidemiologic analysis should be carefully documented so as to indicate the basis for exposure assignment. Thus, the industrial hygienists or health physicists who produce the matrix should maintain a documented file that indicates each job, task, or work area included in the matrix; the exposure value or ranking, by time period; and the data sources that were used to derive the estimates. The source information also should indicate whether a given estimate was based on industrial hygiene or health physics monitoring data, the types of monitoring data (area or personal), whether monitoring was routine or for compliance, the number of samples taken, the ranges and the means or medians, as well as the dates of sampling, and whether the estimate was based on best judgment. Maintaining such a file may seem burdensome, but it provides useful documentation of the study procedures that can facilitate future analyses of the data.

The exposure matrix that can be applied to work history data for the entire study population generally represents the lowest common denominator of exposure data precision. For example, it may be possible to estimate quantitative cumulative exposures for half of the study population, and ordinal estimates can be derived for the remainder. In this instance, an analysis including all workers would be limited to an evaluation of disease rates with respect to ordinal exposure levels. However, the exposure assessment inventory would permit secondary, more exacting analyses of exposure–effect relationships for the subset of workers with quantified exposure estimates.

Prospective Exposure Monitoring

Prospective monitoring of the workplace environment is a logical accompaniment to prospective health surveillance. The data sources shown for historical exposure reconstruction in Table 2–2 are the same as those for prospective monitoring. One valuable addition would be data on previous employment, which is more easily obtained in prospective than historical studies. The critical question is, "How are the resources for prospective exposure monitoring to be spent?" Some aspects of this question are settled automatically. For example, updating personnel files is an ongoing, necessary process in most industries, and periodic compliance sampling for designated toxic substances is mandated by governmental regulatory agencies. These generalizations apply more to large than to small facilities, however.

Decisions as to the types and quantities of additional exposure data to be collected prospectively should be guided by judgments about the health outcomes most likely to warrant epidemiologic study and the possible causative agents. Feasibility of data collection and storage and cost are also important considerations. It may be tempting to devise an exposure monitoring program in which concentrations for a large number of potential toxins are measured routinely, but the costs may be prohibitive, especially when the laboratory assays are elaborate and time-consuming. Moreover, even when existing resources permit a voluminous data collection effort, data storage may become unwieldly, the availability of sophisticated computer systems notwithstanding (Whyte, 1983). Invariably, one has to adopt a compromise strategy that falls between the extremes of "measure and record everything" and "start monitoring only when a significant health hazard is noted." Sampling routinely for a limited number of substances, and timing the sampling so that unnecessary measurements are avoided, can prevent an information overflow. (Some redundant measurements may be necessary for determining reliability.) This minimalist approach may preclude obtaining data on exposure concentrations for some substances that may ultimately warrant study, but qualitative exposure estimation may still be possible if job history, materials usage, and other plant records are maintained carefully.

Table 2–6. Sources of occupational exposure data in community-based studies

1. Personal interviews
2. Hospital records
3. Disease registry records
4. Death certificates
5. Census data

3.2. Community-Based Studies

Occupational exposure effects can also be examined in studies conducted in the general population. Case–control studies of hospitalized patients or of patients identified from disease registers and surveys of occupations recorded on death certificates are some
examples of this type of investigation. (Community- and registry-
based studies are described further in Chapters 3 and 6.) Some of
the common exposure data sources are listed in Table 2–6. In general, exposure data are less detailed in such studies than in industry-
based studies either because of a lack of exposure measurement or
because occupational exposures may be of secondary research interest. Nonetheless, such studies can provide valuable leads for more
intensive investigations of specific occupational groups.

Perhaps the crudest approach to evaluating associations of disease risk with occupations in a community-based study is to compare
disease rates between geographic areas rated according to the
extent of industrial activities of various types. Data on industrial
location and production can be obtained from census or Labor
Department publications. This approach is known as an *ecological
study* because the units of "exposure" pertain to geographical areas
rather than to individuals. Ecological studies have well-recognized
shortcomings, such as lack of exposure specificity and biases due to
selective migration (Morgenstern, 1982). Ecological studies are
most informative when particular industries are highly concentrated
geographically, but such studies usually provide the weakest evidence of causality. They will not be discussed further.

An alternative approach is the *death certificate survey,* in which
occupations recorded on death certificates are compared between
persons dying from specific diseases and all remaining deaths (Milham, 1983). This method is essentially a case-control study (see
Chapter 3). The occupations can be categorized simply by type (e.g.,
farmers, machinists, health care providers) or by specific exposures
(e.g., asbestos, arsenic, electrical fields). The principal limitation of
death certificate studies is that the occupation listed on a death cer-

tificate often represents only the final or "usual" job and may be a poor indicator of lifetime exposure. Also, reporting of occupation by next of kin can be a source of error (Steenland and Beaumont, 1984).

In some U.S. cities commercial city directories provide information on occupation and industry of employment for residents of working age (18 years and older). Identification of specific employers is an improvement over death certificate data, which generally provide only type of industry and occupation (Roush et al., 1982; Steenland et al., 1987).

In England and Wales linking of census data with social class and occupational data contained on death certificates permits the calculation of disease rates for specific occupational groups. Rates can be computed for over 200 *occupation units,* which distinguish such jobs as firemen and policemen, or for 20–30 *occupation orders,* which are groupings of occupation units (Office of Population Censuses and Surveys, 1978). This method of job categorization has been adapted for use in other countries (Pearce and Howard, 1987).

Methods for categorizing occupations with respect to specific agent exposures have been devised for use in community-based case–control studies (Hoar et al., 1980; Pannett et al., 1985; Siemiatycki et al., 1986). These approaches involve compiling lists of industries and component jobs and linkage with exposure ratings for classes of agents or, in some cases, specific substances.

Example 2.4

Hoar and co-workers (1980) devised a system of exposure rating for use in community-based studies of cancer etiology. In this system, five-digit occupation codes were generated, where the first two digits reflect Standard Industrial Codes assigned by U.S. Department of Commerce (1970) and the last three digits designate tasks or industrial processes (U.S. Department of Labor, 1965). For example, knitters and tailors in the textile industry would be assigned codes of 10–789, where 10 indicates the textile industry and 789 designates knitting or tailoring tasks. Known and suspected chemical carcinogens and related substances were then linked to the five-digit occupation codes following a comprehensive literature review of industrial processes and chemical carcinogens. Where possible, an ordinal exposure rating indicating "heavy," "moderate," or "light" was assigned to an occupation–agent combination. Table 2–7 presents an example of the exposure rating for specific chemicals encountered in carpentry occupations in the construction industry. A computer file containing the exposure ratings, by occupation, was ultimately generated and has since been used in several epidemiologic studies. Hinds et al. (1985) applied an adapted version of this rating scheme in their study of occupational risk factors for lung cancer. The rating was simplified to a 0,1,2

Table 2–7. Linkage of occupations with exposure ratings for chemical carcinogens: carpentry in the construction industry

Agent	Exposure rating
Azo compounds	
Oil orange SS	Moderate
Phenols	
Creosote	Moderate
Aromatic hydrocarbons	
Coal tar and pitch	Moderate
Petroleum, coke tar, and pitch	Moderate
Aliphatic compounds	
Water in soluble carbon polymers	Light
Polysiloxanes	Light
Metals	
Chromium	Heavy
Minerals	
Asbestos	Moderate
Physical agents	
Wood dust	Heavy
Ultraviolate radiation	Moderate

Source: Hoar et al. (1980).

scale, denoting, respectively, "no," "light," and "heavy" exposure. Some results of their analysis with respect to suspected lung carcinogens are presented in Table 2–8.

Exposure linkage systems of the type described earlier may not provide sufficient detail when there are specific hypotheses to be tested in a community- or registry-based study. Instead, questioning study subjects about the frequency and duration of contact with certain substances may be more informative.

Table 2–8. Relative risks for lung cancer associated with exposure to specific substances: example of exposure data in a community-based case–control study

	Relative risk[a]	
Agent	Low–moderate exposure	Heavy exposure
Coal tar and pitch	1.15	1.94
Petroleum, coke pitch, and tar	1.18	2.04
Arsenic	1.16	1.24
Chromium	1.51	0.87
Asbestos	1.02	12.06
Nickel	1.66	1.56
Beryllium	1.62	1.57

Source: Hinds et al. (1985).

[a]Odds ratio relative to non-exposed category, adjusted for smoking habits.

Example 2.5

In a case–control study by Hoar et al. (1986), non-Hodgkin's lymphoma cases and controls selected from the community were questioned about the frequency and duration of use of phenoxy herbicides as part of a series of questions regarding farming practices. Subjects were asked also to identify names and locations of companies where herbicides were purchased. The investigators contacted the suppliers to verify reported herbicide purchases. Table 2–9 shows comparative data on the duration and frequency of use of one herbicide, 2,4-dichlorophenoxyacetic acid. Increasing gradients of risk for non-Hodgkin's lymphoma were detected with both duration and frequency of use.

Exposure data obtained by self-reporting may be prone to reporting bias if the subjects have particular reasons to give erroneous answers. (See Chapter 4 for a discussion of sources of bias.) Questionnaires and in-person interviews generally offer more detailed exposure information in community-based studies than routinely recorded data that may be abstracted from hospital records or death certificates. In any case, it is nearly impossible to derive quantitative estimates of intensity, cumulative exposure, or dose in community-based studies. These objectives are more readily achieved in industry-based studies.

4. CLASSIFICATION OF EXPOSURE LEVELS

The unifying concept of all occupational epidemiologic research is the comparison of disease rates between groups of individuals classified according to exposure levels to estimate dose–response relationships. Methods for analyzing the data from various epidemiologic designs are described in Chapters 5–7. In this section we consider briefly the approaches for summarizing exposure data to be used in the analysis. We focus attention on the following topics: (1) classifying exposures specifically for biological targets and (2) combining exposure data from sources that differ in type and quality.

4.1. Exposure Classification for Specific Biological Targets

Many toxic substances can enter the body by more than one route, although typically one route is predominant. Thus, although we might be interested in estimating a worker's potential exposure delivered from all relevant routes, we are usually restricted in this

Table 2-9. Non-Hodgkin's lymphoma in relation to duration and frequency of 2,4-dichlorophenoxyacetic acid use: example of community-based study

	Cases	Controls	Relative risk[a]
Never farmed	37	286	1.0
Duration of use (years)			
1–5	3	16	1.3
6–15	7	22	2.5
16–25	8	15	3.9
>25	6	17	2.3
Frequency of use (days/year)			
1–2	6	17	2.7
3–5	4	16	1.6
6–10	4	16	1.9
11–20	4	9	3.0
>20	5	6	7.6

Source: Hoar et al. (1986).
[a]Odds ratio relative to "Never farmed" category.

effort because of incomplete knowledge of uptake and metabolism or by meager measurement resources. As a result, body burden and dose estimates suffer from imprecision. The imprecision is proportional to the contribution of the unmeasured exposures (e.g., from various routes not considered). Biological monitoring for exposures is advantageous because it permits estimation of doses or budens from exposures through all relevant portals of entry. If concentrations measured in one environmental medium (e.g., air) are directly proportional to those in the unmeasured media (e.g., liquid), then the shape of the exposure–response relationship will be valid, but the effect per unit concentration of the measured environmental medium will be overestimated because total exposure is underestimated. Thus, problems of exposure misclassification arise when direct proportionality does not hold.

To illustrate, consider classification of trichloroethylene (TCE), which is a solvent used for degreasing and cleaning. The principal route of absorption from occupational exposures is inhalation of vapors (Browning, 1965), although percutaneous absorption of the liquid form also can occur, resulting in significant exposure (Sato and Nakajima, 1978). Air concentrations of TCE can be readily measured. However, without performing pharmacokinetic studies, which are not practical in most instances, it is virtually impossible to derive quantitative estimates of dermal uptake. An exposure classification scheme relying on airborne concentrations of TCE would be acceptable for an epidemiologic study of, say, neurotoxicity or liver toxicity, if air concentrations and dermal concentrations were directly proportional to each other. However, air and dermal exposures are not always directly proportional. For example, dermal exposures may exceed air levels for workers who come into contact with liquid TCE, and the opposite may be true for workers who are only in contact with TCE vapors. As a result, dose estimates based on air concentration measurements would be incorrect for workers handling the liquid form.

Where possible, separate exposure ratings for jobs and tasks within an industry should be constructed for each of the important routes of exposure. As mentioned earlier, it is uncommon to have measurements available for more than one exposure route. Consequently, measurement data may have to be combined with ordinally assigned ratings based on task descriptions and judgment. If an overall exposure rating scheme is desired (e.g., to reflect "systemic doses"), then the data can be combined into a crude overall classification scheme using ordinal rankings. Alternatively, the integrity of the quantitative measurement data can be preserved by stratification with respect to the ordinally ranked variables. To illustrate, consider again the problem of assigning exposure ratings for trichloroethylene where air concentrations are available but where dermal exposures can only be ranked as "low," "moderate," and "high." Workers would be classified first into categories of dermal exposure and then assigned their average values of airborne TCE intensity or cumulative exposure levels. Cross-classification of exposure levels can become quite complicated when there are multiple exposure routes or when workers move between levels over time.

4.2. Combining Exposure Data from Various Sources

The types and quality of exposure data often vary in epidemiologic studies. Data may vary within one plant, especially when the study spans long time periods. Data may also vary when combined from multiple occupational settings, such as an industrywide analysis that includes numerous facilities (Marsh, 1987).

There are several ways to handle diverse sets of exposure data. The most extreme (purist) approach is to restrict the study to workers with the most detailed measurement values. This is most justifiable when the study objective is to obtain the most valid estimate of the effect per unit of exposure, as would be the case if the results were to be used for risk assessment. In general, the precision of derived risk estimates is proportional to the number of subjects studied; however, validity is also improved by reducing measurement error in the exposure data. Thus, an analysis restricted to workers with quantitative exposure data reduces measurement error, but at the expense of study size. Therefore, the loss in numbers of subjects (and, hence, precision) from the exposure–response analyses needs to be considered against the potential gain in quantitative exposure information (and, hence, validity).

At the other extreme, one might include in the study all subjects with the minimum usable exposure information. The hazard of this approach is that exposure misclassification may result, thus compromising the study's validity. For example, consider a study of coronary heart disease incidence among workers exposed to carbon disulfide in three plants producing viscose rayon. At one plant the exposure data consist of measured concentrations of carbon disulfide from which cumulative exposures can be estimated. At the second plant limited area sampling data permit workers to be classified into "low," "moderate," and "high" exposure groupings, where approximate estimates of average concentrations can be made for the three categories. At the third plant no measurement data exist, although workers could be assigned into ordinal exposure categories based on a subjective rating of job assignments. If we follow the first approach, then the analysis would be limited to workers from the first plant. The second approach would involve including workers from all three plants and categorizing them according to a common scheme of ordinally ranked exposure strata. This second method would diminish the precision of the study results if "low," "moderate," and "high" represent different true concentrations at the three sites, although this approach would not introduce bias into the study if the scaling of the ratings is the same at all facilities (e.g., "moderate" is twice as intense as "low" at each plant). The lack of measurement data for the third plant prevents a verification of the appropriateness of pooling data across all facilities. A compromise strategy is to include all workers for whom exposure estimates can be combined on at least a semiquantitative basis. In this example, we would combine data from the first two plants because some numerical scaling can be applied to both; workers from the third plant would be excluded, however.

No universally accepted guidelines exist for data pooling. The extent to which investigators are willing to combine diverse sets of exposure data depends on how much variability exists in the data and on the objectives of the research. In general, we recommend that the subset of subjects with the most detailed and accurate expo-sure data be analyzed separately. The results will be informative and will give some indication, albeit approximate, of the findings that would have been seen if data of similar detail and scope had been available for all study subjects.

5. SUMMARY

Estimation of exposure– or dose–response relationships between occupational exposures and disease risks requires that the work-place environment be characterized as thoroughly and precisely as possible. Identification of the types, sources, and routes of exposure is the first step in understanding potential health hazards. Next, environmental concentrations for specific substances are estimated from available data sources. Ultimately, these concentrations are linked with workers' employment histories to derive dose estimates, either on an overall (total body) basis or for individual biological targets. Doses, which are the amounts of substances that reside within target sites during specified time intervals, cannot be esti-mated directly in most instances. Instead, we have to rely on expo-sure concentrations as surrogates for dose rates. Cumulative expo-sure, which combines concentrations with durations, is the most commonly used surrogate for dose. Exposure concentration and cumulative exposure are valid surrogate measures, provided that they are directly proportional to dose rates and doses, respectively.

In industry-based studies, directly measured environmental con-centrations obtained from industrial hygiene or health physics mon-itoring surveys are the best sources for dose estimation. However, monitoring data may not represent true average concentrations when sampling is performed strictly to satisfy compliance testing requirements; data from compliance sampling often overestimate typical (average) exposure levels. Ordinal rankings of jobs, tasks, or work areas are necessitated when measurement data are not availa-ble. Employment personnel records are the most common link between environmental data and estimates for individual workers. Biological monitoring can provide ancillary information.

Community-based studies of occupational risk factors tend to yield less accurate exposure data than industry-based studies. Sources of data in these studies include death certificates, hospital and disease registry records, and questionnaires. Questionnaires generally offer the most detailed occupational history data in community-based studies and are particularly useful when the responses can be verified by other data sources, such as employment records.

Combining exposure data of varying degrees of detail and accuracy from multiple sources is an issue that must be confronted in some studies. When the research objective is to derive valid approximations of dose–response relationships for risk assessment, it is justifiable to restrict the analysis to workers for whom the most accurately quantified data are available. The loss in study subjects would have to be counterbalanced by at least a commensurate reduction of measurement error in order for this approach to be worthwhile. More permissive strategies allow for data pooling and an analysis using less accurate exposure estimates. Data pooling should be guided by judgments as to how likely exposure ratings from differing sources will be in agreement. Inappropriate pooling will result in bias caused by exposure misclassification.

Glossary

burden   Amount of a substance residing in the body (or organ) at a point in time.
concentration   Amount of a substance per unit of environmental medium; also termed *intensity.*
cumulative exposure   Summation of products of concentrations and the time intervals during which they occurred.
dose   Amount of a substance that resides in a biological target during some specified time interval.
exposure   Presence of a substance in the workplace environment.
job–exposure matrix   Classification of substance concentrations or exposure ratings for individual work areas, jobs, or tasks; often includes a time dimension.
retention   Persistence of substances in the body; influenced by rates of uptake, metabolism, and clearance.

References

Acheson ED, Gardner MJ, Winter PD, and Bennett C (1984): Cancer in a factory using amosite asbestos. *Int J Epidemiol* 13:3–10.
Ballantyne B (1985): Evaluation of hazards from mixtures of chemicals in the occupational environment. *J Occup Med* 27:85–94.
Blair A, Stewart P, O'Berg M, et al. (1986): Mortality among workers exposed to formaldehyde. *J Natl Cancer Inst* 76:1071–1084.
Browning E (1965): *Toxicology and Metabolism of Industrial Solvents.* Amsterdam: Elsevier.
Checkoway H, Mathew RM, Hickey JLS, et al. (1985a): Mortality among workers in the Florida phosphate industry. II. Cause-specific mortality relationships with work areas and exposures. *J Occup Med* 27:893–896.
Checkoway H, Mathew RM, Shy CM, et al. (1985b): Radiation, work experience

and cause-specific mortality among workers at an energy research laboratory. *Br J Ind Med* 42:525–533.

Cralley LV, and Cralley LJ (1982): *Patty's Industrial Hygene and Toxicology*, 3rd rev. ed., Vol. 3. New York: Wiley-Interscience.

Dement JM, Harris RL, Symons MJ, and Shy CM (1983): Exposures and mortality among chrysotile asbestos workers. Part I: Exposure estimates. *Am J Ind Med* 4:399–419.

Esmen NA (1979): Retrospective industrial hygiene surveys. *Am Ind Hyg Assoc J* 40:58–65.

Fraser P, Booth M, Beral V, et al. (1985): Collection and validation of data in the United Kingdom Atomic Energy Authority mortality study. *Br Med J* 291:435–439.

Gamble JF, and Spirtas R (1976): Job classification and utilization of complete work histories in occupational epidemiology. *J Occup Med* 18:399–404.

Hinds MW, Kolonel LN, and Lee J (1985): Application of a job-exposure matrix to a case-control study of lung cancer. *J Natl Cancer Inst* 75:193–197.

Hoar SK, Morrison AS, Cole P, and Silverman DT (1980): An occupational and exposure linkage system for the study of occupational carcinogenesis. *J Occup Med* 22:722–726.

Hoar SK, Blair A, Holmes FF, et al. (1986): Agricultural herbicide use and risk of lymphoma and soft-tissue sarcoma. *JAMA* 256:1141–1147.

International Commission on Radiological Protection (1972): *ICRP Publication 19: The Metabolism of Compounds of Plutonium and Other Actinides*, Oxford.: Pergamon Press.

Jarvholm B, and Sanden A (1987): Estimating asbestos exposure: a comparison of methods. *J Occup Med* 29:361–363.

Lauwerys RR (1983): *Industrial Chemical Exposures: Guidelines for Biological Monitoring*. Davis, CA: Biomedical Publications.

Marsh GM (1987): A strategy for merging and analyzing work history data in industry-wide occupational epidemiological studies. *Am Ind Hyg Assoc J* 48:414–419.

Milham S (1983): *Occupational Mortality in Washington State*. DHHS (NIOSH) Publication No. 83-116. Washington D.C.: U.S. Institute for Occupational Safety and Health.

Morgenstern H (1982): Uses of ecologic analysis in epidemiologic research. *Am J Pub Health* 72:1336–1344.

Moses MR, Lilis KD, Crow J, et al. (1984): Health status of workers with past exposure to 2,3,7,8-tetrachlorodibenzo-*p*-dioxin in the manufacture of 2,4,5-trichlorophenoxyacetic acid: comparison of findings with and without chloracne. *Am J Ind Med* 5:161–182.

Newhouse ML, Berry G, and Wagner JC (1985): Mortality of factory workers in East London 1933–80. *Br J Ind Med* 42:4–11.

Office of Population Censuses and Surveys (1978): *Occupational Mortality, 1970–1972. Dicennial Supplement*. London: Her Magesty's Stationery Office.

Pannett B, Coggon D, and Acheson ED (1985): A job-exposure matrix for use in population based studies in England and Wales. *Br J Ind Med* 42:777–783.

Pearce NE, and Howard JK (1987): Occupation, social class and male cancer mortality in New Zealand, 1974–1978. *Int J Epidemiol* 15:456–462.

Pifer JW, Hearne FT, Friedlander BR, and McDonough JR (1986): Mortality study of men employed at a large chemical plant, 1972 through 1982. *J Occup Med* 28:438–444.

Roggli VL, Pratt PC, and Brody AR (1986): Asbestos content of lung tissue in asbestos associated diseases: a study of 110 cases. *Br J Ind Med* 43:18–28.

Roush GC, Kelly JA, Meigs JW, et al. (1982): Scrotal cancer in Connecticut metalworkers: sequel to a study of sinonasal cancer. *Am J Epidemiol* 116:76–85.

Sato A, and Nakajima T (1978): Differences following skin or inhalation exposure in the absorption and excretion kinetics of trichloroethylene and toluene. *Br J Ind Med* 35:43–49.

Shapiro J (1981): *Radiation Protection: A Guide for Scientists and Physicians,* 2nd ed. Cambridge, MA: Harvard University Press.

Siemiatycki J, Richardson L, Gerin M, et al. (1986): Associations between several sites of cancer and nine organic dusts: results from an hypothesis-generating case–control study in Montreal, 1979–83. *Am J Epidemiol* 123:235–249.

Smith TJ, Peters RM, Reading JC, and Castle HC (1977): Pulmonary impairment from chronic exposure to sulfur dioxide in a smelter. *Am Rev Respir Dis* 116:31–39.

Steenland K, and Beaumont JJ (1984): The accuracy of occupation and industry data on death certificates. *J Occup Med* 26:288–296.

Steenland K, Burnett C, and Osorio AM (1987): A case–control study of bladder cancer using city directories as a source of occupational data. *Am J Epidemiol* 126:247–257.

Stewart PA, Blair A, Cubit DA, et al. (1986): Estimating historical exposures to formaldehyde in a retrospective mortality study. *Appl Ind Hyg* 1:34–41.

Takahashi W, Pfenninger K, and Wong L (1983): Urinary arsenic, chromium and copper levels in workers exposed to arsenic-based wood preservatives. *Arch Environ Health* 18:209–214.

U.S. Department of Commerce, Bureau of the Census (1970): *Classified Index of Industries and Occupations.* Washington, D.C.: Library of Congress.

U.S. Department of Labor (1965): *Dictionary of Occupational Titles, Vol I: Definition of Titles, Vol II: Occupational Definitions.* Washington, D.C.: U.S. Government Printing Office.

Vainio H (1985): Current trends in the biological monitoring of exposure to carcinogens. *Scand J Work Environ Health* 11:1–6.

Whitwell F, Scott J, and Grimshaw M (1977): Relationship between occupations and asbestos-fibre content of the lungs in patients with pleural mesothelioma, lung cancer and other diseases. *Thorax* 32:377–386.

Whyte AA (1983): A survey of occupational health information system approaches. *Ann Am Conf Gov Ind Hyg* 6:21–27.

Wilkins JR, and Reiches NA (1983): Epidemiologic approaches to chemical hazard assessment. *Hazard Assessment of Chemicals: Current Developments* 2:133–189.

3 Overview of Study Designs

1. OVERVIEW

This chapter provides an overview of the various study designs used in occupational epidemiology. Chapters 5–7 present in detail methods for planning, implementing, and interpreting the results of such studies. This chapter describes the relative advantages and limitations of the various design options in reference to the types of health conditions to be investigated.

The discussion emphasizes the connections between various study designs. These connections pertain primarily to the causal inferences that can be drawn from occupational epidemiology studies and secondarily to the temporal sequencing of data collection and observation of health outcomes. As we will show, all occupational epidemiology studies are conceptually the same insofar as the objective is to examine relationships between causal exposures and health risks, where exposure necessarily precedes the health outcome. The distinctions between study designs are primarily attributable to variations in the availability of data and the feasibility of study conduct.

2. CASE SERIES

Historically, the recognition of an apparently excessive number of cases of disease among a worker population has been the motivation for conducting formal epidemiologic investigations to assess whether the excess is due to occupational hazards. When inquiry goes no further than mere identification and reporting of a disease cluster, the study is referred to as a *case series* report. Disease cluster reporting frequently emanates from workers or physicians who perceive an unusual occurrence of a certain disease or injury among the workforce as a whole or among some segment of the workforce (e.g., job category).

Example 3.1

In 1974 two physicians (Creech and Johnson, 1974) noted three cases of hepatic angiosarcoma among workers at a vinyl chloride polymerization factory. Angiosarcoma of the liver is a very rare disease in the United States under any circumstance. Thus, the occurrence of even a small number of cases provided reasonable evidence to implicate the characteristic exposure, vinyl chloride, as the etiologic factor. Subsequent epidemiologic investigations of a more formal nature (Waxweiler et al., 1976) confirmed the suspected association.

Case series reports are particularly informative in situations where there are occurrences of very rare conditions for which there are few, if any, established causal factors. When there is only one clearly established risk factor for a disease, such as hepatic angiosarcoma and vinyl chloride (Example 3.1) or asbestos and malignant mesothelioma (IARC, 1980), the occurrence of even one case can sometimes be invoked as prima facie evidence of exposure to the putative causal agent.

Apparent disease clusters can be misleading occasionally because the frequency of occurrence of a rare disease is expected to follow a random distribution in space and time, and a random distribution necessarily includes clusters of events. This means that the frequency of disease ordinarily does not follow a uniform pattern over time. Enterline (1985) demonstrated very effectively with a table of random digits that there are clusters embedded within the random distribution. The implications of this phenomenon are that workers, industrial medical staff, and epidemiologists need to be aware that some apparent disease clusters may be unremarkable events that may have little or nothing to do with hazardous exposures.

3. COHORT STUDIES

The study of diseases less rare than hepatic angiosarcoma or malignant mesothelioma typically requires more formal epidemiologic methods. Cohort studies, among all of the epidemiologic study designs, are most accepted by the scientific community. This is because cohort studies generally include the entire available study population. Also, cohort studies most closely resemble the standard experimental strategy of administration of a toxin to disease-free subjects, follow-up over time, and observation of adverse health effects among exposed and non-exposed groups.

Occupational cohort studies require the enumeration and follow-up of a population of workers, with the objective being to estimate the risks of various diseases among the worker cohort relative to background risks among persons not exposed to the same environmental factors. The terminology for cohort studies regrettably has become confusing, as epidemiologic nomenclature is not standardized (Last, 1983). Throughout this book we distinguish between two types of cohort studies, *prospective* and *historical* designs. Both types of cohort study share common design characteristics of follow-up of a cohort of workers selected on the basis of exposure status and observation of disease frequency over time.

3.1. Prospective Cohort Studies

In a prospective cohort study the cohort is enumerated at the time the study is being conducted (i.e., the present), and follow-up proceeds into the future. The rates of disease occurrence among the cohort usually are compared with prevailing rates in the national or regional (e.g., state or province) population to determine which diseases are occurring more or less frequently among the workers. Comparisons can also be made between subgroups of the cohort classified according to exposure type or level. Often the comparisons of disease rates in the cohort with rates in the national or regional population take the form of Standardized Mortality (Morbidity) Ratios (SMRs), which express the ratio of the observed number of cases of a given disease among the cohort to the number of cases expected among the cohort, where the latter is based on rates among the reference population.

Example 3.2

Schottenfeld and colleagues (1981) performed a prospective cohort study of the incidence and mortality from cancer and other diseases among a cohort of petroleum industry workers from 19 companies in the United States. This investigation was motivated by concerns about possible disease excesses related to exposures to benzene, coke operation emissions, and chemicals associated with asphalt. A worker population census was conducted in which actively employed workers and living annuitants were enumerated. The cohort consisted of 76,336 white and Spanish surname males who were employed at any time during January 1, 1977 to December 31, 1979. Data on cancer incidence were obtained from a cancer reporting system developed for the study, and mortality data were obtained from death certificates. SMRs for cancer incidence were derived from comparisons of site-specific cancer observed and expected numbers of cases, where the expected numbers were estimated from rates published by the National Cancer Institute Surveillance, Epidemiology and End Results program (Young et al., 1981).

Table 3-1. Cancer incidence among U.S. petroleum industry workers

Cancer site	Refinery workers			Petrochemical workers		
	Obs	Exp	RR[a]	Obs	Exp	RR[a]
All cancers	240	278.7	0.86	44	50.9	0.86
Colon	28	24.1	1.16	6	4.3	1.40
Rectum	7	14.0	0.50	3	2.4	1.23
Stomach	5	8.6	0.58	0	1.5	0
Larynx	12	9.4	1.28	3	1.6	1.83
Lung	55	67.6	0.81	11	11.7	0.94
Leukemia	11	7.6	1.45	0	1.5	0
Multiple myeloma	2	3.1	0.64	3	0.5	5.52
Hodgkin's disease	4	3.6	1.10	1	0.9	1.06
Non-Hodgkin's lymphoma	7	9.6	0.73	0	1.9	0
Kidney	8	8.5	0.94	2	1.6	1.28
Prostate	21	24.8	0.85	5	3.9	1.28
Bladder	10	17.7	0.57	3	3.1	0.96

Source: Schottenfeld et al. (1981).

[a]Standardized incidence ratio, based on U.S. incidence rates.

Table 3-1 displays observed and expected cancer incidence for the years when follow-up occurred, 1977–79. The results are presented separately for refinery and petrochemical workers. The numbers of observed cases for many cancer sites are small (<5), although there are suggestions of relative excesses of laryngeal cancer and multiple myeloma among the petrochemical workers.

Prospective cohort studies, although theoretically desirable approaches for studying cause-and-effect relationships, are infrequently used in occupational studies of cancer and other chronic diseases. This is because prospective cohort studies of diseases that have long induction and latency periods require very long periods of follow-up of large populations, thus engendering substantial costs of time, money, and effort. These costs become prohibitive when the health outcome of interest is a "rare" disease. By rare, we mean that less than 5 (or more typically less than 1) percent of the population will develop the disease during the study period. For example, most cancers, even the more common types, such as lung or colon cancer, occur at rates on the order of 50–200 per 100,000 persons per year.

One means of avoiding the problem of excessively prolonged follow-up of a cohort is to include a very large population in the study, as Schottenfeld et al. (1981) did in their study of petroleum industry workers (Example 3.2). The difficulty that arises here is that studying a larger number of workers for a shorter time is costly.

Sometimes, however, a prospective cohort study is the method of choice. Perhaps the best example is the study of changes in health status or physiologic functions that occur over a relatively brief span of time and are consequences of occupational exposure. The time span can be several years, as in a study of pulmonary function decline among firefighters (Musk et al., 1979), or it can be as brief as a single work shift, as in a study of pulmonary function changes during the course of a day in relation to cotton dust exposure (Merchant et al., 1973).

Example 3.3

Toluene diisocyanate (TDI) is recognized as a respiratory irritant capable of causing pulmonary impairment and immunologic disturbances in exposed persons. Diem et al. (1982) used the opportunity of the opening of a new TDI manufacturing plant to obtain baseline measurements and subsequent determinations of health status among workers at the plant. The investigators obtained health data on respiratory symptoms, pulmonary function, and immunologic tests for 168 workers first hired in 1973, and they added similar data for these workers and 109 newly hired workers during the succeeding four years. Their study was accompanied by an industrial hygiene monitoring survey that provided environmental measurements of TDI. Health data were obtained from study subjects at annual intervals.

Table 3–2 gives the results of the average annual change in forced expiratory volume in one second (FEV_1) for workers classified according to cumulative exposure levels (ppb-months of TDI), and stratified by smoking categories and average FEV_1/height^3 (in meters). The findings indicate a consistent effect of cumulative TDI exposure, with the most pronounced differences occurring among nonsmokers.

Example 3.3 illustrates the utility of a prospective cohort design for examining effects of occupational exposures on physiologic

Table 3-2. Average annual change (mL/yr) in forced expiratory volume in 1 second (FEV_1) among workers exposed to toluene diisocyanate.

| | FEV₁ level | | | |
| Smoking category | $FEV_1/ht^3 \geq 550$ exposure (ppb-months) | | $FEV_1/ht^3 < 550$ exposure (ppb-months) | |
	≤68.2	>68.2	≤68.2	>68.2
Never	1	−37	−18	−57
Previous	−12	−15	−32	−35
Current	−26	−37	−46	−57

Source: Diem et al. (1982).

changes during a reasonably short time period. (Five years may appear to be a long time interval, but most epidemiologic studies, irrespective of design, seldom can be completed in less than two years.)

Medical surveillance of occupational populations is a special application of the prospective cohort design. Here a currently enumerated cohort is followed into the future, and measurements of health status and the occurrence of diseases of interest are recorded. In fact, both Examples 3.2 and 3.3 are types of medical surveillance; the former is concerned with cancer incidence and mortality, and the latter focuses on specific physiologic responses. Diem et al.'s study in Example 3.3 is an especially effective use of prospective surveillance in that the cohort contained all workers first hired at a new facility, thus permitting a clear picture of health effects that probably could be ascribed to the workplace. More commonly, surveillance programs are initiated on a cohort of workers with varying lengths of past employment and exposures (Pell et al., 1978).

The focus of prospective surveillance can be very narrow, such as the pulmonary effects of a particular substance, or it may be wide, such as monitoring the morbidity and mortality patterns for a wide range of health outcomes.

3.2. Historical Cohort Studies

The goal of many occupational epidemiology studies is to detect altered rates of diseases of low incidence. Prospective cohort studies are relatively inefficient for this purpose, whereas the *historical cohort* design offers a very useful alternative for studying such conditions. In a historical cohort study, a cohort of workers is enumerated as of some time in the past, and the cohort is then followed over historical time to estimate disease rates for comparative analyses. Thus, the investigator is afforded the luxury of following and making observations on a cohort for periods extending across decades without incurring the tremendous monetary and time expenses usually involved in prospective studies.

The basic study design features of historical cohort studies are identical to those of prospective cohort studies. The rates of disease among a population initially free of disease are estimated for the follow-up interval. Comparisons of these rates are then made against prevailing rates in a non-exposed population, such as the national or regional population, and secondarily, comparisons are made between subgroups of the cohort, classified according to exposure type or level.

Example 3.4

Berry and Newhouse (1983) assembled a historical cohort of 13,425 workers employed during the years 1941–80 in a factory that produces asbestos-containing friction materials. The cohort consisted of 9,087 men and 4,338 women workers. Follow-up was conducted for the years 1942–80, during which time 1,339 male and 299 female workers died. Mortality comparisons were made on a cause-specific basis by means of contrasts of observed numbers of deaths among the cohort against expected numbers, based on death rates for England and Wales during the years of follow-up.

Table 3–3 contains the observed and expected numbers of deaths for selected diseases among workers who had achieved at least ten years of employment. These results pertain to the time period of ten and more years after the ten years of exposure were achieved. The findings reported for respiratory and gastrointestinal cancers are particularly noteworthy insofar as they suggest no substantial hazards from asbestos exposure in this particular setting.

The advantage of the historical cohort design should be evident from Example 3.4, where the investigators were able to study a cohort of nearly 14,000 workers traced for some 40 years. Achieving similar results in a prospective design would be impossible.

Historical cohort studies do have drawbacks, however. The first is that data required to reconstruct a historical cohort may not be available or may be incomplete. For example, it might be desirable to examine the mortality patterns of underground metals miners employed during the early years of the twentieth century, when exposures likely were poorly controlled, but employment records necessary for cohort reconstruction may not have been archived until the 1950s. Interviewing plant personnel or management can provide information on relative exposure rankings for various jobs

Table 3–3. Observed and expected mortality among asbestos friction materials manufacturing workers

Cause of death	Men			Women		
	Obs	Exp	Obs/Exp	Obs	Exp	Obs/Exp
All causes	1339	1361.8	0.98	299	328.0	0.91
Lung and pleural cancer	151	139.5	1.08	8	11.3	0.71
Gastrointestinal cancer	103	107.2	0.96	29	27.4	1.06
Other cancers	77	87.7	0.88	51	60.0	0.85
Other causes	1008	1027.4	0.98	211	229.3	0.92

Source: Berry and Newhouse (1983).

and tasks. However, use of interview information may introduce bias into the study if exposure judgments are influenced by knowledge of the occurrence of disease among workers in certain jobs. Another limitation, which will be discussed at greater length in Chapter 5, is that historical cohort studies usually are restricted to the investigation of fatal diseases. Data on mortality are routinely recorded in most countries, but data on nonfatal diseases are available only when special efforts have been made to document workers' health; comparative morbidity data for non-exposed populations are seldom available.

3.3. Subcohort Analysis

Occupational cohort studies in which disease rate comparisons are made with rates in an external comparison (non-exposed) population, such as the national population, indicate which diseases occur more or less frequently among the workforce. The next level of analysis involves the identification of specific high-risk exposures or jobs. This endeavor requires subdividing the cohort into groups defined on the basis of commonality of exposure level or job type. Comparisons of disease rates between component subgroups of a cohort are referred to as *subcohort analyses*. A subcohort analysis can be performed in either a prospective or historical cohort study.

Example 3.5

In 1962 Lloyd and Ciocco (1969) initiated a historical cohort mortality study of 59,072 steelworkers from seven plants in the United States. Follow-up was conducted for the years 1953–62. Preliminary analyses revealed excess rates of lung cancer among the cohort in comparison with the local county population, and a roughly twofold excess among workers in the coke plant relative to the entire steelworker cohort (Lloyd et al., 1970).

Subcohort analyses were performed to identify further high-risk groups within the cohort (Lloyd, 1971). Table 3–4 gives the lung cancer mortality results for subcohorts of coke plant workers, defined on the basis of job assignment and duration of employment. Relative risk estimates (SMRs) were computed using the rates among all steelworkers for comparison. The greatest excesses occurred among workers employed for five or more years in coke oven jobs (SMR = 3.55), and in particular, among the subcohort of employees who worked for five or more years at the topside of the coke ovens (SMR = 10.00). These findings suggest a strong etiologic link with exposure to the emissions of combustion products from coke ovens.

Subcohort analyses should be performed whenever the available exposure data permit classification of workers into two or more

Table 3-4. Lung cancer mortality among steelworkers in relation to job category

Job category/duration (yr)	Obs	Exp[a]	Obs/Exp
All coke plant/5+	29	13.6	2.13
Noncoke oven/5+	1	5.3	0.19
All coke oven/5+	27	7.6	3.55
Coke oven, never topside/5+	6	4.1	1.46
Coke oven, topside/<5	6	2.1	2.86
Coke oven, topside/5+	15	1.5	10.00

Source: Lloyd (1971).

[a]Expected deaths based on rates for all steelworkers.

quantitative or qualitative categories. One may have to perform sub-cohort analyses for selected diseases if resources are limited (e.g., computer costs may be a limiting factor). In this instance, subcohort analyses should be conducted for diseases for which there are over-all mortality or morbidity excesses, as well as for diseases that are of a priori interest because of findings from previous research. A thor-ough subcohort analysis with respect to job or exposure history requires a large effort by the investigators and is usually costly. In the steelworkers study from Example 3.5, the coding of work history records for 59,000 cohort members involved a major investment of money and personnel effort. Fortunately, there are alternative epi-demiologic methods suitable for investigating associations between diseases and specific exposures in an occupational setting. The case–control design is the best developed of these and is considered next.

4. CASE–CONTROL STUDIES

The main reason for the high cost of evaluating associations of dis-ease with exposures in an occupational cohort study is that the cohort design requires obtaining exposure data on a large number of subjects of which only a small proportion typically develops the disease(s) of interest. The case–control design reduces costs by lim-iting exposure assessment to cases of disease and a sample of the cohort that generated the cases.

Case–control studies provide estimates of relative risks (odds ratios). This is accomplished by comparing the past exposure his-tories of persons with the disease(s) of interest (cases) with those of persons who were free of disease(s) at the times the cases occurred (controls). The case–control design was originally developed as a convenient alternative to prospective cohort studies of chronic diseases (Cornfield, 1951; Mantel and Haenszel, 1959). Thus, case–control studies mitigate the difficulties of following a large cohort (and obtaining exposure data for all subjects) by selecting persons who already have developed the disease of concern. The cost efficiency of the case–control approach is especially attractive because, when used properly, case–control studies yield research findings that are as valid as those obtained from cohort studies (Miettinen, 1976; Liddell et al., 1977; Cole, 1979).

4.1. Industry-Based (Nested) Case–Control Studies

Case–control studies have been particularly useful for investigations of specific workplace hazards that cannot be studied efficiently with cohort and subcohort analyses. For example, if we are interested in studying the possible relationship between exposures to organic solvents and leukemia among a cohort of 10,000 workers in the chemical industry who were employed during a 30-year period, it might be possible to reconstruct the exposure profiles for all 10,000 cohort members and then to conduct leukemia mortality rate comparisons between subcohorts classified with regard to exposure level. A more efficient alternative would be to restrict the analysis to the leukemia deaths, identified during follow-up of the cohort, and a sample of other workers who were free of leukemia at the times when the leukemia deaths occurred.

Example 3.6

From Example 3.4 we saw that the results of Berry and Newhouse's (1983) historical cohort mortality study of asbestos friction materials manufacturing workers evidenced no overall suggestion of a lung cancer excess. The predominant type of asbestos used in the plant was chrysotile, which is generally considered to have less carcinogenic potential than the other two major commercial fiber types, amosite and crocidolite (Craighead and Mossman, 1982). However, there were two brief periods when crocidolite asbestos was used in the production of railway blocks, although only a minority of the workforce was believed to have been exposed to crocidolite. In order to determine whether there had been localized hazards resulting from crocidolite exposure, the investigators conducted a case–control study of pleural mesothelioma. (The mesotheliomas are the cancers most clearly linked to asbestos exposure.) The ten cases of mesothelioma were each matched with four worker controls with respect to gender, year started in the factory, birth year, length of survival (as long as the case), and period of employment at the factory when crocidolite was in use. The results of the case–control analysis are shown in

Table 3–5. Case–control analysis of pleural mesothelioma
and crocidolite asbestos exposure in a friction materials plant

	Exposure to crocidolite			
	Definite	Fringe	None known	Total
Cases	8	1	1	10
Controls	3	7	30	40

Source: Berry and Newhouse (1983).

Table 3–5. Eight of the ten cases, compared with three of the 40 controls, had had "definite" contact with crocidolite asbestos. This finding has particular significance in view of the lack of overall cancer mortality risks among the cohort. The specific association with crocidolite would have gone undetected had the investigators not performed an in-depth analysis.

Case–control studies of the type exemplified in Example 3.6 are frequently referred to as "nested," in that they are embedded within the framework of an occupational cohort (Kupper et al., 1975). Nested case–control studies have gained popularity in occupational epidemiology, as the advantages of studying multiple workplace exposures in an efficient manner have become better recognized.

Example 3.7

Wilcosky and co-workers (1984) conducted a nested case–control study of rubber industry solvent exposures in relation to a number of malignant diseases. A historical cohort study of 6,678 male rubber industry workers from one plant previously had demonstrated mortality excesses of non-Hodgkin's lymphomas (lymphosarcoma and reticulosarcoma), lymphocytic leukemia, stomach cancer, and prostate cancer (McMichael et al., 1974). The cases in Wilcosky's study were deaths from these diseases, and controls were a 20-percent random sample of the cohort. Jobs within the industry were rated with respect to 20 different solvents, including benzene, which historically has been the most strongly suspected carcinogen (Aksoy, 1980). As shown in Table 3–6, several solvents bore strong statistical associations with lymphosarcoma and lymphocytic leukemia, the most prominent of which were carbon tetrachloride and carbon disulfide. No consistent associations emerged for either stomach or prostate cancer.

4.2. Registry-Based Case–Control Studies

If a well-defined occupational cohort cannot be enumerated, a case–control study may be based on a particular disease registry. The "registry" could consist of a population-based disease registry

Table 3–6. Case–control comparisons of solvent exposures among rubber industry workers

	Cancer site							
	Stomach		Prostate		Lympho-sarcoma		Lymphocytic leukemia	
Solvent	Obs	RR[a]	Obs	RR	Obs	RR	Obs	RR
Gasoline	18	1.0	20	1.0	6	1.2	9	5.3
Specialty naphthas	18	1.1	18	0.9	6	1.4	8	2.8
Benzene	12	1.3	11	0.7	6	3.0	4	2.5
Ethanol	8	1.1	8	1.0	1	—	4	2.0
Carbon tetrachloride	7	0.8	12	1.3	6	4.2	8	15.3
Xylene	3	0.5	8	1.5	4	3.7	4	3.2
Carbon disulfide	8	1.2	11	1.5	6	5.6	7	8.9
Ammonia	2	2.1	1	—	0	—	1	—
Ethyl acetate	1	—	5	1.9	1	—	3	5.3
Acetone	1	—	4	1.7	1	—	3	6.8
Hexane	11	1.2	13	1.5	6	4.0	7	4.0
Solvent "A"[b]	15	1.4	13	1.0	6	2.6	7	2.8
Isopropanol	14	1.4	12	1.0	6	2.9	6	1.8
Phenol	6	1.4	2	0.4	0	—	1	—
VM&P naphtha	3	1.1	4	1.6	1	—	3	2.9
Trichloroethylene	5	1.0	3	0.6	3	2.4	2	0.8
Heptane	6	1.3	3	0.6	3	2.3	2	0.9
Toluene	1	—	3	2.6	0	—	2	3.0
Dipentene	2	1.3	0	—	0	—	1	—
Perchloroethylene	1	—	1	—	1	—	1	—

Source: Wilcosky et al. (1984).

[a]Relative risk (odds ratio).

[b]Proprietary mixture of toluene and other solvents.

that includes all cases of specific disease categories, such as cancer or birth defects. Alternatively, cases might be drawn from an ad hoc registry based on records collected for other purposes, such as hospital admissions, insurance claims, or disability pension awards. Controls may be obtained from the source population for the registry. If the source population is difficult to enumerate or if there are concerns about possible bias from selecting healthy controls, controls may be sampled from registrants with other diseases. Studies of this general description can be thought of as registry based.

Example 3.8

Pearce et al. (1986) investigated the associations between occupational exposures to agricultural chemicals and non-Hodgkin's lymphoma in New Zealand. The expo-

Table 3–7. Case–control study of non-Hodgkin's lymphoma and occupations and activities involving potential exposure to chlorophenols

Occupation or activity	No. of cases exposed	Other cancer controls		General population controls	
		No. exposed	RR	No. exposed	RR
Fencing as farmer	33	43	1.9	71	1.9
Fencing contractor	4	6	1.4	5	6.1
Sawmill or timber merchant	10	23	0.9	32	0.7
Meat works	19	23	1.9	39	1.9
Pelt department in meat works	4	4	2.3	6	4.1
Tannery	2	3	1.3	9	0.5

Source: Pearce et al. (1986).

sures of greatest interest were the phenoxyherbicides and chlorophenols, and chemical and microbiological agents associated with meat works. The cases were 83 males aged 20–69 years when diagnosed with non-Hodgkin's lymphoma who were identified from the files of the New Zealand Cancer Registry. Two sets of controls were selected. The first consisted of 168 males with cancers of other types, also identified from the cancer registry; the second set was made up of 228 males randomly chosen from the New Zealand electoral roll. Cases and controls were similar with respect to herbicide exposures, although strong associations with fencing and meat works emerged (Table 3–7). The authors postulated that possible causative exposures were arsenic and sodium pentachlorophenate in fencing and 2,4,6-trichlorophenol and/or zoonotic viruses in meat works.

Registry-based case–control studies of occupational exposures are frequently performed when it is not possible or feasible to assemble a cohort of workers in a particular occupation or profession (Houten et al., 1976). Farmers (as in Example 3.8) and auto mechanics are two such examples. In most situations registry-based case–control studies provide less detailed exposure data (often only an industry or job title) and hence are less informative with respect to characterizing exposure–response relationships than case–control studies nested within occupational cohorts. Often the best use of registry-based studies is for screening hypotheses regarding occupational exposures that may warrant more intensive inquiry in subsequent industry-based studies.

5. PROPORTIONATE MORTALITY STUDIES

Sometimes it is impossible to enumerate a cohort either for prospective or historical analysis but information exists on disease occurrence among members of the worker population. The most common situation is when death certificates are available for deceased company employees or union members but personnel information that would be needed to conduct a cohort or nested case–control study is incomplete. An indication of relative disease frequencies among workers can be obtained by means of comparisons of the proportional distributions of causes of death among workers with the corresponding proportions among a reference population. This type of design is known as a *proportionate mortality study*.

Example 3.9

Dalager and colleagues (1980) compared the distributions of cause of death between 202 male painters who had been employed at two aircraft maintenance bases, and the U.S. male population for the years 1959–77. The motivation for this study was a concern about possible carcinogenic effects of zinc chromates contained in paint. The analysis involved contrasts of observed numbers of deaths from specific causes among the painters with expected numbers, where the expected numbers were derived by applying the proportional distribution of deaths, by cause, among U.S. males to the total (202) deaths among the painters. These ratios are termed Proportionate Mortality Ratios (PMRs). Additionally, the investigators compared the distributions of site-specific cancer deaths as proportions of all cancer deaths in the painters and U.S. males, thus yielding Proportionate Cancer Mortality Ratios (PCMRs). Dalager et al. observed an overall PMR of 1.84 and a PCMR of 1.46 for respiratory cancer. Table 3–8 gives the results for respiratory cancer according to length of employment in the painting trade.

PMR studies have the attractive feature of providing results relatively quickly. However, the validity of a PMR study depends on whether the deaths included are generally representative of all deaths that would be identified if follow-up of the full cohort had been conducted. For example, if deaths from a particular cause were recorded preferentially because they were compensible or of

Table 3–8. Proportionate mortality from respiratory cancer among white male painters

Duration of employment (yr)	Proportionate mortality			Proportionate cancer mortality	
	Obs	Exp	PMR	Exp	PCMR
<5	9	6.4	1.41	7.2	1.25
5–9	6	3.0	2.00	4.0	1.50
≥10	6	2.0	3.00	3.2	1.88

Source: Dalager et al. (1980).

particular concern, then the PMR for that cause would probably appear to be elevated, even if the actual rate of disease in the cohort were not excessive. In practice, there is seldom any way to determine if this type of bias is at play, apart from the observation of an obviously anomalous result. A nonrepresentative sample of deaths can also be a problem in cohort or nested case–control studies but is potentially more prominent in proportionate mortality studies because in the latter, mortality data typically are death certificates that are readily available rather than those obtained from follow-up of the cohort.

Even when there is complete ascertainment of deaths, a shortcoming of the PMR approach is that when the PMRs for some diseases are elevated, counterbalancing proportionate mortality deficits will occur for other causes. This occurs because, by definition, the total number of observed deaths from all causes combined will equal the expected number. Several authors have discussed the utility of PMR studies (Kupper et al., 1978; Decoufle et al., 1980; Waxweiler et al., 1981; Wong and Decoufle, 1982; Wong et al., 1985). The commonly held view appears to be that PMRs are good approximations to SMRs obtained from cohort studies when the cohort's all-causes combined SMR is equal to 1.0 (i.e., observed is equal to expected). It should be noted that SMR analyses can also be misleading because of the typical pattern of a depressed all-causes combined mortality in the cohort in comparison with an external (e.g., national) reference population. This phenomenon is known as the *Healthy Worker Effect*. (We discuss the Healthy Worker Effect in Chapter 4.)

Proportionate mortality studies can be used with greater confidence when observed and expected distributions of specific diseases are compared *within* a disease category for which the Healthy Worker Effect is weak or nonexistent. For example, cancer mortality is generally less affected by the Healthy Worker Effect than cardiovascular disease mortality (McMichael, 1976). A commonly applied approach is to compare observed and expected site-specific cancer proportionate mortality, in which the mortality for a particular cancer site is expressed as a proportion of all cancer mortality. Here the Proportionate Cancer Mortality Ratio (PCMR) is the estimate of effect (see Example 3.9).

If the Healthy Worker Effect is of equal strength for the disease(s) of interest and for all causes combined, then the PMR will not be biased (although the SMR may still be biased). In practice, PMRs are computed for a large number of diseases, and mortality from some will be affected differentially by the Healthy Worker Effect. Thus, a reasonable approach to proportionate mortality analysis is to compute proportionate mortality ratios for specific diseases as proportions of the broader disease categories in which they are included (e.g., lung cancer as a proportion of all cancers, ischemic heart disease as a proportion of all cardiovascular diseases).

With minor modifications in the analysis, proportionate mortality studies can also be treated (more validly) as special types of the case–control design. In this situation, the analysis is restricted to deaths from the disease(s) of interest (i.e., cases) and other diseases assumed to be unrelated to the exposure(s) under study (i.e., controls). Additionally, it is required that the Healthy Worker Effect is equally strong in the diseases compared (Miettinen and Wang, 1981). This situation is discussed in more detail in Chapter 6 in the context of case–control studies using other diseases as controls.

On balance, PMR studies are most suitably used to explore for disease excesses and deficits on preliminary analysis of the available data. When the data are analyzed properly as a case–control study, proportionate mortality analysis yields valid results, provided that the control diseases are unrelated to the exposures of concern and that the Healthy Worker Effect is equally strong in the study (case) and control diseases.

6. CROSS-SECTIONAL STUDIES

Investigations of nonfatal diseases or physiologic responses to workplace exposures necessitate special studies that may involve clinical examinations, symptom surveys, or direct biological or physical measurements. The cross-sectional design is a suitable method for these purposes.

In an occupational cross-sectional study the prevalence of disease or related symptoms is compared between groups of workers classified with respect to exposure status. (Comparisons with an external reference population are made less frequently.) Prevalence refers to the number of cases of disease or the level of impairment existing at the time the study is being conducted.

Example 3.10

Smith et al. (1980) compared renal function, as estimated by urinary excretion of beta$_2$-microglobulin, among groups of workers exposed to varying levels of air-

Table 3–9. Urinary excretion of Beta$_2$-microglobulin according to exposure levels among cadmium-exposed workers

	Low exposure ($N = 11$)		High exposure ($N = 16$)	
	geometric mean	(SD)[a]	geometric mean	(SD)[a]
Beta$_2$-microglobulin (g/creatinine)	13.3	(4.62)	64.8	(6.05)
Beta$_2$-microglobulin (g/24 hr)	36.6	(4.37)	168.8	(5.46)

Source: Smith et al. (1980).

[a]Geometric standard deviation.

borne cadmium dust in a foundry. Two comparison groups were defined as a low-exposure group of 11 supervisory and laboratory personnel and a highly exposed group of 16 production workers. The findings in Table 3–9 show markedly elevated excretion rates of beta$_2$-microglobulin in the highly exposed group.

The particular advantage of cross-sectional studies is that they permit the study of conditions (e.g., kidney function in Example 3.10) for which data would not ordinarily be collected on a routine basis. Cohort and case–control studies usually focus on fatal diseases or other severe, overt states of impaired health (e.g., cancer, coronary heart disease, fatal accidents).

The most prominent shortcoming of many cross-sectional studies is that they typically include only currently employed workers; thus, retirees and other workers who were forced to terminate employment prematurely because of ill health, possibly attributable to their occupational exposures, go unstudied. Such persons may be the most relevant subjects for investigating delayed or progressive health consequences of exposure.

7. CONNECTIONS BETWEEN STUDY DESIGNS

The unifying feature of all epidemiologic study designs is that in each approach the investigator is examining the population's (cohort's) disease occurrence experience over some specified time interval (Miettinen, 1985). The cohort itself is termed the *base population,* and its experience over time forms the *study base* (Miettinen, 1982; Axelson, 1983). Person-years of observation are the familiar units that comprise the study base. The particular segment of the study base available for observation (e.g., from the cohort's inception to the end of follow-up in a cohort study, or the prior exposure patterns of cases and controls in a nested case–control study) is the distinguishing characteristic of a study.

Figure 3–1 is a simple representation of the causal sequence of exposure and subsequent health outcome. If we had the opportunity to conduct a prospective cohort study on workers, with enumeration occurring at time A and follow-up extending to time B, then data collection would start in the present and the health outcome would occur at some point in the future. As we discussed earlier, the historical cohort design offers a more cost- and time-efficient method for accomplishing the same objectives as a prospective cohort study. If a historical cohort study were to be conducted, then we would begin data collection (cohort enumeration and exposure assessment) at time B, but the follow-up interval would still be from A to B, where A is some point in the past.

The perception of the timing of a study (prospective or historical) is determined solely by when the investigator enters the picture. For example, if point A in Figure 3–1 were January 1, 1960, and point B were January 1, 1985, then whether the cohort study would be considered as prospective or historical would depend on when the investigator enumerated the cohort and began follow-up. If the research activities began in 1960, then the study would be considered as prospective, whereas if data collection began in 1985, then the study would be considered historical. In either case, the temporal relationship of exposure and health outcome would be the same. There might also be a situation where the cohort was enumerated at point A but for some reason (e.g., lack of funding) follow-up was not done until point B. Here again the cohort's disease experience and the inferences that could be drawn would be the

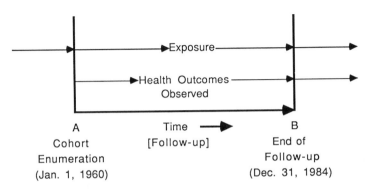

Figure 3–1. Temporal sequence of exposure and health outcomes.

same as in the more typical prospective or historical cohort approaches.

Perhaps more relevant than when follow-up is actually conducted is the timing of collection of exposure data. For example, the plant management may have begun exposure data collection in 1960 and continued collection through 1985. In this instance, a historical cohort study started in 1985 would be as valid as a prospective cohort study initiated in 1960, provided that there were no differences in losses to follow-up. If, however, exposure data for the study period (1960–85) were reconstructed in 1985, then a historical cohort study would be inferior to the prospective cohort study if exposure reconstruction was hindered by incomplete or missing data. The important point is that the differences in these approaches, with regard to their relative informativeness, depend strictly on the amount and quality of data that can be obtained and on feasibility.

The distinction between a cohort and a case–control design is one of studying the entire cohort's experience over time versus sampling from this experience. In a case–control study, the epidemiologist studies cases that have already occurred and samples a comparison group of workers who were free of disease at the times when the cases' diseases were identified. The logical direction from exposure to health outcome is the same for the case–control and cohort designs. The reduced size of the case–control study will not compromise the validity of results unless there has been a biased selection of cases or controls.

As is discussed in Chapter 6, specific guidelines for control selection in case–control studies exist to ensure that the findings, theoretically, are identical to those that would be derived from a cohort study of the entire worker population. Moreover, there are suitable methods (e.g., latency analysis) for determining the temporal relationships between exposure and disease; these methods are applicable to both cohort and case–control studies. Latency analysis is discussed in Chapters 5 and 6.

The proportionate mortality design, when analyzed appropriately, is a case–control study (Miettinen and Wang, 1981). The main distinction between proportionate mortality and nested case–control studies is that proportionate mortality studies ordinarily include deaths from an external reference population, whereas in nested case–control studies, controls are selected from the base cohort and may include living workers. Nevertheless, the comparisons of exposure between cases and controls in both designs are conceptually similar.

The case series is essentially a case–control study without controls. Thus, although the case series is an incomplete design, causal inference is not qualitatively different from that obtainable from other, more rigorous methods.

Selection of subjects in a cross-sectional study generally is made with respect to workers' exposure profiles, and health outcome is determined at the time of the study. (As is discussed in Chapter 7, subject selection can also be made with respect to current disease status without changing the interpretation of the findings.) The design of cross-sectional studies appears most likely to create dilemmas in distinguishing the timing of exposure and health outcome because both are determined simultaneously. Again, we point out that the timing of an epidemiologic study only has meaning in relation to when the investigator is conducting the research.

If we refer to Figure 3–1, the cross-sectional study would be represented adequately, with both exposure and outcome measured at point B. The temporal relationship between exposure and disease is the same as that in a cohort or case–control study. Any ambiguity of exposure and outcome sequencing should, in principle, be resolvable by carefully ascertaining the timing of occurrence of the two. This issue is by no means unique to cross-sectional studies, as valid inferences from cohort or case–control studies require similar efforts to establish the timing of cause and effect. It should be noted that cross-sectional studies measure disease prevalence rather than incidence, as in the other designs. Thus, findings from cross-sectional studies may be influenced by factors that affect disease duration. An example might be very intense dust exposure leading to rapid progression and disability or death; in this case a cross-sectional study would underestimate disease frequency.

We can therefore conclude that all of these study designs share a common direction and that they are generally distinguished only by the convenience of the sampling strategy. To illustrate, consider Figure 3–2, which depicts the employment and health experiences of two hypothetical workers. Both workers are hired at point A and retire at point C. Worker 1 develops the disease under study at point B and ultimately dies from this condition at point D. Worker 2 remains free from the disease throughout the period of the study to point E. We can consider worker 1's condition at point B to be the nonfatal form of his disease, which is not sufficiently severe to

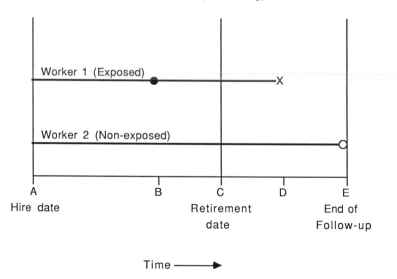

Figure 3–2. Employment and disease history for two hypothetical workers (● = disease onset; x = death from disease of interest; o = free of disease of interest at end of follow-up).

force retirement. These two workers are further distinguished by the fact that worker 1, but not worker 2, had experienced an exposure that caused his disease.

If we were to adopt a cohort study approach, then it is evident that worker 1 would be included in the "exposed" subcohort; he would also be counted as a case in an incidence study or a death in a mortality study. Worker 2 would be a member of the "non-exposed" subcohort as a noncase. Comparisons of incidence and/ or death rates between the two subcohorts would then be performed accordingly.

In a case–control analysis, worker 1 would be a case and worker 2 would be eligible to be a control (i.e., he was free of disease at the time when worker 1's case was detected, either at point B or D). Here the comparisons would consist of contrasts of exposure to the specific factor(s) that caused disease in worker 1.

A cross-sectional study of disease including these two workers would only demonstrate a difference in prevalence if the study were conducted after point B; before the onset of worker 1's disease there would be equal disease prevalences among exposed and non-exposed workers. After point B and up to point D, when worker 1 dies, there would be a demonstrable difference in prevalence. The time sequencing of either a cohort or case–control study would be similarly influential. If a cohort study did not extend to point *B*, then there would be an apparent lack of effect of exposure, as the disease rates in the exposed and non-exposed workers would be equal. Conducting a case–control study nested within a cohort study that terminated before point *B* would, of course, be uninformative, as no cases would be available for study.

The foregoing remarks about the conceptual (theoretical) equivalences of each study design should not be construed to imply that all approaches are equally suitable for the investigation of any health outcome. Indeed, there are decided advantages and disadvantages to the various approaches that are determined largely by logistical considerations.

8. SUMMARY

Formal epidemiologic research into occupational health hazards is often motivated by observations of apparent clusters of disease that are perceived to constitute excesses. Case series reports can be virtually conclusive in their own right when the health outcome seen is a very rare disease or an uncommon manifestation of a relatively common condition. Disease clusters can be misleading, however, because most diseases tend to follow a random occurrence distribution in time and space (e.g., area within a plant) wherein clusters of events are to be expected.

The "natural" epidemiologic study design is the cohort study. Here a worker population, presumed free of disease at the outset, is followed over time, and its disease rate patterns are contrasted with those of non-exposed reference populations, such as the national population. In addition, when data on exposures permit classification of worker subcohorts, disease rate comparisons can be made between these subcohorts in an effort to evaluate exposure–response relationships. Cohort studies can be considered as either prospective (follow-up begins at the time of the research and proceeds into the future) or historical (follow-up is conducted for time periods before the research is conducted). The distinction between prospective and historical cohort studies is not conceptual, as the designs are identical. Instead, the timing of the conduct of the research in relation to the actual occurrence of follow-up differentiates the two strategies. Practical considerations will dictate which of the two approaches is most suitable for a given situation. In general, prospective cohort studies of chronic diseases with long induction and latency intervals are too expensive and time-consuming for routine use. Historical cohort studies have the advantage, typically, of being more cost-efficient, but they can be limited by the absence or sparseness of cohort enumeration (personnel) and exposure data for times in the distant past.

Nested case–control studies involve comparisons of the exposure profiles of workers who developed the disease of interest (cases) with other workers who were apparently free of the disease at the times when the cases were identified (controls). Case–control studies nested within cohort studies are especially valuable designs because they can accomplish the same objectives as subcohort disease rate comparisons but have a reduced burden of data collection and processing.

Another type of occupational case–control study is the registry-based design, where cases—identified from hospitals, population-based disease registers, or other community sources—are compared with controls with respect to occupational factors. Registry-based studies generally are less informative with respect to specific exposure data than nested case–control studies. However, registry-based studies will be the option of choice for studies of occupational groups that are difficult or impossible to enumerate as cohorts (e.g., agricultural workers).

Nonfatal health effects or physiologic consequences of exposure are frequently investigated by cross-sectional studies. In this design, disease prevalence or physiologic status is compared between workers classified on the basis of current or, in some circumstances, lifetime occupational exposure levels.

The common feature of all these study designs is that the direction of each study is from exposure (presumed cause) to health outcome (effect). Study designs differ only with regard to the nature of the sampling of subjects from the study base, which is the health experience of workers over time. Logistical considerations, such as disease induction and latency intervals, or the availability of past exposure data, determine which design option is most suitable for a particular epidemiologic study.

Glossary

base population   The worker population (cohort) to be studied.
case–control study   Comparison of exposure histories of workers with disease (cases) with those of workers free of disease at the times when the cases occurred (controls).

case series   Report of a number of cases of disease occurring in a worker population.

cross-sectional study   Comparison of disease prevalence among groups of workers, or comparisons of exposures among prevalent cases and workers free of disease.

disease cluster   Occurrence of an apparently excessive number of cases of disease in a worker population.

healthy worker effect   A depressed mortality from all causes combined often observed among occupational cohorts compared with national or regional populations.

historical cohort study   Follow-up of worker cohort from the past to the present, and determination of disease rates during that time period.

nested case–control study   Case–control study in which cases and controls are selected from a defined occupational cohort.

proportionate mortality study   Comparisons of distributions of specific diseases (among all diseases) between the cohort and reference population.

prospective cohort study   Follow-up of worker population from the present into the future and determination of disease rates during that time period.

registry-based case–control study   Case–control study in which cases are selected from hospitals or other disease registers and controls are selected from the same register or from the community at large.

reference population   Population with which exposed cohort is compared; external reference population usually the national or regional population; internal reference population usually the least exposed segment of the cohort.

study base   The person-time of observation and associated disease rates of the study (base) cohort of workers.

subcohort   A segment of the cohort, usually defined on the basis of exposure type or level.

References

Aksoy M (1980): Different types of malignancies due to occupational exposure to benzene: a review of recent observations in Turkey. *Environ Res* 23:181–190.

Axelson O (1983): Elucidation of some epidemiologic principles. *Scand J Work Environ Health* 9:231–240.

Berry G, and Newhouse ML (1983): Mortality of workers manufacturing friction materials using asbestos. *Br J Ind Med* 40:1–7.

Cole P (1979): The evolving case–control study. *J Chron Dis* 32:15–27.

Cornfield J (1951): A method of estimating comparative rates from clinical data. Application to cancer of the lung, breast and cervix. *J Natl Cancer Inst* 11:1269–1275.

Craighead JE, and Mossman BT (1982): The pathogenesis of asbestos-related diseases. *N Engl J Med* 306:1446–1455.

Creech JL, and Johnson MN (1974): Angiosarcoma of liver in the manufacture of polyvinyl chloride. *J Occup Med* 16:150–151.

Dalager NA, Mason TJ, Fraumeni JF, et al. (1980): Cancer mortality among workers exposed to zinc chromate paints. *J Occup Med* 22:25–29.

Decoufle P, Thomas TL, and Pickle LW (1980): Comparison of the proportionate mortality ratio and the standardized mortality risk measures. *Am J Epidemiol* 111:263–269.

Diem JE, Jones RN, Hendrick DJ, et al. (1982): Five-year longitudinal study of workers employed in a new toluene diisocyanate manufacturing plant. *Am Rev Respir Dis* 126:420–428.

Enterline PE (1985): Evaluating cancer clusters. *Am Ind Hyg Assoc J* 46:B10–13.

Fox AJ, and Collier PF (1976): Low mortality rates in industrial cohort studies due to selection for work and survival in the industry. *Br J Prev Soc Med* 30:225–230.

Houten HA, Bross IDJ, and Viadanna E (1976): Hospital admission records: a source for identifying occupational groups at risk of cancer. *Ann NY Acad Sci* 71:384–387.

International Agency for Research on Cancer (1980): *Biological Effects of Mineral Fibres.* IARC Scientific Publications No. 30. Lyon, France: International Agency for Research on Cancer.

Kupper LL, McMichael AJ, and Spirtas R (1975): A hybrid epidemiologic study design useful in estimating relative risk. *J Am Stat Assoc* 70:524–528.

Kupper LL, McMichael AJ, Symons MJ, and Most BM (1978): On the utility of proportional mortality analysis. *J Chron Dis* 31:15–22.

Last JM (ed) (1983): *A Dictionary of Epidemiology.* Oxford: Oxford University Press.

Liddell FDK, McDonald JC, and Thomas DC (1977): Methods of cohort analysis: appraisal by application to asbestos mining. *J R Stat Soc (A)* 140:469–491.

Lloyd JW (1971): Long-term mortality study of steelworkers. V. Respiratory cancer in coke plant workers. *J Occup Med* 13:53–68.

Lloyd JW, and Ciocco A (1969): Long-term mortality study of steelworkers. I. Methodology. *J Occup Med* 11:299–310.

Lloyd JW, Lundin FE, Redmond CK, et al. (1970): Long-term mortality study of steelworkers. IV. Mortality by work area. *J Occup Med* 12:151–157.

Mantel N, and Haenszel W (1959): Statistical aspects of the analysis of data from retrospective studies of disease. *J Natl Cancer Inst* 22:719–748.

McMichael AJ (1976): Standardized mortality ratios and the "healthy worker effect": scratching beneath the surface. *J Occup Med* 18:155–168.

McMichael AJ, Spirtas R, and Kupper LL (1974): An epidemiologic study of mortality within a cohort of rubber workers. *J Occup Med* 16:458–464.

Merchant JA, Lumsden JL, Kilburn KH, et al. (1973): An industrial study of the biological effects of cotton dust and cigarette smoke exposure. *J Occup Med* 15:212–221.

Miettinen OS (1976): Estimability and estimation in case-referent studies. *Am J Epidemiol* 103:226–235.

Miettinen OS (1982): Design options in epidemiologic research: an update. *Scand J Work Environ Health* 8(Suppl 1):7–14.

Miettinen OS (1985): *Theoretical Epidemiology: Principles of Occurrence Research.* New York: John Wiley & Sons.

Miettinen OS, and Wang J-D (1981): An alternative to the proportionate mortality ratio. *Am J Epidemiol* 114:144–148.

Musk AW, Smith TJ, Peters JM, and McLaughlin E (1979): Pulmonary function in firefighters. Acute changes in ventilatory capacity and their correlates. *Br J Ind Med* 36:29–34.

Pearce NE, Smith AH, Howard JK, et al. (1986): Non-Hodgkin's lymphoma and exposure to phenoxyherbicides, chlorophenols, fencing work and meat works employment: a case–control study. *Br J Ind Med* 43:75–83.

Pell S, O'Berg MT, and Karrh BW (1978): Cancer epidemiologic surveillance in the DuPont Company. *J Occup Med* 20:725–740.

Schottenfeld D, Warshauer ME, Zauber AG, et al. (1981): A prospective study of morbidity and mortality in petroleum industry employees in the United States—a preliminary report. In: Peto R, and Schneiderman M (eds): *Quantification of Occupational Cancer, Banbury Report No. 9.* Cold Spring Harbor, NY: Cold Spring Harbor Laboratory, pp. 247–260.

Smith TJ, Anderson RJ, and Reading JC (1980): Chronic cadmium exposures associated with kidney function effects. *Am J Ind Med* 1:319–337.

Waxweiler RJ, Stringer W, Wagoner JK, and Jones J (1976): Neoplastic risk among workers exposed to vinyl chloride. *Ann NY Acad Sci* 271:40–48.

Waxweiler RJ, Haring MK, Lettingwell SS, and Halperin WH (1981): Quantification of differences between proportionate mortality ratios and standardized mortality ratios. In: Peto R, and Schneiderman M (eds): *Quantification of Occupational Cancer, Banbury Report No. 9.* Cold Spring Harbor, NY: Cold Spring Harbor Laboratory, pp. 379–389.

Wilcosky TC, Checkoway H, Marshall EG, and Tyroler HA (1984): Cancer mortality and solvent exposures in the rubber industry. *Am Ind Hyg Assoc J* 45:809–811.

Wong O, and Decoufle P (1982): Methodologic issues involving SMR and PMR in occupational studies. *J Occup Med* 24:299–304.

Wong O, Morgan RW, Kheifets L, and Larson SR (1985): Comparison of SMR, PMR and PCMR in a cohort of union members potentially exposed to diesel exhaust emissions. *Br J Ind Med* 42:449–460.

Young JL, Percy CL, Asire AJ, et al. (1981): *Surveillance, Epidemiology and End Results: Incidence and Mortality Data. 1973–77.* National Cancer Institute Monograph No. 57. NIH Publication No. 80-2330. Bethesda, MD: U.S. Department of Human Health Services.

4 Issues of Study Design and Analysis

1. OVERVIEW

General issues of the design and analysis of epidemiologic studies have been explored in several well-known texts (e.g., Kleinbaum et al., 1982; Rothman, 1986). This chapter is intended not to substitute for these texts but to give a brief overview of the most important design and analysis issues in occupational epidemiology. Our objective is to provide a basis for the more detailed discussion in the chapters that follow. We start by outlining the distinction between issues of precision, which involve random error, and issues of validity, which involve systematic error. The major validity issues—selection bias, information bias, and confounding—are then defined and illustrated. Finally, we discuss the estimation of joint effects and the related concept of effect modification.

2. PRECISION AND VALIDITY

2.1. Precision

Random error can occur in any epidemiologic study. It is often referred to as "chance," although it can perhaps more reasonably be regarded as ignorance. For example, suppose that 50 lung cancer deaths occurred among 10,000 asbestos-exposed workers aged 35–39 years during one year. If each worker had exactly the same cumulative exposure to asbestos fibers, we might expect two subgroups of 5,000 workers each to experience 25 deaths during the one-year period. However, just as 50 tosses of a coin do not usually produce exactly 25 heads and 25 tails, usually there will not be exactly 25 deaths in each group. This occurs because of differences in exposure to other risk factors for lung cancer and differences in individual susceptibility between the two groups. Ideally, we should attempt to gather information on all known risk factors

72

and to adjust for them in the analysis. However, other, unknown or unmeasurable risk factors will always occur; hence, the disease rates in particular subgroups will fluctuate about the average. This will occur even if each subgroup has exactly the same exposure history.

Even in an experimental study, in which subjects are randomized into exposure groups, "random" differences in background risk will occur between the compared groups. These differences will diminish in importance as the study size increases, however. In occupational epidemiology studies there is no guarantee that differences in background risks between the exposure groups will balance each other as the study size increases, but it is necessary to make this assumption in order to proceed with the study (Greenland and Robins, 1986). Hence, any occupational epidemiology study involves the assumption that the background fluctuation in disease rates is "random" in that it arises merely because a subgroup has effectively been sampled "at random" from the overall cohort, rather than because of systematic differences in unknown risk factors between subgroups of the cohort. If random error can be reduced by increasing the study size, then the precision of the effect estimate will be increased (i.e., its confidence limits will be narrower).

A second factor that can affect precision is the size of the comparison group relative to the study group (i.e., the ratio of non-exposed to exposed persons in a cohort study, or of controls to cases in a case–control study). For example, a cohort study of 10,000 persons with 1 exposed and 9,999 non-exposed will not be as informative as a study with 5,000 persons exposed and 5,000 non-exposed. When the study factor has no effect, a 1:1 ratio is most efficient for a given total study size. When there *is* an effect, a larger ratio may be more efficient. The optimal ratio is rarely greater than 2:1 (Walter, 1977), but a larger average ratio across strata may be desirable to ensure an adequate ratio in each stratum of the analysis.

The ideal study would be infinitely large, but practical considerations limit the number of subjects that can be included. Given these limits, it is desirable to find out, before starting, whether the study is large enough to be informative. One method is to calculate the "power" of the study. This depends on five factors: (1) the accepted level of statistical significance (e.g., $p = .05$), (2) the outcome proportion in the study group (i.e., the disease rate in the exposed group in a cohort study or the exposure prevalence among cases in a case–control study), (3) the outcome proportion in the comparison group, (4) the number of study subjects, and (5) the relative size of the two groups. Note that the outcome proportion in the study group can be estimated using the outcome proportion in the comparison group and the expected size of the effect. The standard normal deviate corresponding to the power of the study (derived from Rothman and Boice, 1982) is then

$$Z_\beta = \frac{N_2^{1/2}|P_1 - P_2|B^{1/2} - Z_\alpha B}{K^{1/2}} \qquad (4.1)$$

where Z_β = standard normal deviate corresponding to a given statistical power

Z_α = standard normal deviate corresponding to a p-value considered "statistically significant"

N_2 = number of persons in the reference group (i.e., the non-exposed group in a cohort study or the controls in a case–control study)

P_1 = outcome proportion in study group

P_2 = outcome proportion in the reference group

A = allocation ratio of reference to study group (i.e., the relative size of the two groups)

$B = (1 - P_2)(P_1 + (A - 1)P_2) + P_2(1 - P_1)$

$C = (1 - P_2)(AP_1 - (A - 1)P_2) + AP_2(1 - P_1)$

$K = BC - A(P_1 - P_2)^2$

Related approaches are to estimate the minimum sample sizes required to detect statistically significant effect estimates (e.g., relative risk) of specified magnitudes (Beaumont and Breslow, 1981) and to estimate the minimum detectable statistically significant effect estimate for a fixed study size (Armstrong, 1987).

Occasionally, the outcome is measured as a continuous rather than a dichotomous variable (e.g., blood pressure). In this situation the standard normal deviate corresponding to the study power is

$$Z_\beta = \frac{N_2^{1/2}(\mu_1 - \mu_2)}{s(A + 1)^{1/2}} - Z_\alpha \qquad (4.2)$$

where μ_1 = mean outcome measure in study group

μ_2 = mean outcome measure in reference group

s = estimated standard deviation of outcome measure

The power is not the likelihood that the study will estimate the size of the effect correctly. Rather, it is the likelihood that the study will yield a statistically significant finding in the expected direction when an effect of the postulated size exists. The observed effect could be greater or less than expected but still be statistically significant. The overemphasis on statistical significance is the source of many of the limitations of power calculations. One limitation is that the significance level is an arbitrary boundary. Also, issues of confounding, misclassification, and effect modification are frequently ignored in power calculations (although appropriate methods are available; see, e.g., Schlesselman, 1982; Greenland, 1983), and the size of the expected effect is often just a guess. More information can be provided by calculating a family of power curves for various study sizes and effect levels, but limitations remain nevertheless.

Estimating the expected precision can also be useful (Rothman, 1986). This can be done by "inventing" the results, based on the same assumptions used in power calculations, and carrying out an analysis by calculating effect estimates and confidence limits. This approach has particular advantages when the exposure is expected to have no effect, since the concept of power is not applicable, but precision is still of concern. However, this approach should be used with considerable caution, because the results may be misleading unless they are interpreted carefully (Greenland, 1987). In particular, a study with an expected lower limit equal to a particular value (e.g., 1.0) has only a 50-percent chance of yielding an observed lower confidence limit above that value.

Example 4.1

Consider a proposed study of 5,000 exposed persons and 5,000 non-exposed persons followed for a period of one year. Suppose that on the basis of mortality rates in a comparable group of workers, the expected number of lung cancer deaths is 25 in the non-exposed group and 50 in the exposed group. Then

$z_\alpha = 1.645$ (if a one-tailed significance test, for a p-value of .05, is to be used)

$N_2 = 5,000$

$P_1 = 0.010 \ (= 50/5000)$

$P_2 = 0.005 \ (= 25/5000)$

Using equation (4.1), the standard normal deviate corresponding to the power of the study to detect a statistically significant lung cancer excess in the exposed group is

$$Z_\beta = \frac{(5,000)^{1/2}(0.010 - 0.005)(0.0149)^{1/2} - 1.645 \times 0.0149}{(0.000197)^{1/2}} = 1.32$$

From tables for the (one-sided) standard normal distribution, it can be seen that this corresponds to a power of 91 percent. This means that if 100 similar studies of this size were performed, then we would expect 91 of them to show a statistically significant ($p < .05$) lung cancer excess in the exposed group.

An alternative approach is to carry out a standard analysis of the hypothesized results. If we make the preceding assumptions, then the relative risk would be 2.0, with a 90-percent confidence interval of 1.4–3.0. This approach has only an indirect relationship to the power calculations. For example, if the lower 90-percent confidence limit is 1.0, then the power for a one-tailed test (of $p < .05$) would be only 50 percent. Nevertheless, the confidence limit approach gives the same general conclusion as the power calculation: that the study will have reasonably adequate power if the true relative risk is 2.0. It also provides the additional information that it is quite likely that the observed relative risk could be as large as 3.0 or as low as 1.4. This may be quite acceptable if the aim of the study is merely to show an increased risk, but may not be acceptable if the aim is to measure the risk precisely, such as for purposes of risk assessment. In the latter instance a larger study would probably be required.

In practice, the study size is determined by the number of available subjects and by available resources. The former constraint is particularly relevant in occupational studies because the number of persons who have worked in a particular factory or industry usually sets an upper limit on the number of available study subjects. Within these limitations it is desirable to make the study as large as possible, taking into account the trade-off between including more subjects and gathering more detailed information about a smaller number of subjects. Hence, power calculations can serve only as a rough guide as to whether a study that is feasible is large enough to yield precise information. Even if such calculations suggest that a particular study would have very low power, the study may still be worthwhile if exposure information is collected in a form that permits the study to contribute to the broader pool of information concerning a particular exposure–disease relationship. For example, one important development has been the initiative of the International Agency for Research on Cancer (IARC) in organizing international collaborative studies such as that of occupational exposure to man-made mineral fibers (Simonato et al., 1986). This study involved pooling the findings from individual cohort studies of 13 European factories. Most of the individual cohorts were too small to be informative in themselves, but each contributed to the overall pool of data.

Once a study has been completed, there is little value in retrospectively performing power calculations, since the confidence limits of the observed measure of effect provide the best indication of the range of possible values within which the true effect may lie. In the remainder of this chapter, random error is ignored; the discussion concentrates on avoiding systematic error.

2.2. Validity

Systematic error, or *bias,* occurs if there is a difference between what the study is actually estimating and what it is intended to estimate. Systematic error is thus distinguished from random error in that the former would be present even with an infinitely large study, whereas random error can be reduced by increasing the study size. There are many different types of bias, but three general forms have been distinguished: selection bias, information bias, and confounding.

3. SELECTION BIAS

3.1. Definition

Selection bias is any bias arising from the procedures by which the study subjects were chosen from the entire population that theoretically could be studied (Rothman, 1986). The potential total pool of data includes every person who ever worked in a particular occupation or industry, with each person followed to the end of life. Most studies use a subset of this person-time experience, and hence bias may occur. For example, if a national population registry (or some surrogate for this, such as the United States Social Security Administration) were not available, then it might be necessary to attempt to contact each worker or his next of kin to verify vital status. Bias could occur if the response rate was higher in the most heavily exposed persons who had been diagnosed with disease than in other persons.

Although we should recognize the possible biases arising from subject selection, it is important to note that epidemiologic studies need not be based on representative samples to avoid bias. For example, in a cohort study persons who develop disease might be more likely to be lost to follow-up than persons who did not develop disease; however, this would not affect the relative risk estimate, provided that loss to follow-up applied equally to the exposed and non-exposed populations (Criqui, 1979). On the other hand, case–control studies have differing selection probabilities as an integral part of their design, in that the selection probability of diseased persons is usually close to 1 (provided that most persons with disease are identified), whereas that for nondiseased persons is substantially less.

3.2. The Healthy Worker Effect

The Healthy Worker Effect is perhaps the most common selection bias in occupational studies. This phenomenon is characterized typically by lower relative mortality, from all causes combined, in an occupational cohort (McMichael, 1976) and occurs because relatively healthy individuals are likely to gain employment and to remain employed. Including the person-time experience of every person who ever worked in a particular factory or industry minimizes bias because healthy persons remain in employment, but it does not remove the bias resulting from initial selection of healthy persons into employment. The same issues of bias apply to other study designs (such as case–control and cross-sectional studies) that involve sampling from the cohort's experience over time.

These effects were first described by William Ogle in 1885 (quoted in Fox and Collier, 1976), when he outlined the two major difficulties encountered in studying the occupational distribution of mortality. One is that "some occupations may repel, while others attract, the unfit at the age of starting work." The other is the "considerable standard of muscular strength and vigor to be maintained" by those who pursued various occupations. In 1902 Latham (quoted in Alderson, 1972) discussed the effects of the demands of the job on entry into and exit from occupations and described the plight of a man compelled by ill health to change from skilled worker to cabdriver to street hawker before becoming unemployed.

At least three factors are involved in the Healthy Worker Effect (Fox and Collier, 1976): the selection of healthy members from the source population, the survival in the industry of healthier men, and the length of time the population has been followed. The Healthy Worker Effect may also be exacerbated by various methodological errors such as considering subjects lost to follow-up as alive at the end of the study (Vena et al., 1987). Wilcosky and Wing (1987) have suggested that other mechanisms may also play a role, including the selection of economically advantaged workforces for epidemiologic studies. Tola and Hernberg (1983) have commented that, because of the multifaceted nature of the Healthy Worker Effect, it is doubtful whether such a crude summary term is useful at all, and that one should perhaps try to make distinctions between the different

Table 4-1. Cause-specific relative risks for white male workers at an energy research laboratory compared with U.S. white men, 1943-77

Cause of death	Obs	Exp	Relative risk[a]
All cancers	194	250.0	0.78
Arteriosclerotic heart disease	344	459.9	0.75
Cerebrovascular disease	62	76.9	0.81
Diabetes mellitus	10	18.3	0.55
Nonmalignant respiratory diseases	42	69.2	0.61
Digestive system diseases	26	72.0	0.36
Genitourinary system diseases	15	18.2	0.82
Diseases of blood-forming organs	2	3.1	0.65
Motor vehicle accidents	36	60.2	0.60
Suicide	39	40.2	0.97
All causes	966	1320.0	0.73

Source: Checkoway et al. (1985).

[a]Obs/Exp.

underlying factors. These issues are further discussed in Section 5.3 of this chapter, where we examine methods for minimizing the Healthy Worker Effect.

Example 4.2

Table 4-1 gives the findings of a cohort study of mortality among 8,375 white males who worked for at least one month during the period 1943-72 at an energy research laboratory (Checkoway et al., 1985). Follow-up was conducted for the period 1943-77. For every disease category the observed number of deaths was less than that expected, on the basis of national mortality rates. In most studies the Healthy Worker Effect is weaker for cancer than for other causes of death. For example, Fox and Collier's (1976) study found a relative risk of 0.75 for all causes, 0.91 for all cancers, 0.77 for circulatory disease, and 0.63 for respiratory disease. However, in this study the authors found that the Healthy Worker Effect was nearly as strong for cancer (SMR = 0.78) as for all causes of death (SMR = 0.73).

3.3. Minimizing Selection Bias

If selection bias has occurred in the enumeration of the study group, it may still be possible to avoid bias by choosing an appropriate comparison group. For example, if the study cohort consists primarily of active or recently active workers, then it would not be appropriate to use national mortality rates as a comparison because of the Healthy Worker Effect. However, bias may be avoided, or at least minimized, by choosing a more appropriate comparison group, such as active or recently active workers from another industry who do not have the same exposures. The choice of comparison groups is discussed in more detail in Chapter 5.

4. INFORMATION BIAS

Information bias involves misclassification of the study subjects with respect to disease or exposure status. It is customary to consider two types of misclassification: nondifferential and differential misclassification.

4.1. Nondifferential Information Bias

Nondifferential information bias occurs when the *likelihood of misclassification is the same for both groups compared.* This can occur if exposed and non-exposed persons are equally likely to be misclassified according to disease outcome or if diseased and nondiseased persons are equally likely to be misclassified according to exposure.

One special type of nondifferential information bias occurs when the study outcome is not well defined and includes a wide range of etiologically unrelated outcomes (e.g., all deaths). This may obscure the effect of exposure on one specific disease since a large increase in risk for this disease may only produce a small increase in risk for the overall group of diseases under study. A similar bias can occur when the exposures are incorrectly defined, sometimes due to the inclusion of exposures that could not have caused the disease because they occurred after or shortly before diagnosis. It could be argued that these phenomena do not represent information bias because these are not errors in measurement. However, they do involve information bias in the sense that the etiologically relevant exposure (or disease) has not been measured appropriately.

Nondifferential misclassification of exposure will bias the effect estimate toward the null value (Copeland et al., 1977). Hence, it is of particular concern in studies that show no association between exposure and disease.

Example 4.3

In many occupational cohort studies some exposed persons are classified as non-exposed, and vice versa, because of errors or deficiencies in routinely collected employee records. Table 4–2 illustrates this situation with hypothetical data from a study of lung cancer incidence in asbestos workers. Suppose the true incidence rates are 100 per 100,000 person-years in the exposed group and 10 per 100,000

Table 4-2. Hypothetical data from a cohort study in which 15 percent of exposed persons and 10 percent of non-exposed persons are incorrectly classified

	Actual		Observed	
	Exposed	Non-exposed	Exposed	Non-exposed
Deaths	100	10	$85 + 1 = 86$	$9 + 15 = 24$
Person-years	100,000	100,000	$85,000 + 10,000 = 95,000$	$90,000 + 15,000 = 105,000$
Incidence rate per 100,000 person-years	100	10	91	23
Rate ratio	10.0		4.0	

person-years in the non-exposed group, and the relative risk is thus 10.0. If 15 percent of exposed persons are incorrectly classified, then 15 of every 100 deaths and 15,000 of every 100,000 person-years will be incorrectly allocated to the non-exposed group. Similarly, if 10 percent of non-exposed persons are incorrectly classified, then 1 of every 10 deaths and 10,000 of every 100,000 person-years will be incorrectly allocated to the non-exposed group. As a result, the observed incidence rates per 100,000 person-years will be 91 and 23, respectively, and the observed relative risk will be 4.0. Because of nondifferential misclassification, incidence rates in the exposed group have been biased downward, and incidence rates in the non-exposed group have been biased upward.

4.2. Differential Information Bias

Differential information bias occurs when the likelihood of misclassification of exposure is different in diseased and nondiseased persons or the likelihood of misclassification of disease is different in exposed and non-exposed persons. This can bias the observed effect estimate either toward or away from the null value. For example, in a nested case–control study of lung cancer, with a control group selected from among nondiseased members of the cohort, the recall of occupational exposures in controls might be different from that of the cases. In this situation, differential information bias would occur, and it could bias the odds ratio toward or away from the null, depending on whether members of the cohort who did not develop lung cancer were more or less likely to recall such exposure than the cases.

Example 4.4

Table 4–3 shows data from a hypothetical case–control study in which 70 of the 100 cases and 50 of the 100 controls have actually been exposed to some chemical. The true odds ratio (Chapter 6) is thus $(70/30)/(50/50) = 2.3$. If 90 percent (63) of the 70 exposed cases but only 60 percent (30) of the 50 exposed controls are classified correctly, then the observed odds ratio would be $(63/37)/(30/70) = 4.0$. This example provides a simple illustration of differential information bias. How-

---

Table 4-3. Hypothetical data from a case-control study in which 90 percent of exposed cases and 60 percent of exposed controls are correctly classified

	Actual		Observed	
	Exposed	Non-exposed	Exposed	Non-exposed
Cases	70	30	63	37
Controls	50	50	30	70
Odds ratio	2.3		4.0	

ever, it should be noted that there is inadequate information to indicate whether differences in recall have been a source of serious bias in occupational studies (Axelson, 1985).

As can be noted from Example 4.4, information bias can drastically affect the validity of a study. Given limited resources, it is often more desirable to reduce information bias by obtaining more detailed information on a limited number of subjects than to reduce random error by including more subjects. However, a certain amount of information bias is unavoidable, and it is usually desirable to ensure that it is nondifferential, as the bias is then in a known direction (toward the null value).

Example 4.5

In the case–control study of lung cancer in Example 4.4, the information bias could be made nondifferential by selecting controls from cohort members with other types of cancer, or other diseases, so that their recall of exposure would be more similar to that of the cases. As before, 63 (90 percent) of the exposed cases would recall exposure, but now 45 (90 percent) of the 50 exposed controls would recall their exposure. The observed odds ratio would be $(63/37)/(45/55) = 2.1$. This estimate is still biased in comparison with the correct value of 2.3. However, the bias is nondifferential, is much smaller than before, and is in a predictable direction toward the null. However, it should be noted that making a bias nondifferential does not always make it smaller (see Example 4.3).

4.3. Assessment of Information Bias

Information bias is usually of most concern in historical cohort studies or case–control studies when information is obtained by personal interview. Despite these concerns, relatively little information is generally available on the accuracy of recall of exposures. Two studies (Baumgarten et al., 1983; Brisson et al., 1988) showed good accuracy of job history data obtained by interview. In both studies, the subjects accurately identified employers for more than 80 percent of the person-years considered, although Brisson et al. (1988) found that recall was less accurate for the period 12–28 years (74 percent) than for the period 0–11 years (89 percent) prior to the interview. In both studies, validity was poorer among persons who had worked in numerous jobs, but the extent of concordance did not differ substantially by age or education level. Furthermore, a study of the association between pleural plaques and asbestos exposure (Jarvholm and Sanden, 1987) suggests that subjects' own estimates of exposure may be more accurate than expert estimates based on classification of occupational titles.

When possible, it is important to attempt to validate the classification of exposure or disease (e.g., by comparing interview results with other data sources, such as employer records) and to assess the potential magnitude of bias due to misclassification of exposure. These issues are discussed in more detail in the context of specific study designs (see Chapters 5–7).

5. CONFOUNDING

5.1. Definition

Confounding occurs when the exposed and non-exposed groups are not comparable because of inherent differences in background disease risk (Greenland and Robins, 1986). This usually occurs because of differences in exposures to other risk factors. Confounding can thus be thought of as a mixing of the effect of the study factor with the effects of other risk factors. In general terms, to be a confounder a factor must be associated with both exposure and disease, even in the absence of the study exposure.

More explicitly, if no other biases are present, three conditions are necessary for a factor to be a confounder (Rothman, 1986). First, the factor must be associated with disease, even in the absence of the exposure under study. It should be noted that even surrogates for causal factors, such as social class or age, may be regarded as potential confounders, even though they are not direct causal factors.

Second, a confounder must be associated with exposure in the study base (the cohort's person-time experience), not merely among the cases. In case–control studies this means that a confounder must be associated with exposure among the controls. An association can occur among the cases simply because the study factor and a potential confounder are both risk factors for the disease, but this does not cause confounding in itself.

Finally, the potential confounder must not be an intermediate step in the causal pathway between exposure and disease. In this situation there is no mixing of effects, but only one effect, and controlling for such an intermediate factor will make it impossible to measure this effect. For example, in a study of colon cancer among clerical workers, it would be inappropriate to control for low physical activity if it was considered that reduced physical activity was a

Table 4–4. Lung cancer mortality rates per 100,000 person-years at risk in a cohort of asbestos insulation workers compared to those in other blue-collar occupations

	Rate in smokers	Rate in nonsmokers	Pooled rate if 30 percent smoke	Pooled rate if 60 percent smoke
Asbestos	590	58	218	377
Nonasbestos	120	11	44	76
Rate ratio	4.9	5.2	5.0	5.0
Rate difference	470	47	174	301

Source: Hammond et al. (1979).

consequence of being a clerical worker, and hence a part of the causal chain leading from clerical work to colon cancer. On the other hand, if low physical activity itself was of prime interest, then this should be studied directly, and clerical work would be regarded as a potential confounder if it also involved exposure to other risk factors for colon cancer. Evaluating this type of possibility requires information external to the study to determine whether a factor is likely to be a part of the causal chain.

Example 4.6

Table 4–4 presents data from a cohort study of 12,051 North American male asbestos insulators with at least 20 years of exposure who were followed from 1967 to 1976 (Hammond et al., 1979). The mortality pattern of these workers was compared with that of 73,763 male blue-collar workers who were enrolled in a prospective cohort study and followed from 1967 to 1972. It can be seen from Table 4–4 that for both smokers and nonsmokers, the lung cancer mortality rate in asbestos insulators is approximately five times that in other blue-collar workers. Hence, if the asbestos insulators and other blue-collar groups contain the same percentage of smokers, then the overall relative risk (for asbestos exposure) will be approximately five times. Suppose, however, that only 30 percent of the insulators were smokers compared with 60 percent of other blue-collar workers. Then the lung cancer death rate in the asbestos workers would be $0.70 \times 58 + 0.30 \times 590 = 218$ per 100,000 person-years, whereas the rate in other blue-collar workers would be $0.40 \times 11 + 0.60 \times 120 = 76$. The rate ratio would then be $218/76 = 2.9$, which is still elevated but much less than the correct figure of approximately 5.0. Smoking operates as a confounder in this example, because it is predictive of disease in the absence of asbestos exposure (Table 4–4) and is associated with asbestos exposure in the study base.

5.2. Relationship of Confounding to Selection and Information Bias

Selection bias, information bias, and confounding are not always clearly differentiated. In particular, selection bias and confounding can be viewed as separate aspects of the same phenomenon. One approach is to consider any bias that can be controlled in the analysis as confounding (Rothman, 1986). Other biases can then be categorized according to whether they arise from the selection of study subjects (selection bias) or their classification (information bias).

5.3. The Healthy Worker Effect Revisited

The relationship between selection bias and confounding is typified by the Healthy Worker Effect, which was discussed in the context of selection bias. An alternative viewpoint is offered by Monson (1980), who argues that the Healthy Worker Effect occurs through confounding by the factor of "good health status" that is associated with the outcome (death) and with the exposure (employment in the industry). Information on good health status is rarely obtainable, but it is usually possible to characterize the Healthy Worker Effect according to the timing of the events on which it operates: employment in the industry and termination of employment. Figure 4–1 illustrates the employment history of a hypothetical worker and specifies four time-related factors that delimit the operation of the Healthy Worker Effect: age at first employment, duration of employment, length of follow-up, and age at risk. We will review the relationship of these factors to the Healthy Worker Effect in order to illustrate their importance as potential confounders in occupational studies.

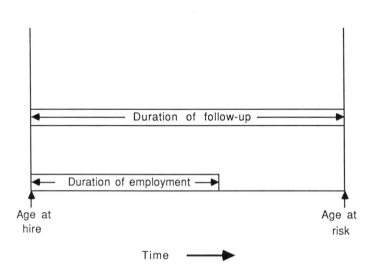

Figure 4–1. Employment history of a hypothetical worker.

Table 4–5. Relative risks for all causes of mortality by length of follow-up

Study	Type of comparison	Follow-up (yr)				
		0–4	5–9	10–14	≥15	Total
Fox and Collier (1976)	External	0.37	0.63	0.75	0.94	0.75
Gilbert[a] (1982)	Internal	0.63	0.93	1.01	1.03	1.00

[a]Follow-up groups do not exactly correspond to those in heading.

The mortality of employed persons, relative to the general population, is lowest during the period immediately after starting employment (Table 4–5). In their cohort study of polyvinyl chloride production workers, Fox and Collier (1976) found that the all-causes mortality of men within five years of entering the industry was as low as 37 percent of that expected. For circulatory disease and respiratory disease it was as low as 21 percent whereas for cancer it was 45 percent. The effect decreased with length of time since entry into the cohort and had almost disappeared after 15 years of follow-up, and the relative risks were 0.94 for all causes mortality and 1.12, 0.91, and 0.93 for cancer, circulatory disease, and respiratory disease mortality, respectively. A study by Gilbert (1982) that used an internal comparison group found a similar, but weaker, pattern (Table 4–5). Many other studies have also found relatively low relative risks for the early years of follow-up, with relative risks slowly approaching 1.0 as follow-up continued (Pearce et al., 1986).

Although the relative mortality advantage of employed persons diminishes with length of follow-up, it is most pronounced in workers with the longest duration of employment. This latter association is attributable to the survival in the industry of relatively healthier persons. For example, Gilbert's (1982) study of workers at the Hanford nuclear facility found an elevated all-causes mortality in short-term workers (see Table 4–6) and in terminated workers.

In Fox and Collier's (1976) study the survival effect was measured by separating men who survived 15 years according to whether they were still in the industry. The mortality rate among those who left was approximately 50 percent higher than those still in the industry

Table 4–6. Relative risk for all causes of mortality by duration of employment

Study	Type of comparison	Duration of employment (yr)				
		0–1	2–4	5–9	10–14	≥15	Total
Gilbert (1982)	Internal	1.15	0.92	0.97	0.94	0.92	1.00

for all causes, cancer, circulatory disease, and respiratory disease and was approximately three times higher for lung cancer. Vinni and Hakama's (1980) study of a random sample of 20,000 persons from the total Finnish population considered associations between changes in occupations from 1960 to 1970 and mortality during 1971–75. Those staying in the same occupational category during the period 1960–70 had 20 percent lower overall mortality than those who did not. However, the latter group was not homogeneous; the investigators reported relative risks of 0.70 for persons changing to another occupational category between 1960 and 1970, 1.00 for persons retiring at the usual age of 65 years during the same period, and 1.30 for persons retiring early. Similarly, a study in Denmark (Olsen and Sabroe, 1979) found mortality rates to be 65 percent higher in persons leaving the Danish carpenters' union compared with persons entering the union, but mortality was much lower for persons leaving for a higher-paid job compared with persons leaving for other reasons. Delzell and Monson (1981) also found excess risks among early retirees, particularly during the first year following early retirement. Thus, the Healthy Worker Effect is strongest during active employment and rapidly disappears following the cessation of employment, particularly if this occurs before the usual retirement age. Wen and Tsai (1982) have thus commented that the Healthy Worker Effect is most characteristic of actively employed workers and would be more accurately addressed as the "active worker effect."

Table 4–7 shows data from several investigations that have examined the relative mortality advantage of employed persons at different levels of age at risk (i.e., the age at any point in follow-up). McMichael (1976), in a study of male rubber industry workers, found an all-causes relative risk of 0.81 at ages 40–54 years, whereas the relative risk for the 75 years and over age group was 1.13. Similar patterns have also been observed by Fox and Collier (1976) and Delzell and Monson (1981).

Table 4–7. Relative risks for all causes of mortality by age at risk

Study	Type of comparison	Age at risk (yr)				
		<55	55–64	65–74	≥75	Total
Fox and Collier (1976)	External	0.64	0.79	0.96	0.60	0.75
McMichael et al. (1976)	External	0.81	0.89	0.95	1.13	0.98
Delzell and Monson (1981)	External	0.8	0.9	0.9	1.0	0.9

Table 4-8. Relative risks for all causes of mortality by age at hire

Study	Type of comparison	Age at hire (yr)				
		25–44	45–54	55–64	65–74	Total
Fox and Collier (1976)	External	0.45	0.37	0.32	0.23	0.37

Note: This paper does not explicitly present risks by age at hire. These data represent relative risks by age at death during the first five years of hire.

Two studies have presented relative risks according to age at hire. Musk et al. (1978), in a study of mortality among firefighters, found all-causes relative risks of 0.92 for persons hired before age 40 and 0.88 for persons aged 40 years or more at hire. Fox and Collier's (1976) study presented data for the first five years after hire with relative risks of 0.45 and 0.23 for the 25–44- and 65–74-year age groups, respectively (Table 4–8). This suggests that the relative mortality advantage of employed persons may be greater with increasing age at hire—the opposite pattern to that for age at risk. This hypothesis is plausible, since, if a certain level of health is required to gain employment, then the proportion of persons attaining the required level is likely to be smaller in the older age groups. Therefore, gradients of health between workers and the general population are likely to increase with increasing age at hire.

The association of the time-related factors depicted in Figure 4–1 with various health outcomes has important implications for the design and analysis of occupational epidemiology studies because it suggests that the use of an internal comparison group will not eliminate bias if the exposure groups differ according to the time-related factors under consideration. For example, if exposure occurs in jobs assigned primarily to short-term, transient workers, then bias may occur if the crude mortality rates for exposed persons are compared with those for a non-exposed workforce with longer average duration of employment because the transient workers may have different background disease risks attributable to unfavorable life-style factors. This phenomenon may be reflected in the findings of a study by Peto et al. (1985) of lung cancer in asbestos textile factory workers that show the highest relative risks in long-term workers and in persons who had worked for less than one year. It might be hypothesized that the excess in long-term workers is due to asbestos exposure, whereas the latter effect might be due to life-style-related confounding. Of course, if workers with adverse life-styles are preferentially assigned to the most heavily exposed jobs, then a bias in an internal exposure–response analysis is present. This bias will occur even if such workers are not short-term or transient workers. An analytic method to minimize this type of bias has been developed (Robins, 1986; 1987), although it requires complex computations.

Bias may also occur if exposure levels at a factory have been reduced over time as a result of changes in control measures, work practices, or changes in production. The more recently employed workers, who would have a lower level of exposure, might have been followed for a shorter period of time and hence have lower mortality rates than those employed in a previous period. In other words, the time-related factors depicted in Figure 4–1 are predictive of disease in occupational cohorts and will be confounders if they are also associated with exposure. Calendar year may also be a confounder if disease incidence and exposure patterns vary over time.

Apart from age at risk, the strongest predictors of disease in occupational studies appear to be calendar year and length of follow-up. Furthermore, duration of employment is strongly correlated with cumulative exposure, and it may be difficult to separate their effects. In general, adjustment for duration of employment is not warranted. Age at hire is a direct function of age at risk and length of follow-up, and further adjustment for this factor is not appropriate.

It should be stressed, however, that adjustment for factors such as length of follow-up may minimize confounding due to the Healthy Worker Effect but may not eliminate more complex biases associated with it. In particular, Robins (1986) has shown that bias may occur if risk factors for disease are also determinants of employment status (and hence of subsequent exposure). For example, if smokers terminate employment early (perhaps because of smoking exacerbating the effects of the study exposure on disease symptoms, such as respiratory tract irritation), then smokers who have increased disease risks due to their smoking will have lower cumulative exposures than nonsmokers. Such bias would be difficult to detect if smoking information were not available. More generally, when a confounding factor (such as termination of employment) determines subsequent exposure and is determined by previous exposure, then standard analyses that estimate disease incidence as a function of cumulative exposure can underestimate the true exposure effect, even when adjustment is made for the confounder. However, the likelihood of such biases occurring is seldom clear, and adjustment for factors such as length of follow-up (but not duration of employment) may still be warranted even if it will not completely eliminate bias.

5.4. Other Confounders

Other confounders commonly addressed in occupational studies include age, gender, and ethnicity. Cigarette smoking is the major potential life-style confounder in studies of smoking-related diseases. However, Axelson (1978) has shown that differences in smoking status are unlikely to account for relative risks for lung cancer of greater than 1.5 or less than 0.7 in studies involving a comparison with national mortality rates. Furthermore, Siemiatycki et al. (1988) have found that confounding by cigarette smoking is likely to be minimal when an internal comparison group is used.

An indirect approach to controlling for life-style confounders is to control for social class, which is strongly related to mortality (Pearce et al., 1985; Pearce and Howard, 1986), in part because of its association with such factors as smoking, diet, exercise, housing, and access to health care. Appropriate information is often not available in occupational studies, but it may be possible to construct a social class scale based on education, income, or job category. Such analyses should be conducted with caution, however, as crudely constructed social class measures may be poor surrogates for life-style factors. Moreover, other occupations in the same social class may also involve occupational risk factors for the study disease. Control for life-style is not appropriate if modification of life-style is an intermediate step in the causal pathway leading from occupation to disease. For example, in a study of psychosocial aspects of work and their relationships to disease, control for cigarette smoking would not be appropriate if it was felt that the psychosocial work-related factors caused disease through increased cigarette smoking. In this context, it has been argued that "smoking behaviour cannot be taken as a fundamental cause of ill-health, it is rather an epiphenomenon, a secondary symptom of deeper underlying features of economic society" (DHSS, 1980).

Finally, most occupations involve exposure to more than one potential risk factor, and the possibility of confounding by other occupational exposures must be considered in the context of each study. For example, studies of cancer and pesticide exposures in farmers ideally should take into account the other potential carcinogens to which farmers are exposed, such as solvents, oils, fuels, dusts, paints, welding fumes, zoonotic viruses, microbes, and fungi (Blair, 1985). However, controlling for such exposures may be difficult when they are highly correlated, making it difficult to separate their effects. Previous or subsequent employment in industries other than the one under study likewise can be an important potential confounder.

5.5. Assessment of Confounding

The assessment of confounding involves the use of a priori knowledge about the potential confounder, together with assessment of the extent to which the effect estimate changes when the factor is controlled in the analysis. Most epidemiologists prefer to make a decision based on the latter criterion, although this approach can be misleading, particularly if there is misclassification of exposure (Greenland and Robins, 1985). The decision to control for a presumed confounder can certainly be made with more confidence if there is supporting prior knowledge that the factor is generally predictive of disease.

When necessary information is not available to control confounding directly, it is still desirable to assess its potential strength. For example, the assessment of potential confounding by cigarette smoking is of particular concern in occupational studies of cancer because smoking information is rarely available for all study subjects (although, as noted earlier, smoking is usually a relatively weak confounder in occupational studies). One approach is to conduct an analysis of smoking-related diseases other than the disease of primary interest (Steenland et al., 1984). If mortality from such diseases (e.g., nonmalignant respiratory disease) is not elevated, this may suggest that any excess for the disease of interest is unlikely to be due to smoking.

Axelson (1978) has presented a useful indirect approach to assessing confounding in occupational cohort studies. This is based on the relation

$$I = I_0(1 - P_{CF}) + I_{CF}P_{CF} \qquad (4.3)$$

where I = overall incidence rate in the cohort
I_{CF} = incidence in those exposed to confounder
I_0 = incidence in those not exposed to confounder
P_{CF} = proportion of cohort exposed to confounder

Equation (4.3) can be used to evaluate the possible confounding effect of a factor such as smoking with regard to lung cancer by assessing the range of overall incidence rates that could be obtained with various smoking frequencies (see Example 4.7).

Checkoway and Waldman (1985) have presented an extension of this method to case–control studies. This involves the relation

$$\frac{I_2}{I_1} = R_C = \frac{(R-1)P_2 + 1}{(R-1)P_1 + 1} \tag{4.4}$$

where I_1 = incidence rate in the nonexposed category with "standard" exposure to confounder

I_2 = incidence rate in an exposed population with different exposure to confounder

P_1 = proportion (among those whose confounding status is known) of controls not exposed to the study factor but exposed to the confounder

P_2 = proportion (among those whose confounding status is known) of controls exposed to the study factor who are exposed to the confounder

R = relative risk associated with exposure to the confounder

R_C = relative risk due to confounding

Example 4.7

Suppose that a cohort study of lung cancer involves a comparison with national mortality rates in a country where 50 percent of the population are nonsmokers, 40 percent are moderate smokers with a ten-fold risk of lung cancer (compared to nonsmokers), and 10 percent are heavy smokers with a twenty-fold risk of lung cancer. Then, using equation (4.3), it can be calculated that the national lung cancer incidence rate will be 6.5 (= $0.50 \times 1.0 + 0.40 \times 10 + 0.10 \times 20$) times the rate in nonsmokers. Suppose that it was considered most unlikely that the cohort under study contained more than 50 percent moderate smokers and 20 percent heavy smokers. Then the incidence rate in the study cohort would be 9.4 times the rate in nonsmokers. Hence, the observed incidence rate would be biased upward by a factor of 9.4/6.5 = 1.4 due to confounding by smoking. Table 4–9 gives a range of such calculations presented by Axelson (1978) using data from Sweden. The last column indicates the likely bias in the observed rate ratio due to confounding by smoking. (A value of 1.00 indicates no bias.)

Table 4–10 illustrates Checkoway and Waldman's (1985) case–control extension of this approach to a hypothetical study of 100 cases and 200 controls. Information on exposure to the study factor can be determined for all subjects, but exposure information for some confounding factor is incompletely ascertained. A relative risk of 3.0 is assumed for the confounding factor from previous investigations. The crude odds ratio (see Chapter 6) is $(50 \times 130)/(50 \times 70) = 1.86$. The estimated odds ratio due to confounding associated with exposure to the study factor is

$$\frac{(3-1)(30/50) + 1}{(3-1)(40/90) + 1} = 1.16$$

This suggests that the odds ratio estimate was biased upward by a factor of 1.16.

Table 4-9. Estimated crude rate ratios in relation to fraction of smokers in various hypo-thetical populations

	Population fraction (%)		Bias in relative risk
Nonsmokers	Moderate smokers[a]	Heavy smokers[a]	
100	—	—	0.15
80	20	—	0.43
70	30	—	0.57
60	35	5	0.78
50	40	10	1.00[b]
40	45	15	1.22
30	50	20	1.43
20	55	25	1.65
10	60	30	1.86
—	65	35	2.08
—	25	75	2.69
—	—	100	3.08

Source: Axelson (1978).

[a]Two different risk levels are assumed for smokers: 10 times for moderate smokers and 20 times for heavy smokers.

[b]Reference population with rates similar to those in the general population in countries such as Sweden.

5.6. Control of Confounding

Two possible errors arise from confounding. These occur when no attempt is made to control for a confounder, and when one controls for a nonconfounder. The former error is potentially more serious because it results in a biased effect estimate, whereas controlling for a nonconfounder does not usually bias the effect estimate but may reduce its precision.

Table 4-10. Hypothetical example of case–control distributions accord-ing to exposure to a study factor and a confounding factor[a]

Exposure to study factor	Exposure to confounding factor			
	Yes	No	Unknown	Total
Cases				
Yes	20	20	10	50
No	20	10	20	50
Controls				
Yes	30	20	20	70
No	40	50	40	130

Source: Checkoway and Waldman (1985).

[a]A rate ratio of 3.0 is assumed for the confounding factor, as determined from previous investigations.

Misclassification of a confounder leads to a loss of ability to control confounding, although control may still be useful, provided that misclassification of the confounder is nondifferential (Greenland, 1980). Misclassification of exposure poses a greater problem because factors that influence misclassification may appear to be confounders, but control of these factors may increase the net bias (Greenland and Robins, 1985). In general, control of confounding requires careful use of prior knowledge, as well as inference from the observed data.

Confounding can be controlled in the study design, in the analysis, or both. Control at the design stage involves three main methods (Rothman, 1986). The first is randomization (i.e., random allocation to exposure categories), but this is not an option in occupational studies. A second method of control at the design stage is to restrict the study to narrow ranges of values of the potential confounders (e.g., by restricting the study to white males aged 35–54 years). This approach has a number of conceptual and computational advantages but may severely restrict the number of potential study subjects and the informativeness of the study, because effects in younger or older workers will not be observable.

A third method of control involves matching study subjects on potential confounders. For example, in a cohort study one would match a white male non-exposed subject aged 35–39 years with an exposed white male aged 35–39 years. This will remove confounding in a cohort study but is seldom done, because it may be very expensive. Matching can also be expensive in case–control studies. Moreover, matching does not remove confounding, but merely facilitates its control in the analysis. Matching may actually reduce precision in a case–control study if it is done on a factor that is associated with exposure, but the matching factor is not a risk factor for the disease of interest. However, matching on a strong risk factor usually increases the precision of effect estimates. Some of the practical advantages of matching in case–control studies are discussed in Chapter 6.

Confounding can also be controlled in the analysis, although it may be desirable to match on potential confounders in the design to optimize the efficiency of the analysis. The analysis ideally should control simultaneously for all confounding factors. Control of confounding in the analysis involves stratifying the data according to the levels of the confounder(s) and calculating an effect estimate that summarizes the information across strata of the confounder(s).

For example, controlling for age (grouped into five categories) and gender (with two categories) might involve grouping the data into the 10 (= 5 × 2) confounder strata and calculating a summary effect estimate which is a weighted average of the stratum-specific effect estimates.

It is usually not possible to control simultaneously for more than two or three confounders in a stratified analysis. For example, in a cohort study, finer stratification often leads to many strata containing no exposed or no non-exposed persons. Such strata are uninformative; thus, fine stratification is wasteful of information. This problem can be mitigated to some extent by the use of mathematical modeling that allows for simultaneous control of more confounders by "smoothing" the data across confounder strata. Mathematical modeling is discussed in Chapter 8.

6. ESTIMATING JOINT EFFECTS

6.1. Joint Effects

Estimating the joint effect(s) of two or more factors is often an analytic goal. For example, Checkoway et al. (1988) estimated the joint effect of exposure to alpha and gamma radiation on lung cancer mortality among workers exposed to uranium at a nuclear materials fabrication plant. They found a rate ratio of 4.60 for cumulative exposure to more than 5 rem of both alpha and gamma radiation compared to cumulative exposure to less than 1 rem of both radiation types.

If two factors are independent (i.e., there are no cases of disease caused *only* by the joint effect of the two factors), then their effects will be *additive* (Rothman, 1986). Most analyses of occupational studies involve relative risk measures, which assume that the risk factors involved have *multiplicative* effects. However, it is still possible to calculate the separate and joint effect(s) of two or more factors and assess the findings on an additive scale.

Example 4.8

Consider the data in Table 4–4. The relative risks for each stratum, relative to persons with no exposure to asbestos or cigarette smoke (obtained by dividing each cell by 11), can be presented as follows:

Smoking

		Yes	No
Asbestos	Yes	53.6	5.2
	No	10.9	1.0

The observed joint relative risk is 53.6, whereas it would be $1 + (5.2 - 1) + (10.9 - 1) = 15.1$ if the effects of the two factors were additive. The fact that the joint effect is more than additive has two important implications. In the public health context, it indicates that it is more important to prevent asbestos exposure in smokers than in nonsmokers, as intervention will prevent approximately 43 lung cancer cases in smokers for every four lung cancer cases prevented in nonsmokers. In scientific terms, nonadditivity suggests that asbestos and smoking take part in at least one common causal process.

It is difficult to learn much more from such data without using a specific causal model. For example, the Armitage–Doll multistage model of carcinogenesis (Armitage and Doll, 1961) might be used to examine the interrelationships of asbestos and smoking (Thomas, 1983). If smoking data were not available, then it might still be desirable to examine the asbestos effect in light of this model. This latter approach is illustrated in Chapter 10.

6.2. Effect Modification

It should also be noted that the examination of joint effects of two or more factors often is discussed in the context of *effect modification*, which occurs when the estimate of the effect of the study factor depends on the level of another factor in the study base (Miettinen, 1974). The term *statistical interaction* denotes a similar phenomenon in the observed data. We will use the term *effect modification* in the subsequent discussion. However, both effect modification and statistical interaction are merely statistical concepts that depend on the methods used. In fact, all secondary risk factors modify either the rate ratio or the rate difference, and uniformity over one measure implies nonuniformity over the other (Koopman, 1981; Steenland and Thun, 1986); for example, an apparent additive joint effect implies a departure from a multiplicative model.

Example 4.9

The data presented in Table 4–4 provide an example of effect modification. If the rate difference is used, then smoking clearly modifies the effect of asbestos exposure since the rate difference (for asbestos exposure) is 470 per 100,000 person-years at risk in smokers and 47 per 100,000 person-years at risk in nonsmokers. However, if the rate ratio is used, then the effect of asbestos exposure is about five times in both smokers and nonsmokers. Asbestos exposure thus appears to multiply the lung cancer death rate by about five times, and this effect is not modified by smoking if a multiplicative effect measure (such as the rate ratio) is used. However, smoking does modify the effect of asbestos exposure if an additive effect measure (such as the rate difference) is used. Another way of stating this is that there is no interaction (i.e., departure from an assumed model) of smoking with asbestos exposure on a multiplicative scale, but there is an interaction on an additive scale.

When the assessment of joint effects is a fundamental goal of the study, it can be accomplished by calculating stratum-specific estimates, as in Example 4.8. On the other hand, it is less clear how to proceed when effect modification is occurring, but assessment of joint effects is not an analytical goal. Some authors (e.g., Kleinbaum et al., 1982) argue that it is not appropriate in this situation to calculate an overall estimate of effect summarized across levels of the effect modifier. However, it is common to ignore this stipulation if the differences in effect estimates are not pronounced.

Glossary

allocation ratio   Relative size of comparison group to study group.

bias   See *systematic error.*

cohort   The population to be followed.

comparison group   Non-exposed group in a cohort study, or control group in a case–control study; also known as the reference group or reference series.

confidence limits   A range of values for the effect estimate within which the true effect is thought to lie, with the specified level of confidence.

confounder   A variable that, if not controlled, produces distortion in the estimated effect of the study exposure; in the absence of misclassification, such a variable will be associated with the study exposure and predictive of risk among the non-exposed. A confounder must not be an intermediate step in the causal pathway from exposure to disease.

effect estimate   The estimate of the effect of the study factor on disease—for example, the risk ratio, rate ratio, odds ratio, rate difference, or risk difference.

expected number   The number of cases or deaths that would have occurred in the study cohort had the rates in the non-exposed population prevailed.

Healthy Worker Effect   Lower mortality in occupational cohorts than external comparison populations; usually attributed to selection for employment of fit-test members of the population.

information bias   Bias arising from the misclassification of disease or exposure status.

odds   The ratio of the proportion of a group experiencing an event to the proportion not experiencing the event.

odds ratio   The ratio of two odds.

power   The likelihood that a study will yield a statistically significant finding in the expected direction (when there is an actual effect).

precision   The stability of an estimate of effect, as reflected in its confidence interval.

rate difference   Difference in disease rates between two populations.

rate ratio   Ratio of disease rates in two populations.

relative risk   A general term to denote the rate ratio, risk ratio, or odds ratio.

response rate   The proportion of intended study subjects for whom information ‘was obtained.

risk   The average probability of developing disease during some specified time interval.

risk difference   Difference of disease risks in two populations.

risk factor   A factor that is associated with an increased likelihood of disease or death.

risk ratio   Ratio of risks in two populations.

selection bias   Bias arising from the manner in which the study subjects were chosen from the entire population that theoretically could be studied.

systematic error   Error that occurs if there is a difference between what a study is actually estimating and what it is intended to estimate.

variance   A measure of the stability of the effect estimate that indicates the amount of variation in the estimate that would be obtained if similar studies were repeated a large number of times.

Notation

Z_α Standard normal deviate corresponding to p-value that will be considered statistically significant

Z_β Standard normal deviate corresponding to study power

N_1 Number of persons in study group

N_2 Number of persons in comparison group

A Allocation ratio of comparison group to study group

P_1 Outcome proportion in study group

P_2 Outcome proportion in comparison group

References

Alderson MR (1972): Some sources of error in British occupational mortality data. *Br J Ind Med* 29:245–254.

Armitage P, and Doll R (1961): Stochastic models for carcinogenesis. In: Proceedings of the 4th Berkeley Symposium on Mathematical Statistics and Probability: Biology and Problems of Health, Vol 4. Berkeley, CA: University of California Press, pp. 19–38.

Armstrong B (1987): A simple estimator of minimum detectable relative risk, sample size, or power in cohort studies. *Am J Epidemiol* 125:356–358.

Axelson O (1978): Aspects on confounding in occupational health epidemiology. *Scand J Work Environ Health* 4:85–89.

Axelson O (1985): The case-referent study—some comments on its structure, merits and limitations. *Scand Work Environ Health* 11:207–213.

Baumgarten M, Siemiatycki J, and Gibbs GW (1983): Validity of work histories obtained by interview for epidemiologic purposes. *Am J Epidemiol* 118:583–591.

Beaumont JJ, and Breslow NE (1981): Power considerations in epidemiologic studies of vinyl chloride workers. *Am J Epidemiol* 114:725–734.

Blair A, Malker H, Cantor KP, et al. (1985): Cancer among farmers: a review. *Scand J Work Environ Health* 11:397–407.

Breslow NE, and Day NE (1980): *Statistical Methods in Cancer Research. Vol I: The Analysis of Case–Control Studies.* Lyon, France: International Agency for Research on Cancer.

Brisson C, Vezina M, and Bernard PM (1988): Validity of occupational histories obtained by interview for epidemiologic purposes. Unpublished manuscript.

Checkoway H, and Waldman GT (1985): Assessing the possible extent of confounding in occupational case–referent studies. *Scand J Work Environ Health* 11:131–133.

Checkoway H, Mathew RM, Shy CM, et al. (1985): Radiation, work experience, and cause specific mortality among workers at an energy research laboratory. *Br J Ind Med* 42:525–533.

Checkoway H, Pearce N, Crawford-Brown DJ, and Cragle DL (1988): Radiation doses and cause-specific mortality among workers at a nuclear materials fabrication plant. *Am J Epidemiol* 127:255–266.

Copeland KT, Checkoway H, McMichael AJ, and Holbrook RH (1977): Bias due to misclassification in the estimation of relative risk. *Am J Epidemiol* 105:488–495.

Criqui MH (1979): Response bias and risk ratios in epidemiologic studies. *Am J Epidemiol* 109:394–399.

Delzell E, and Monson RR (1981): Mortality among rubber workers: IV. General mortality patterns. *J Occup Med* 23:850–856.

DHSS (1980): Report of a research working group. *Inequalities in Health.* London: Department of Health and Social Services.

Fox AJ, and Collier FF (1976): Low mortality rates in industrial cohort studies due to selection for work and survival in the industry. *Br J Prev Soc Med* 30:225–230.

Gilbert ES (1982): Some confounding factors in the study of mortality and occupational exposures. *Am J Epidemiol* 116:177–188.

Greenland S (1980): The effect of misclassification in the presence of covariates. *Am J Epidemiol* 112:564–569.

Greenland S (1983): Tests for interaction in epidemiologic studies: a review and a study of power. *Stat Med* 2:243–251.

Greenland S (1987): On sample-size and power calculations for studies using confidence intervals. Unpublished manuscript.

Greenland S, and Robins JM (1985): Confounding and misclassification. *Am J Epidemiol* 122:495–506.

Greenland S, and Robins JM (1986): Identifiability, exchangeability and epidemiological confounding. *Int J Epidemiol* 15:412–418.

Hammond E, Selikoff I, and Seidman H (1979): Asbestos exposure, cigarette smoking, and death rates. *Ann NY Acad Sci* 33:473–489.

Jarvholm B, and Sanden A (1987): Estimating asbestos exposure: a comparison of methods. *J Occup Med* 29:361–363.

Kleinbaum DG, Kupper LL, and Morgenstern H (1982): *Epidemiologic Research:*

Principles and Quantitative Methods. Belmont, CA: Lifetime Learning Publications.

Koopman JS (1981): Interaction between discrete causes. *Am J Epidemiol* 13:716–724.

McMichael AJ (1976): Standardized mortality ratios and the "healthy worker effect": scratching below the surface. *J Occup Med* 18:165–168.

Miettinen OS (1974): Confounding and effect modification. *Am J Epidemiol* 100:350–353.

Monson RR (1980): *Occupational Epidemiology.* Boca Raton, FL: CRC Press.

Musk AW, Monson RR, Peters JM, et al. (1978): Mortality among Boston firefighters, 1915–1975. *Br J Ind Med* 35:104–108.

Olsen J, and Sabroe S (1979): Health selection among members of a Danish trade union. *Int J Epidemiol* 8:155–159.

Pearce NE, and Howard JK (1986): Occupation, social class and male cancer mortality in New Zealand 1974–78. *Int J Epidemiol* 15:456–462.

Pearce NE, Davis PB, and Smith AH (1985): Social class, ethnic group and male mortality in New Zealand 1974–1978. *J Epidemiol Community Health* 39:9–14.

Pearce NE, Checkoway H, and Shy CM (1986): Time-related factors as potential confounders and effect modifiers in studies based on an occupational cohort. *Scand J Work Environ Health* 12:97–107.

Peto J, Doll R, Hermon C, et al. (1985): Relationships of mortality to measures of environmental asbestos pollution in an asbestos textile factory. *Ann Occup Hyg* 29:305–355.

Robins JM (1986): A new approach to causal inference in mortality studies with a sustained exposure period—application to the healthy worker survivor effect. *Math Modeling* 7:1393–1512.

Robins JM (1987): A graphical approach to the identification and estimation of causal parameters in mortality studies with sustained exposure periods. *J Chronic Dis* 40 (Suppl 2):139S–161S.

Rothman KJ (1986): *Modern Epidemiology.* Boston, MA: Little, Brown & Co.

Rothman KJ, and Boice JD (1982): *Epidemiologic Analysis with a Programmable Calculator.* Boston, MA: Epidemiology Resources.

Schlesselman JJ (1982). *Case-Control Studies: Design, Conduct, Analysis.* New York: Oxford University Press.

Siemiatycki J, Wacholder S, Dewar R, et al. (1988): Smoking and degree of occupational exposure: are internal analyses in cohort studies likely to be confounded by smoking status? *Am J Ind Med* 13:59–69.

Simonato L, Fletcher AC, Cherrie J, et al. (1986): *Scand J Work Environ Health* 12(Suppl 1):34–47.

Steenland K, and Thun M (1986): Interaction between tobacco smoking and occupational exposures in the causation of lung cancer. *J Occup Med* 28:110–118.

Steenland K, Beaumont J, and Halperin W (1984): Methods of control for smoking in occupational cohort mortality studies. *Scand J Work Environ Health* 10:143–149.

Thomas DC (1983): Statistical methods for analyzing effects of temporal patterns of exposure on cancer risks. *Scand J Work Environ Health* 9:353–366.

Tola S, and Hernberg S (1983): Healthy worker effect. In: Chiazze L, Lundin FE, Watkins D (eds). *Methods and Issues in Occupational and Environmental Epidemiology,* Ann Arbor, MI: Ann Arbor Science Publishers.

Vena JE, Sultz HA, Carlo GC, et al. (1987): Sources of bias in retrospective cohort mortality studies: a note on treatment of subjects lost to follow-up. *J Occup Med* 29:256–261.

Vinni K, and Hakrama M (1980): Healthy worker effect in the total Finnish population. *Br J Ind Med* 37:180–184.

Walter SD (1977): Determination of significant relative risks and optimal sampling procedures in prospective and retrospective studies of various sizes. *Am J Epidemiol* 105:387–397.

Wen CP, and Tsai SP (1982): Anatomy of the healthy worker effect—a critique of summary statistics employed in occupational epidemiology. *Scand J Work Environ Health* 8(Suppl 1):48–52.

Wilcosky T, and Wing S (1987): The healthy worker effect: selection of workers and workforces. *Scand J Work Environ Health* 13:70–72.

5 Cohort Studies

1. OVERVIEW

Cohort studies of occupational populations provide the most direct approach for evaluating overall patterns of health and disease. This chapter contains a description of the study design and analysis features that are specific to occupational cohort studies.

As was shown in Chapter 3, every epidemiologic study is based on a particular population's experience over time. The cohort design has the advantage, relative to other study designs, that ideally it includes all of the relevant person-time experience of the population under study. In contrast, other study designs involve sampling from that experience. However, problems pertaining to feasibility constraints and validity of data are potentially as prominent in cohort studies as in other designs.

The specific features of cohort studies to be presented in this chapter include cohort definition, follow-up procedures, choice of comparison populations, and methods of data analysis. Examples from the published literature are used to illustrate issues of design and analysis. In particular, a cohort study of mortality among asbestos textile manufacturing workers, conducted by Dement and colleagues (1983a,b), is discussed in some detail in this and in subsequent chapters.

2. BASIC COHORT DESIGN

2.1. Design Options: Prospective and Historical

Cohort studies can be classified according to the temporal sequence of conduct. The investigator may follow a currently enumerated population into the future; this strategy is commonly referred to as a *prospective cohort study.* Alternatively, one may follow a historical cohort, enumerated as of some prior time, to the present. The latter

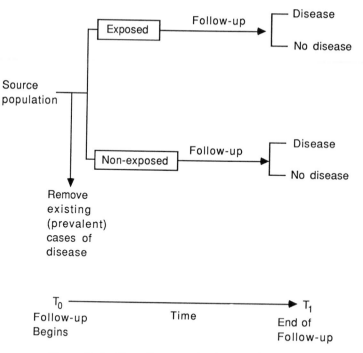

Figure 5–1. Flow diagram of cohort study design.

approach is termed a *historical cohort study*. Historical cohort studies have also been referred to as *retrospective cohort studies* (Last, 1983). For purposes of clarity, we use the terms *prospective* and *historical* cohort studies to denote, respectively, studies where follow-up proceeds into the future or where it has taken place from the past to the present. Some studies combine features of both prospective and historical designs.

The common elements of each of these types of cohort study are (1) the identification of a study population, or cohort, of persons exposed to the factors of interest, (2) the identification of a comparison (reference) population, (3) follow-up of the cohort over time, and (4) comparisons of disease rates between the cohort and a reference population. Figure 5–1 depicts schematically the basic design of a cohort study. In a prospective cohort study, t_0 would be present and t_1 would be some point in the future. In a historical cohort study, t_0 would be a point in the past, and t_1 would represent the present or some time close to the present.

Historical cohort studies are far more common than prospective studies in occupational epidemiology; therefore, we focus most attention on the design and conduct of the former. However, the basic methodological features of all cohort studies are the same.

Thus, the discussion of historical cohort studies pertains also to the other types of cohort study.

2.2. Defining and Following the Study Cohort

Cohort Definition

An occupational cohort can be defined in several ways. The simplest situation is when the investigator selects as cohort members all workers ever employed in one factory or manufacturing complex. A second option is to include in the cohort workers from multiple plants operated by different companies but engaged in the same industrial processes. International studies that combine occupational populations from similar facilities located in different countries are extensions of this approach. The European cohort study of workers exposed to man-made mineral fibers is one such example (Saracci, 1986). A third cohort definition is to study members of a trade union or professional organization that includes workers from numerous plants or worksites who share a common set of occupational exposures. Examples of the last type are cohort studies of cancer mortality among meatworks union members (Johnson et al., 1986) and reproductive hazards experienced by dental technicians (Cohen et al., 1980). A fourth, special type of cohort consists of registered cases of occupational diseases. Here interest would be in studying mortality from the registered disease as well as the incidence of and mortality from other diseases. Examples of the fourth type of cohort are mortality studies among pneumoconiosis cases registered in the Swedish Pneumoconiosis Register (Westerholm, 1980) and Canadian asbestosis cases receiving compensation awards (Finkelstein et al., 1981).

The advantage of the first option, restricting the cohort to workers from one facility, is that characterization of exposures may be more consistent and precise when work history and environmental data are obtained from a single source than when multiple sources of varying levels of completeness and quality are used. However, pooling cohort members from multiple facilities, as is done in the second and third options, may be necessary to increase the study size.

Selection of Study Populations

Figure 5–2 illustrates the possible cohort selection options for a historical cohort study with depictions of hypothetical individual workers. This diagram shows the situation for studying workers from a

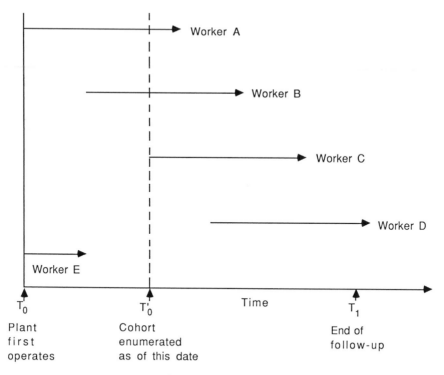

Figure 5–2. Cohort membership inclusion options.

single plant, but the discussion that follows also applies to the other cohort definition types described earlier. In the ideal case, one would choose to study all workers employed from the beginning of plant operation (i.e., workers A, B, C, D, and E in Figure 5–2). (By analogy, for a study of union members, this date would correspond to the beginning date of the union, which would not necessarily coincide with the earliest beginning date of the companies and trades included in the union.) Often records for workers that date back to plant beginnings (t_0) are not available, especially for very old plants. As a compromise, one could choose some date (t_0') for which a sufficiently large cohort can be reconstructed from personnel and other records. In this situation, workers A, B, C, and D would qualify for inclusion in the cohort; worker E would not be included because a record of his employment would not exist.

Fixed and Dynamic Cohorts

A further consideration in defining a study population is whether the cohort is fixed or dynamic. A *fixed cohort* is one in which the cohort is restricted to members employed on or hired as of some given date, either the beginning of plant operations, in the ideal circumstance, or the earliest date for which employment records are available. Thus, no workers hired subsequent to that date would be included. By contrast, a *dynamic cohort* includes all workers who would be enumerated in a fixed cohort as well as workers hired subsequently. A dynamic cohort is sometimes referred to as an *open population* (Miettinen, 1985). In the context of Figure 5–2, if the earliest date of available data is t_0', then worker D would not be included in a fixed cohort defined as workers actively employed or hired on t_0'. Worker D would be included in a dynamic cohort, however.

The choice of a fixed or dynamic cohort may be dictated by the availability of data or by special exposure circumstances that occurred during some particular (usually brief) time period. Zack and Suskind's (1980) study of a group of workers exposed to dioxin during an industrial accident at a trichlorophenol manufacturing plant provides an example of where a fixed cohort would be preferred.

More commonly, fixed cohorts are enumerated when data are available for a specified time interval, but not thereafter. Our recommendation is that one should enumerate a dynamic cohort when employee data are available that span a broad time interval, including information on workers hired after cohort inception (t_0'). There are several theoretical and practical reasons for this recommendation. First, human populations are naturally dynamic; births and deaths, which are the analogues of hires and retirements in occupational cohorts, occur continuously. A dynamic (rather than fixed) cohort more closely mimics its source population, which is dynamic. Second, dynamic cohorts usually include more study subjects than fixed cohorts; thus, the effect of exposure on disease can be measured more accurately. However, one can isolate fixed cohorts that are segments, or *subcohorts,* of a dynamic cohort by means of stratification on year or age of hire. The topic of stratification is taken up in some detail later in this chapter.

When the date of cohort inception, corresponding to the date of follow-up commencement, is later than the date of a plant's first operation (i.e., $t_0' > t_0$), a cohort defined as workers active on that date, t_0' (and those hired subsequently in the case of a dynamic cohort), will in most instances include workers hired at various times between t_0 and t_0' (viz, workers A and B in Figure 5–2). That is, the workers active at t_0' will represent a heterogeneous mix of persons employed for various lengths of time and who may have experienced varying exposure types and intensities if, as often occurs, exposures had changed over time (Weiss, 1983). Stratification with respect to length of employment and year of first hire should mitigate potential biases resulting from inappropriate pooling of cohort members with dissimilar employment histories.

Cohort Enumeration

The enumeration of a historical cohort requires assembly of personnel employment records or membership listings for unions or professional organizations, depending on the type of cohort under study (Table 5–1). As mentioned previously, the completeness of these data sources often determines the size of the cohort that can be assembled and the length of time the cohort can be followed. For prospective cohort studies, the data needed to enumerate a cohort are obtained from personnel records of workers active on the starting date of the study, as well as data for workers hired subsequently. The cohort may be supplemented with data on retirees, if they are to be included in the cohort.

Plant personnel records that contain dates of first and last employment and the various jobs held, with their associated dates, are the best source for cohort enumeration for plant- or industry-based cohorts. These records are also a principal source of exposure assignment data. Union membership listings and medical or insurance claims records are ancillary data sources for enumeration; these listings are better used for cross-checking plant personnel records than as primary enumeration sources because they tend to be less complete than personnel records.

Marsh and Enterline (1979) have described a procedure for verifying the completeness of cohort enumeration in the United States using Internal Revenue Service quarterly earnings reports (Form 941A). These earnings reports list all workers for whom social security payments were made by the employees and employers for each

Table 5–1. Data sources for cohort enumeration and verification

Source	Primary use
1. Plant personnel records	Cohort enumeration
2. Union membership listings	Cohort enumeration
3. Medical insurance claims	Ancillary source of enumeration
4. Quarterly earnings reports (IRS Form 941A)	Cohort verification

quarter of a year. Thus, the method is relevant for workers who achieved a minimum of three months continuous service in a company but is of limited utility for workers employed in defunct companies or ones that have changed ownership, because requests for the 941A forms must be submitted by the employer.

Cohort Restriction

When enumerating a cohort, the investigator should attempt initially to identify as many workers as possible without imposing arbitrary restrictions. Some restrictions, however, may simplify enumeration. For example, it would be desirable to eliminate plant construction workers under contract from another company so as to focus the study on health effects related to the manufacturing process. Arbitrary exclusions from enumeration of workers considered unlikely to be exposed to the agents of concern (e.g., plant managers or office workers) can be wasteful of information insofar as removal of the least exposed workers ultimately will diminish the precision of observed exposure–response relationships. Decisions regarding exposure status should be deferred until a thorough evaluation of employment and exposure history has been made. In some instances, inspection of complete employment data will reveal that office workers and other "salaried" personnel had held exposed jobs at some time during employment.

Some investigators prefer to restrict dynamic cohorts to workers first employed during a particular time interval (e.g., up until ten years before the end of follow-up), thus allowing for a minimum follow-up duration for all cohort members. This approach is usually adopted to allow for minimum induction and latency times for delayed exposure effects. Restrictions of this type are not necessary at the stage of cohort enumeration if latency analyses are to be performed on the data. We discuss disease latency and related methods of analysis later, in Section 4.4.

Restrictions on gender or race are made ordinarily for convenience. The majority of cohorts studied in the United States are limited to white males because white men tend to predominate in many workforces and because vital status tracing is usually easiest for this group. Changes in marital status and accompanying surname changes complicate follow-up of women workers. In the United States, census and vital statistics recording for nonwhites historically has been less complete and accurate than for whites. In countries where there is complete population registration, such as Sweden,

Finland, and Denmark, these difficulties pose less of a problem for vital status tracing. There is no scientific basis for limiting a cohort to any particular gender or race group. Indeed, including all workers for whom health and exposure data can be obtained enlarges the study size and permits inspection for particular subgroups more or less susceptible to adverse exposure effects (e.g., women in early stages of pregnancy).

A minimum length-of-employment criterion may be imposed in defining the study cohort. The choice is arbitrary, unless dictated by constraints on data availability (e.g., personnel records maintained only for workers employed ten years or longer). Judgments based on the demographic characteristics of the workforce, the types and toxicities of occupational exposures, and cost should guide this decision. For example, if there is an agent in the industrial environment that may pose demonstrable health risks following even brief periods of exposure and if exposures to this agent can occur at any time during employment, then there is justification for not imposing a minimum employment duration restriction on cohort membership. There are real situations where the most intense occupational exposures are most likely to occur during the early years of employment, such as during apprenticeship or on initial assignment to the most heavily exposed work areas. Industrial accidents typically cluster among the least experienced workers (Baker, 1975), for example. However, a cost increment (often substantial) will result from inclusion of all workers when short-term, transient workers, who are difficult to trace, comprise a large proportion of the workforce. Furthermore, as discussed in Chapter 4, short-term workers may have atypical life-styles that make them noncomparable to longer-term workers (Gilbert, 1982).

Minimum employment duration inclusion limits of one month, twelve months, five years, or ten years are the most frequently used. Improved likelihood of follow-up, compatibility of cohort definition with those of other studies of cohorts with similar exposures, or the availability of data for the so-called vested workers, who are eligible for pensions (McMichael et al., 1976), are reasons often cited to justify the selection of a particular minimum value for employment duration. Restricting the study to vested workers may be advantageous, because enumeration and follow-up of workers are facilitated (Collins and Redmond, 1976); however, health effects among workers with short employment durations, and effects possibly related to exposures in more recent years, would go undetected.

Also, selection of vested workers becomes complicated in situations where vestment requirements have changed over time.

There is no simple rule for choosing a minimum employment duration. Decisions need to be made in light of the balance between potential gains in information and study precision achievable by including short-term workers, on the one hand, and the possible introduction of bias and added costs, on the other.

When a minimum employment duration of x years is imposed in a cohort study, follow-up for each worker should be started either at the date at which x years of service has been attained or at t_0', whichever occurs later. The reason for this shift in follow-up commencement date is that, by virtue of the cohort inclusion criterion, it is known that each worker survived for at least x years. Thus, his first x years are effectively free from risk. Failure to account for these x years as "risk-free" would tend to underestimate disease rates in the cohort (Waxweiler, 1980). To illustrate, consider workers A, C, and D in Figure 5–2. Assume that a minimum of one year employment is required for inclusion in the cohort, and that t_0 is 1930 and t_0' is 1945. Additionally, consider the situation where records are available for cohort enumeration only as of t_0'. Thus, follow-up for workers A and B should begin on t_0' because they had achieved one year of employment by that date. Follow-up for workers C and D should begin at the corresponding one-year anniversary dates of hire. Here again, we can see a characteristic feature of a dynamic cohort in that follow-up begins at a time that is specific for each worker.

Follow-up of the Cohort

Epidemiologic cohort studies of mortality are far more common than those of nonfatal diseases; therefore, most of the discussion focuses on mortality studies. It should be appreciated that the only differences between mortality and morbidity cohort studies pertain to the types and sources of health outcome information. The design and analyses are otherwise identical.

The popularity of occupational mortality studies derives from scientific and public health concerns (i.e., assessment of risks of fatal diseases) and from convenience. The fact, location, and cause of death are routinely recorded, and in some instances, computerized, in most developed countries.

Figure 5–3 shows the follow-up and outcome of a historical

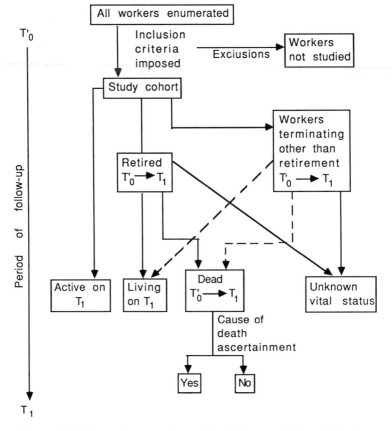

Figure 5–3. Flow diagram of mortality follow-up of historical cohort.

cohort mortality study, beginning with selection of the study cohort from the enumerated workforce and proceeding through to the determination of living or dead status and ascertainment of cause of death for identified deaths. Retirees typically constitute the majority of deaths, but workers leaving the industry prematurely (before age 65 or normal retirement age) can contribute significant numbers of deaths, especially when occupational exposures result in disabling morbidity.

Sources of Vital Status Data

In mortality studies vital status tracing is accomplished by linking cohort members' personal identifiers (name, date of birth, registration number, etc.) with data compiled on a national or regional basis. In the United States the Social Security Administration (SSA) is the most frequently used primary source of vital status data. The SSA will provide information on vital status as of some target date (t_1) by comparing social security numbers of the cohort with those of citizens who are either continuing to make social security payments or actively receiving benefits (i.e., still living) or whose survivors are receiving death benefits. For identified deaths, the SSA will indicate the state in which a death benefit claim was filed, which is usually the state where the death occurred. Vital status tracing using the SSA of course depends on the availability of workers' social security numbers. Most industries maintain employees' social security numbers because they are required to issue employer payments to the SSA. A certain number of workers invariably cannot be traced by this method because of inaccuracies in social security numbers, employment in occupations exempt from SSA payments (e.g., federal government workers), or incompleteness in SSA registration, which occurred most noticeably in the late 1930s, when the SSA system began.

Some states and municipalities maintain death indexes that can be searched for vital status data. Since 1979 a National Death Index for the United States, which can be used for vital status tracing of cohorts, has been compiled and computerized.

Several other sources can be used to verify that a former worker is still alive. These include motor vehicle bureaus, voter registration lists, and the Internal Revenue Service. Ostensibly, a person who receives a motor vehicle license or traffic violation, registers to vote, or files an income tax return is still living.

In Great Britain the Central Record Office of the Ministry of Pensions and National Insurance is the analogous tracing source to the SSA in the United States. Centralized population registers maintained throughout individuals' lives are quite valuable tracing resources in Denmark, Sweden, and Finland (Riihimakii et al., 1982; Lynge, 1985; Gustafsson et al., 1986). Vital status tracing is considerably more difficult in countries that lack national population registers or only maintain regional registers. For example, in their study of workers from a German rock wool factory, Claude and Frentzel-Beyme (1984) determined vital status from multiple inquiries made to worker registration offices and from contacts made at workers' last known addresses or places of birth.

A vital status ascertainment rate of 95 percent or greater is a desirable target, although 90–95-percent tracing is acceptable in large cohort studies. If, for example, tracing is especially poor for workers who quit employment before the normal retirement age and if ill health attributable to the occupational environment is suspected as a reason for early retirement, then an unacceptably low vital status rate may result in an underestimation of disease risks. Workers who terminate employment prematurely may include an important segment of the workforce that experienced the heaviest exposures.

Cause-of-Death Determination

Cause-of-death information for identified deaths can be obtained by requesting copies of death certificates from state or municipal vital statistics offices. Some company medical departments, unions, and professional organizations also maintain copies of death certificates. A 90–95-percent cause-of-death determination rate is a desirable target.

Table 5–2 summarizes the various sources of data on vital status, cause of death and disease incidence.

Coding the causes of death reported on death certificates should be performed by a nosologist trained in the rules specified by the International Classification of Diseases (ICD) volumes compiled by the World Health Organization (WHO, 1967). Revisions to the ICD are made roughly every 10 years, and changes in coding for some causes may influence the mortality findings of the study. One pro-

Table 5–2. Sources of vital status data in cohort studies

Source	Data supplied
1. Social Security Administration (U.S.)	Vital status, year and state of death, if dead
2. National and state death indexes (U.S.)	Date, state, and cause of death
3. Motor vehicle bureaus (U.S.)	Alive status inferred from license or citation issuance
4. Voter registration lists	Alive status inferred from registration
5. National Office of Pensions and Insurance (U.K.)	Vital status, location, and year of death, if dead
6. Population-based disease registers (Sweden and Finland, among others)	Vital status, cause of death, incidence of specific diseases, location, and year of occurrence
7. Vital statistics bureaus	Death certificates
8. Company medical departments and insurance claims records	Death certificates, disease incidence reports
9. Unions and professional organizations	Death certificates, disease incidence reports

cedure to circumvent problems caused by ICD revisions that occur during the period of follow-up is to classify each cause of death according to the ICD revision in effect at the time of death and then to reassign these codes to the corresponding codes in effect at the time when the study is being conducted. The alternative of coding all deaths according to one ICD revision, usually the most recently available one, may result in over- or underestimated mortality rates for some diseases. In practice, the latter approach is most often taken, primarily because there are few nosologists trained to perform coding with multiple revisions of the ICD. The extent of coding bias introduced is generally minimal, although some diseases (e.g., the leukemias and cerebrovascular disease) have undergone considerable coding revisions.

Data on disease incidence, rather than mortality, can be obtained, provided that there are population-based disease registers or that special incidence surveys have been conducted on the workforce. Regional cancer registries in the United States (Young et al., 1981) and national cancer registries in some other countries offer valuable data sources for morbidity studies.

Missing Information

In a cohort mortality study there are two types of workers for whom vital status information may be missing. The first are workers of unknown vital status. Occupational epidemiologists use several approaches to address this issue (Monson, 1980). One option is to delete the untraced workers from the study. This choice is unnecessarily wasteful of information in that some person-time of observation would be excluded from the analysis. A second option is to assume that all the unknowns remain alive at t_1. This approach has the disadvantage of artificially lowering the mortality rates of the cohort if some of the unknowns had, in fact, died before the end of the study. A third method is to assume that all unknowns had died by the end of the study period. This approach inflates the death rates spuriously. Finally, one can count person-years of observation for unknowns up until the dates of last contact, typically the dates of termination from the industry, and make no assumptions regarding their vital status thereafter. The last approach is the most defensible in that it requires no unverifiable assumptions about the mortality experience of cohort members after they were lost to follow-up (Vena et al., 1987). Furthermore, all the available information (i.e., the person-years of observation) is included in the analysis.

Thus, we recommend the last approach for reasons of validity and simplicity.

The second category of workers with missing information is that in which the cause of death is unknown. This situation usually arises when death certificates cannot be located, but it may also occur when cause-of-death information on some death certificates is judged by the nosologist to be inadequate for coding. Two approaches can be adopted for handling unknown cause of death. The first is to leave the deaths in an "unknown" cause-of-death category in the reporting of results. The second is to assume that the distribution of deaths, by cause, among the unknowns is the same as that for the deaths with known causes and to add deaths to the various cause groupings on a proportional basis. Thus, if there are 100 deaths of unknown cause and if 5 percent of the known deaths are from cerebrovascular disease, then one would add five deaths to the observed number for the cerebrovascular disease category. Sometimes this approach results in the addition of fractions of deaths (i.e., when the percentage of deaths from a particular cause among deaths with known causes multiplied by the total number of deaths of unknown cause is not a integer). Fractions of deaths are awkward to explain. We prefer creating an "unknown" cause-of-death category because this approach does not require unverifiable assumptions about the distribution of cause of death among the unknowns.

3. METHODS OF DATA ANALYSIS

This section contains a description of the procedures used to analyze data from cohort studies. We begin by devoting some attention to the basic concepts of person-time, risks, and rates. We follow this discussion with a description of statistical methods for analysis of the data for the entire cohort and for subcohorts defined on the basis of various demographic and exposure characteristics.

3.1. Risks and Rates

Distinctions and Uses

An understanding of the analytic techniques used in occupational cohort studies requires an appreciation of the distinction between disease risks and rates. A *risk* is the probability of developing or dying from a particular disease during a specified time interval. Thus, if we conduct a ten-year follow-up on a cohort of 1,000 workers enumerated at t_0 (or t_0', depending on the availability of data), and observe 30 deaths, then the ten-year risk of death is 30/1,000 workers.

A second approach to quantify the population disease frequency during a specified time period is to compute the number of newly occurring, or *incident,* cases during the time interval of follow-up per number of *person-years of observation.* This quantity is a disease rate. Other terms for a disease *rate* are *incidence density, instantaneous risk,* and *hazard rate.* For simplicity, we use the term *rate* to denote an expression of newly occurring cases per person-time units. A more mathematical explanation of the distinction between risks and rates is given by Elandt-Johnson (1975).

The value of computing disease rates, rather than risks, in occupational cohort studies is that rates take into account the person-time of observation, which is likely to vary between cohort members when deaths (or cases) occur at variable points in time. Hence, this approach considers not only whether disease occurred, but also when it occurred (Clayton, 1982).

Rates are therefore especially applicable for studies of dynamic cohorts, which are far more common than those of fixed cohorts. In a dynamic cohort the person-time of observation (follow-up) will vary as a function of both the time of entry into the cohort, usually taken as t_0' or a worker's date of hire if later than t_0', and the duration of follow-up for subjects remaining alive or free of the disease of interest. By contrast, disease risks are most suitably computed for fixed cohort studies and require certain restrictive assumptions about follow-up time to be applicable for studies where follow-up extends over long periods of time, such as decades (Kleinbaum et al., 1982). In considering methods of data analysis for cohort studies, we limit the discussion to the analysis of disease rates, as illustrated with data from dynamic cohort studies. Methods for analyzing disease risks among fixed cohorts are virtually identical to the methods presented in Chapter 7 on cross-sectional studies.

Computing Person-time of Observation

Computation of person-time data has long been a routine procedure in demography and has become standard practice in epidemiologic studies of dynamic occupational cohorts since the 1950s (Case and Lea, 1955; Doll, 1955). The procedure for computing

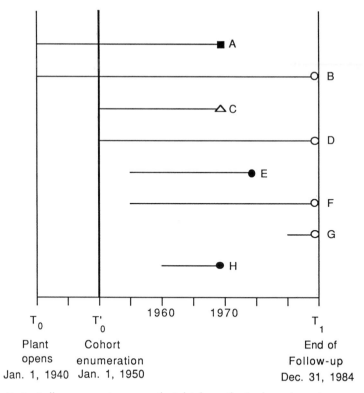

Figure 5-4. Follow-up outcomes of eight hypothetical workers (■ = cancer death, ● = other death, △ = lost to follow-up, o = alive at end of follow-up).

rates with person-years (years are the time units used in most investigations of chronic diseases) as denominators is known as the *modified life table method* (Ederer et al., 1961; Berry, 1983).

The basic notion behind person-time calculations is that each subject alive at the beginning of follow-up is observed for some, usually variable, length of time, and thus contributes person-years of observation until he or she either develops or dies from the disease of interest, dies from another cause, or the end of follow-up occurs. This description of person-time calculation pertains equally to prospective and historical cohort studies.

Figure 5–4 shows schematic representations of eight workers in a hypothetical cohort mortality study where follow-up is from 1950 (t_0') through 1984 (t_1). Two workers, A and B, were first employed on the date when the plant opened (t_0); all others were hired either on t_0' or subsequently. Workers A and C both contribute 20 person-years of observation (1950–1970). However, as we will discuss later, their differences in employment duration and, possibly, age need to be taken into account. Worker A will be counted as a death in the numerator of the death rate. Worker C, who was lost to follow-up after 20 years, also will contribute 20 person-years to the denominator. Workers B and D present situations similar to workers A and C except that, because both B and D were alive at the end of the study, each contributes 35 person-years of observation (1950–1985). The other four workers, E, F, G, and H, were all hired subsequent to t'_0, and person-year counting proceeds in like fashion as for workers A, B, C, and D.

It should be recognized that, to this point, we have considered only length of follow-up and not length of employment. The two are identical only for workers who either die while still actively employed or are still working when the study ends (t_1). (Of course, interruptions in employment from layoffs, illness, or military service create exceptions to this generalization.) If we assume that the follow-up times for workers G and H in Figure 5–4 are also their periods of employment, and if a minimum of ten years of employment is required for inclusion into the cohort, then both of these workers would contribute 0 person-years of observation. Also, follow-up for all other workers would begin at year $t'_0 + 10$ when a ten-year minimum employment duration is imposed.

Inspection of Figure 5–4 further reveals that person-years in a dynamic cohort can be accrued at different calendar years, which may also correspond to different ages for cohort members. Consider workers C and E in Figure 5–4. Worker C was hired at age 30 years in 1950 and was followed to 1970 (20 person-years of observation). Worker E was hired at age 45 years in 1955 and died at age 65 in 1975; he also contributes 20 person-years of observation. There are quite distinct differences in the 20-person-year intervals for these two workers. Worker C's person-year at age 45 years occurred in 1965, which is 15 years after his first employment. For worker E, his person-year at age 45 years occurred in 1955 and was only his first year of employment.

Stratification of Person-years

The epidemiologic method, borrowed from demography, for summarizing person-years across age and calendar years is to stratify the cohort's collective person-years into a cross-classified distribution (Hill, 1972). Age and calendar year are the two most important stratification variables because many diseases are strongly age related, and population rates (even within narrow age categories) vary over time (Jarvholm, 1987). As discussed in Chapter 4, length of employment, age at first employment, and time since first employment also can influence disease rates, primarily as confounders or effect modifiers of the associations between disease and the exposures of interest. Stratum widths for age and calendar year can be as small as one year, although five-year stratum widths are customary. Person-years accumulation is therefore accomplished by summing each cohort member's contribution to every attained category, where the categories are jointly specified by age and calendar year strata.

To illustrate the method of stratification, consider again the hypothetical workers in Figure 5–4. Age strata can be defined as ages 15–19, 20–24, . . . , 80–84; similarly, five-year calendar year strata can be defined as 1950–54, 1955–59, . . . , 1980–84. Suppose that both workers A and B were aged 30 years in 1950. Then each contributes 5 person-years to the 30–34-year age and 1950–54 calendar year jointly classified stratum. (It is convenient, though not necessary, to specify equal widths for age and calendar year strata.) During the interval 1955–59 both workers A and B were aged 35–39 years, and therefore each contributes 5 person-years into the corresponding stratum. For the group of eight workers in this example there is a total of 20 person-years accrued in the 1950–54 calendar year stratum (from workers A, B, C and D), whereas in the 1965–69 period all but one worker (G) contributes 5 person-years each, yielding a total of 35 person-years. In like manner, person-years are summed across age strata. Ultimately, the joint distribution of person-years, by age and calendar year, can be tallied.

This hypothetical example is intentionally simplified so that follow-up times begin and end conveniently at five-year age and calendar year junctures. In actual cohort studies workers will have begun and ended follow-up times at any number of possible ages and time points within calendar years. Fortunately, sophisticated computer programs can accommodate person-years counting for these more complex, yet typical, situations (Monson, 1974; Marsh and Preininger, 1980; Waxweiler et al., 1983).

The process of stratification of person-years can be extended to include these variables and other factors (e.g., race, socioeconomic status, age at hire, duration of employment, cumulative exposure, etc.) by apportioning person-years into a K-dimensional matrix, where K represents the number of stratification variables. The number of person-years in any cell of such a matrix diminishes as the number of variables and associated categories increases. Also, close correlations among variables, such as age at hire and year of hire, will result in many cells with 0 person-years, and hence unstable or incalculable rates, because there will be few workers with extreme values opposite in magnitude (e.g., very old workers with short durations of follow-up).

Stratum-specific incidence or mortality rates are computed by dividing the cohort's total number of cases (deaths) by the number of person-years. Descriptions of appropriate analytic methods follow.

3.2. Stratum-Specific Rates

From the discussion in Section 3.1., it should be clear that the counting of person-years and computation of rates involving stratification on relevant factors (e.g., age, calendar year) will generate a large array of stratum-specific rates. When studying rates for many different diseases among a cohort, the stratum-specific rates may be highly unstable because of small numbers of cases or person-years in individual strata. This type of problem can arise even when the cohort is relatively large (e.g., thousands of workers collectively contributing several hundred thousand person-years of observation), the analysis is limited to broad disease groupings (e.g., all cancers) or stratification is restricted to only two or three factors.

Table 5–3 gives the general layout for data from a cohort study. This is the data layout for the *crude* table when there is no stratification made on age, calendar year, or any other potentially confounding variable. The same basic data layout is used for each stratum in a stratified data presentation; here the cell entries (a, b, N_1, N_2, M, and T) would be indexed by subscripts such as i, j, k, and so on, denoting levels of the various stratification factors. For example, if stratification is performed on age at five levels and calendar year at three levels, then there would be $5 \times 3 = 15$ age/calendar year-specific strata. Age might be indexed by $i = 1, 2, \ldots, 5$, and calendar-year by $j = 1, 2, 3$. Thus, the data table for the second age

Table 5–3. Data layout for a cohort study using rates and person-years

	Exposed	Non-exposed	Total
Cases	a	b	M
Person-years	N_1	N_0	T

group and first calendar year stratum would be a_{21}, b_{21}, and so forth. If particular strata contain very few person-years, then one solution might be to broaden the widths of the strata, while still maintaining the stratification. Earlier we mentioned that five-year stratum widths for age and calendar year are commonly used, in part because national death rates tabulated by vital statistics bureaus or cancer incidence rates reported by disease registries typically are presented on a quinquennial basis. The choice of the five-year stratum width has become standard primarily because a period of five years usually includes large enough numbers of cases and person-years to ensure stability of rates, at least in a national or regional population. If one widens the age strata to, say, 20 years, then, for example, a single rate for workers aged 40 to 59 years is less likely to depict reliably the disease experience in this age group than four age-specific rates for workers aged 40–44, 45–49, 50–54, and 55–59 years.

3.3. Summary Measures of Effect

Standardization

Two approaches that can be taken to summarize rates across strata of a confounder (e.g., age), while maintaining the unique information contained within strata (stratum-specific rates), are to compute either *standardized rates* or *pooled rates*. Several analytic options for standardizing rates are available. These procedures are useful for most analyses of occupational cohort data. More advanced mathematical modeling techniques can be valuable adjuncts to the basic methods described here and are discussed in Chapter 8.

The basic feature of a standardized, or summary, rate is that it is a weighted average of stratum-specific rates. A general expression for a standardized rate (SR) is

$$SR = \frac{\sum_i W_i I_i}{\sum_i W_i} \tag{5.1}$$

where i indexes the strata, the W_i are the stratum-specific weights, and the I_i are the stratum-specific incidence (or mortality) rates.

As can be seen from expression (5.1), the choice of weights determines the type of summary measure. Ideally, one would choose weights that result in the most precise summary estimate of effect. When the rates in two (or more) populations are to be compared, it is important that the rates be standardized using the same set of

weights so that the comparisons are not confounded by the stratifying variable(s). The choice of weights depends on the group to
which inferences are to be made. There are two common practical
alternatives. First, the rates can be standardized to the confounder
distribution of the study (exposed) population. This is done in an
SMR analysis (see the following discussion). Alternatively, the rates
may be standardized to the confounder distribution of the comparison, or reference, population (assumed non-exposed). These two
approaches will be illustrated for the situation of confounding by
age at risk (indexed by i, as before). In either case, the ratio of standardized rates (RR_S) is expressed as

$$RR_S = \frac{\sum_i W_i(a_i/N_{1i})}{\sum_i W_i(b_i/N_{0i})} \tag{5.2}$$

Note that the numerator of expression (5.2) is the standardized rate
in the exposed population, and the denominator is the standardized
rate in the reference population.

In computing an SMR, the W_i are taken from the confounder distribution of the exposed population (i.e., $W_i = N_{1i}$), and expression
(5.2) reduces to

$$SMR = \frac{\sum_i a_i}{\sum_i N_{1i}(b_i/N_{0i})} \tag{5.3}$$

The SMR is thus the ratio of the sum of the observed cases in the
exposed population, relative to the sum of the expected numbers in
the exposed population, where the expected numbers are based on
rates in the reference population.

The alternative method of taking weights from the confounder
distribution of the reference population (i.e., $W_i = N_{0i}$) is exemplified by the standardized rate ratio (SRR) procedure described by
Miettinen (1972). When the SRR is used as the summary rate ratio,
expression (5.2) becomes

$$SRR = \frac{\sum_i N_{0i}(a_i/N_{1i})}{\sum_i b_i} \tag{5.4}$$

The SRR is therefore the ratio of the number of expected cases
in the reference population, based on rates in the exposed group,
to the number of observed cases in the reference population.

Pooling Rates

Another general method of summary rate ratio estimation is pooling, which involves computing a *weighted average of the stratum-specific rate ratios* [rather than the ratio of weighted averages of stratum-specific rates, as in expression (5.2)]. In this case, RR_S takes the form

$$RR_S = \frac{\sum_i W_i(a_i/N_{1i})/(b_i/N_{0i})}{\sum_i W_i} \tag{5.5}$$

The most common choice of weights is that given by the Mantel–Haenszel (1959) method, which uses weights of $b_i N_{1i}/T_i$ (Rothman and Boice, 1979). With these weights, expression (5.5) becomes

$$RR_{M-H} = \frac{\sum_i a_i N_{0i}/T_i}{\sum_i b_i N_{1i}/T_i} \tag{5.6}$$

A related method for summary rate ratio estimation is the *precision weighting* approach, which involves using the inverses of the variances of the stratum-specific rate ratios as the weights in expression (5.5) (Kleinbaum et al., 1982). However, the computations required for precision weighting are more complex than those for RR_{M-H}, and precsion weighting has the disadvantage of yielding unstable summary rate ratios when there are zero cells in some of the stratum-specific tables.

Several points should be made regarding these summary measures of effect. First, all are ratio estimates and therefore express disease frequency on a *multiplicative scale* (Breslow et al., 1983). Thus, their interpretation is made in reference to the null (no effect) value of 1.0. One may prefer rate difference measures that yield absolute estimates of effect, that is, on an *additive scale*. One convenient way of presenting absolute effect estimates is to compute the difference in observed and expected numbers of cases or deaths (e.g., from an SMR or SRR) divided by the person-time of observation (Monson, 1986). Summary measures of rate differences can be derived in a fashion similar to that for rate ratios; however, we will focus on ratio measures because they are more familiar in occupational epidemiology.

The second point is that, for a particular stratum of the confounder, the SMR, SRR, and RR_{M-H} all provide the same unbiased estimate of the rate ratio. This can be demonstrated by recasting expressions (5.2) and (5.5) specifically for just the ith stratum by eliminating the summation. When the rate ratio is constant across all strata of the confounder, all three estimators give the same result. This can be shown by assuming that the rate for the exposed group is equal to some multiple M of the rate in the reference population, that is, $a_i/N_{1i} = M(b_i/N_{0i})$. Substitution into expression (5.2) (for the SMR or SRR) or expression (5.5) (for RR_{M-H}) yields $RR_S = M$, in each instance.

SMR Analysis

SMR analysis is the most widely employed and familiar technique for rate adjustment in occupational cohort studies. In an SMR analysis, the nonexposed group is usually an external reference population. National or regional (e.g., state or province) populations are frequently chosen as reference populations. The advantage of using a national or regional reference population is that the stratum-specific rates in such a population are generally stable, and thus the expected numbers of the SMR can be considered as virtual constants (Gardner, 1986).

The numerator of the SMR is obtained simply by summing the number of cases (deaths) in the cohort across all strata of age, calendar year, and other stratification variables. The denominator of the SMR is then obtained by multiplying the stratum-specific rates in the reference population by the corresponding numbers of person-years in the cohort and then summing over all strata (Berry, 1983). It should be recognized that multiplying the expected rate (cases/person-years) by person-years will yield the expected number of cases. (Disease rates for national or regional reference populations are often reported as annual numbers of cases per 100,000 persons, rather than as person-years. Nonetheless, these quantities are rates if it is assumed that, for any single year, each person in the reference population contributes 1 person-year.) The denominator of the SMR can be thought of as the number of cases that would have occurred in the cohort had the cohort experienced the same stratum-specific rates as the reference population during the specified time interval of the study.

A hypothetical example illustrating the computations for an SMR is shown in Table 5–4. Only one stratification variable, age, at four levels, is considered, so as to simplify the calculations, but the same

Table 5–4. Hypothetical example illustrating calculation of the standardized mortality ratio (SMR)

	Study cohort		Reference population		
	(1)	(2)	(3)	(4)	
		Person-		Exp =	SMR =
Age	Obs	years	Rate per 1,000	(2) × (3)	(1) ÷ (4)
40–49	6	1,200	2.5	3.00	2.00
50–59	27	2,340	6.1	14.27	1.89
60–69	98	3,750	12.4	46.50	2.11
70–79	48	975	25.0	24.38	1.97
Total	179			88.15	2.03

principles apply in analyses involving more than one factor. This example shows that the SMR is 2.03, indicating a 103-percent disease excess in the cohort relative to the reference population.

The validity of the SMR as a summary measure of effect has been the subject of debate among epidemiologists (Gaffey, 1976; Chiazze, 1976; Wong, 1977; Symons and Taulbee, 1981; Breslow et al., 1983). One criticism is that the SMR, like any summary measure, obscures stratum-specific effects (Chiazze, 1976). For example, the SMR will not reveal which age groups experienced the greatest relative disease excesses or deficits.

One often noted shortcoming of SMR analysis is that, if the study involves several exposed groups, such as subcohorts of the main cohort, then comparisons of SMRs between groups will not be appropriate if their confounder distributions differ [i.e., the SMRs do not share a common set of weights (Yule, 1934; Miettinen, 1972; Breslow, 1984)]. For example, comparisons of SMRs between subgroups of the cohort, classified according to duration of employment, may be confounded if the subgroups have different distributions of age or calendar year.

To illustrate the problem of noncomparable SMRs, consider the hypothetical example in Table 5–5. Here SMRs for two cohorts, A and B, are compared, where the SMRs are derived from age-specific rates in the same external reference population. We can see that the age-specific SMRs (and hence the underlying rate ratios) are similar for the two cohorts, whereas the summary SMRs are different. The reason for this discrepancy is that cohort A has a preponderantly older age structure (3,000 of 4,000 person-years in the ≥40-year age stratum), whereas the age structure of cohort B is reversed. Also, the rates in the reference population and in the two cohorts

Table 5–5. Example of confounded comparisons of SMRs

Age	Cohort A				Cohort B				Reference population, rate per 1,000
	Person-years	Obs	Exp	SMR	Person-years	Obs	Exp	SMR	
<40	1,000	25	15	1.67	3,000	75	45	1.67	15.0
≥40	3,000	375	150	2.50	1,000	125	50	2.50	50.0
Total	4,000	400	165	2.42	4,000	200	95	2.11	

increase with age. Thus, the higher summary SMR in cohort A is an artifact of its older age composition.

Approximate confidence interval estimation for the SMR can be obtained by setting limits for the numerator, the observed number of cases, and assuming the denominator to be a constant (Rothman and Boice, 1979). The formula for the lower limit of an SMR is

$$\underline{SMR} = Obs\left[1 - \frac{1}{9\,Obs} - \left(\frac{Z}{3}\right)\left(\sqrt{\frac{1}{Obs}}\right)\right]^3 \Bigg/ Exp \quad (5.7)$$

and the upper limit is given as

$$\overline{SMR} = (Obs + 1)\left[1 - \frac{1}{9(Obs + 1)} + \left(\frac{Z}{3}\right)\left(\sqrt{\frac{1}{Obs + 1}}\right)\right]^3 \Bigg/ Exp$$

$$(5.8)$$

where Obs is the numerator of the SMR, Exp is the denominator of the SMR, and Z is the standard normal deviate specifying the width of the confidence interval (e.g., $Z = 1.96$ for a 95-percent interval). Exact confidence intervals can be computed (especially when the expected number is less than 2), but they require iterative calculations (see Rothman, 1986).

Several methods are available for statistical significance testing for departures of SMRs from 1.0. The simplest computational method is to compute a chi-square test with 1 degree of freedom, which takes the following form

$$\chi^2 = \frac{(Obs - Exp)^2}{(Exp)} \quad (5.9)$$

It is commonly assumed that the observed number of cases or deaths from a particular disease follows a random, or Poisson, distribution in time. Thus, under the null hypothesis, the expected value (Exp) for the total number of cases observed estimates the variance of Obs (Armitage, 1971).

The chi-square test in expression (5.9) is most applicable when the expected value (Exp) is 2 or greater (Bailar and Ederer, 1964). In the example in Table 5–4 the chi-square value is 93.48 $[= (179 - 88.20)^2/88.20]$, and the associated p-value is less than 10^{-5}.

When Exp is less than 2, an "exact" p-value can be computed (Armitage, 1971) from the following formula:

$$p = \sum_{k=a}^{\infty} \frac{e^{-\lambda}\lambda^k}{k!} \tag{5.10}$$

where p is the probability of observing an SMR as large or larger than that detected, a is the total number of cases observed, and λ is the number of cases expected. Note that the summation is taken to infinity. In practice, however, one would sum values beginning with $k = a, k = a + 1, \ldots$, until the increment to p becomes virtually zero.

SMRs based on expected values of less than 2 occur with considerable regularity in occupational cohort studies that encompass many disease outcomes. In most instances, the SMR for an entire cohort for a particular disease should be regarded with caution when the expected value (not the observed) is less than 2, because such a result may be misleading, except when the disease is very rare in non-exposed populations (e.g., malignant mesothelioma). In such instances, the possibility of diagnostic error for rare diseases in both the study cohort and the reference population should be borne in mind.

SRR Analysis

Because of problems associated with the Healthy Worker Effect in studies using an external reference population, investigators increasingly have conducted analyses using *internal reference groups* identified from within the cohort. SMR analysis can still be used for comparisons with an internal reference group. However, the SRR approach is better suited for analyses involving internal reference groups because it avoids the noncomparability problems of SMRs. Statistical aspects of SRR analysis are presented here, and practical applications are demonstrated in Section 3.4 on subcohort analysis.

As noted earlier, the SRR is a summary rate ratio that involves taking weights from the reference group. When there are several "exposed" groups in the study (e.g., subcohorts of workers with increasing exposure levels) and one reference group (i.e., "non-exposed"), the SRRs computed for these groups can be compared validly because they are based on a common set of weights, the confounder person-time distribution of the reference group.

There are several available methods for computing confidence intervals for SRRs (Miettinen, 1976; Greenland, 1982; Flanders, 1984; Rothman, 1986). An approximate confidence interval for an SRR can be calculated using a formula for the approximate variance of the natural logarithm of the SRR [ln(SRR)] (Rothman, 1986), which is given as

$$\text{Var}[\ln(\text{SRR})] = \frac{\sum_i N_{0i}^2(a_i/N_{1i}^2)}{\left[\sum_i N_{0i}(a_i/N_{1i})\right]^2} + \frac{1}{\sum_i b_i} \tag{5.11}$$

Upper and lower confidence limits for an SRR are then obtained by exponentiation as follows:

$$\underline{\text{SRR}}, \overline{\text{SRR}} = \exp\left[\ln(\text{SRR}) \pm Z\sqrt{\text{Var}[\ln(\text{SRR})]}\right] \tag{5.12}$$

A statistical test of the departure of the SRR from the null value can be applied using the Mantel–Haenszel chi-square test, adapted for use with person-time data (Shore et al., 1976; Rothman and Boice, 1979). The test statistic, with one degree of freedom, is

$$\chi^2 = \frac{\sum_i (a_i - N_{1i}M_{1i}/T_i)^2}{\sum_i M_{1i}N_{1i}N_{0i}/T_i^2} \tag{5.13}$$

Mantel–Haenszel Analysis

Mantel–Haenszel summary rate ratios (RR_{M-H}s) are alternatives to the SRR. The SRR can be unstable (thus resulting in imprecise effect measures) when there are unstable stratum-specific rates in the groups compared. In contrast, the stability of the RR_{M-H} only depends on the overall, rather than stratum-specific, number of cases. However, when more than two groups are to be compared, the RR_{M-H} suffers from the same potential problem of noncomparability that hinders SMR analysis. With the RR_{M-H}, the weights depend on the confounder distributions of both groups compared; thus, in an analysis of more than two groups, the weights change, depending on which groups are compared. This problem is not as great as that with an SMR analysis of more than two groups if the same reference group is included in every RR_{M-H} computation.

Confidence intervals for the RR_{M-H} can be derived by using an approximate variance formula of the natural logarithm of RR_{M-H} (Greenland and Robins, 1985), and exponentiating the upper and lower limits as in expression (5.12). The approximate formula for the variance of $\ln(RR_{M-H})$ is

$$\text{Var}[\ln(RR_{M-H})] = \frac{\sum_i M_{1i}N_{1i}N_{0i}/T_i^2}{\left(\sum_i a_iN_{0i}/T_i\right)\left(\sum_i b_iN_{1i}/T_i\right)} \tag{5.14}$$

Thus, the lower and upper confidence limits for RR_{M-H} are

$$\underline{RR_{M-H}}, \overline{RR_{M-H}} = \exp\left[\ln(RR_{M-H}) \pm Z\sqrt{\text{Var}[\ln(RR_{M-H})]}\right] \tag{5.15}$$

The "test-based" method of confidence interval estimation (Miettinen, 1976) is a convenient alternative approach. The form of the test-based confidence interval is given by

$$\underline{RR_{M-H}}, \overline{RR_{M-H}} = RR_{M-H}^{(1 \pm Z/\sqrt{\chi^2})} \tag{5.16}$$

where χ^2 is the Mantel–Haenszel chi-square statistic given in expression (5.13).

The test-based confidence interval estimation method has the advantage of ease of computation but is only applicable to RR_{M-H} and should not be used for the SMR or SRR (Greenland, 1984). Even for RR_{M-H} it is inaccurate when the rate ratio estimate is less than 0.2 or greater than 5.0 (Greenland, 1984). Nonetheless, it performs well within that range, especially closest to the null value, where accuracy is most important (Miettinen, 1977).

4. STRATEGIES OF ANALYSIS

4.1. Overall Cohort Analysis

The first research question addressed in a cohort study is whether the rates of various diseases observed for the study cohort are different from rates found in a comparison population that is presumed to be non-exposed to the workplace agent(s) of concern. In this first level of analysis, the disease frequencies experienced by the entire cohort throughout the study period are examined to provide a general picture of disease excesses and deficits. This type of over-all analysis can therefore be viewed as a method of screening for associations that ultimately will warrant more intensive and formal-ized investigation. From a public health perspective, such an analy-sis describes the cohort's health profile relative to the norm and sug-gests areas for possible intervention.

Example 5.1

An example of an SMR mortality analysis on a cause-specific basis is shown in Table 5–6. These data were obtained in a historical cohort study of workers in the phos-phate mining and fertilizer industry (Checkoway et al., 1985b). The reference pop-ulation is U.S. white males, and SMRs were computed using age and calendar year stratification, with stratum widths of five years for both variables. The numbers for the major cause of death groupings (e.g., all causes, all cancers, cardiovascular dis-eases) are sufficiently large, and thus yield stable SMRs. However, some of the site-specific cancer SMRs (e.g., liver, larynx, Hodgkin's disease) are based on small numbers and are therefore subject to wide fluctuations.

It should be appreciated that the absence of apparent disease excesses in an overall SMR analysis can occur despite localized excess risks in subgroups of the cohort. In some cases, etiologic

Table 5–6. Standardized mortality ratios, by cause of death, among white male phosphate industry workers: 1949–78

Cause of death	Obs	Exp	SMR
All causes	1,620	1,623.8	1.00
Ischemic heart disease	512	552.2	0.93
Vascular lesions of CNS	90	93.75	0.96
Nonmalignant respiratory diseases	73	82.95	0.88
Motor vehicle accidents	132	86.84	1.52
All malignant neoplasms	289	304.3	0.95
Cancer of the oral cavity	11	10.09	1.09
Stomach cancer	9	15.52	0.58
Colon cancer	13	26.00	0.50
Liver cancer	3	5.56	0.54
Pancreas cancer	18	16.36	1.10
Lung cancer	117	95.90	1.22
Larynx cancer	3	4.55	0.66
Prostate cancer	17	14.78	1.15
Bladder cancer	7	7.87	0.89
Kidney cancer	6	7.89	0.76
Lymphosarcoma and reticulosarcoma	7	7.69	0.91
Hodgkin's disease	1	5.88	0.17
Leukemia and aleukemia	15	13.51	1.11

Source: Checkoway et al. (1985b).

associations may only emerge upon more refined analyses. Subgroup, or subcohort, analysis is discussed in Section 4.2.

Stratified Analysis

We have already stressed the importance of stratification on age and calendar year in the discussion of statistical methods. Stratification can be extended to include factors additional to age and calendar year. The most important of these factors are (1) age at hire, (2) year of hire, (3) year of birth, (4) length of employment, (5) time since first exposure, and (6) length of follow-up (see Chapter 4). Accordingly, we might compute separate SMRs for strata defined by one or more of these factors, while also maintaining stratification with respect to age and calendar year. The principles of SMR analysis, including invalid comparisons of SMRs when there are dissimilar distributions of confounders, described previously for the more simple situations apply here as well. The objective of this type of analysis is to examine disease frequency contrasts between subgroups of the cohort, defined by stratification on one or more of these variables.

When evaluating the effects of any one of these factors, ideally one would like to control for the others, in addition to age (or age at risk, as it is sometimes called) and calendar year. There are practical difficulties with this approach, however. First, these stratification variables are highly intercorrelated. For example, if one knows age at hire and age, then time since first exposure is also known, because it is the difference of the two. Similarly, age at hire is determined by year of birth and year of hire. Interdependence of factors therefore precludes simultaneous control. This problem is referred to as *multicollinearity* in statistics (see Chapter 8).Furthermore, simultaneous stratification on multiple factors in an SMR analysis will result in many cells with few or no person-years, thus necessitating a mathematical modeling approach.

A common strategy for assessing SMRs computed according to these influential factors is to stratify on age, calendar year, and one (or at most two) of the remaining variables. This approach has the limitation of potentially confounded comparisons of SMRs but can give informative results in some instances.

Example 5.2

Table 5–7 shows SMRs for lung cancer among phosphate industry workers (Checkoway et al., 1985b), adjusted for age and calendar year, and stratified on each of

Table 5-7. Standardized mortality ratios for lung cancer among white male phosphate industry workers: 1949-78, according to selected stratification variables

Variable	Obs	SMR
Length of employment (yr)		
1–4	29	1.36
5–9	17	1.18
10–19	29	1.09
20–29	25	1.05
30–39	15	1.88
≥40	2	0.80
Years since first employment		
1–4	8	1.48
5–9	7	0.76
10–19	36	1.28
20–29	35	0.96
30–39	21	1.71
≥40	10	2.08
Age at hire (yr)		
<20	4	1.29
20–29	29	1.23
30–39	45	1.38
40–49	32	1.18
≥50	7	0.71
Year of hire		
Before 1930	7	1.19
1930–39	11	1.67
1940–49	49	1.23
1950–59	29	1.03
1960–69	19	1.57
1970 or later	2	0.59

Source: Checkoway et al. (1985b).

four other factors: length of employment, years since first employment, age at hire, and year of hire. The patterns of the SMRs stratified on these factors are irregular. Nevertheless, we can note that the largest SMRs for the longest strata of years since first employment and the youngest age at hire strata are consistent in suggesting a long lapse time between exposure onset and lung cancer mortality. The trend with length of employment, however, does not indicate a strong exposure–response association.

Example 5.3

Table 5–8 provides an example of cross-classification of SMRs according to two factors (in addition to age and calendar year). These data are SMRs for lung cancer from a historical cohort mortality study of metal tradesmen (Beaumont and Weiss, 1980). The SMRs, which are jointly stratified according to length of employment and time since first employment, fill up only the top right half of the table because length of employment cannot exceed time since first employment. The SMRs in the margins of Table 5–8 are similar to those presented in Table 5–7 from the preced-

Table 5–8. Lung cancer SMRs according to length of employment and years since first employment among metal trades union members

Length of employment (yr)	Years since first employed					
	3–9	10–19	20–29	30–39	≥40	Total
3–9	0.59	1.43	1.84	2.06	—[a]	0.98
10–19		0.88	1.83	1.20	0	1.16
20–29			0.93	2.16	—	1.18
30–39				1.52	1.68	1.55
≥40					1.34	1.34
Total	0.59	0.98	1.26	1.69	1.42	1.17

Source: Beaumont and Weiss (1980).

[a]Zero person-years in the stratum.

ing example. One particular feature of the data in Table 5–8 deserves comment. The SMRs directly adjacent to the diagonal from top left to bottom right, which are for workers who died shortly after employment, are somewhat higher than those in the remainder of the table. One possible explanation for this result is that illness, which may have led to excessive mortality, may also have resulted in premature retirement. Other authors have remarked on this phenomenon (Delzell and Monson, 1981; Gilbert, 1982).

In an analysis comparing incidence or mortality between subgroups of the cohort, classified by, say, age at hire or length of employment, confounding of the type just described could occur unless other predictors of disease are controlled. Thus, we are faced with an apparent dilemma: multiway stratification may control for confounding from a number of factors, but it may also yield unstable results because of small numbers. One obvious approach is to examine the distributions of other potential confounders between categories of the main stratification variable(s) before attempting to compute a summary measure that takes into account these other factors. For example, if we are going to compare SMRs between strata of employment duration but are concerned about possible confounding from year of hire, we could compare the distributions of year of hire between the employment duration strata. Similarity of distributions would give some assurance that the comparisons would not be confounded, and we would then be justified in ignoring year of hire in the analysis.

The situation becomes more complex as the number of potential confounders increases. Thus, if we are concerned about age at hire and time since first exposure, in addition to year of hire, then we would need to compare the distributions of all three variables between employment duration strata. In fact, we might need to compare the joint distributions of these factors between groups if there were reason to suspect that confounding may occur because of some complex pattern of variables. Furthermore, as mentioned previously, simultaneous control of all potential confounders in a cohort analysis is impossible because of the direct numerical dependence between subsets of these variables.

Difficulties associated with the simultaneous control of multiple potential confounders are by no means unique to occupational cohort studies. A reasonable strategy to adopt is to decide in advance which factors are of particular interest and which are less important. The latter can be ignored in the analysis if their control is likely to offer a limited gain in insight. This approach is a gamble to some extent, as unanticipated confounding or effect modification may be ignored to the detriment of the study.

Choice of Reference Populations

The Healthy Worker Effect poses a major problem with cohort studies involving comparisons with a national or regional external reference population. Several approaches for circumventing bias caused by the Healthy Worker Effect are available. One strategy is to compare disease rates among the cohort with rates in an external reference population also consisting of employed (and retired) workers. Such a reference population may be identified from national census data when information on employment is recorded. Data of this sort exist in Great Britain (Fox and Goldblatt, 1982) but are available in few other countries.

Alternatively, the reference population might be selected from among employees in an industry other than the one under study. For example, Hernberg et al. (1970), in their study of cardiovascular diseases among viscose rayon factory workers, selected as a comparison group workers at a paper mill not exposed to the suspected etiologic factor, carbon disulfide. Comparing disease rates between two industrial populations has the potential advantages of minimizing bias from the Healthy Worker Effect and achieving control of confounding from other factors, such as social class. However, relative excesses or deficits of disease among the study cohort may be difficult to interpret if the reference worker cohort is exposed to the same agents or to agents that cause the diseases of interest. To illustrate, consider a cohort study of lung cancer incidence among uranium miners in which asbestos insulation workers are chosen as the reference group. In this instance, an excess of lung cancer among the uranium miners would be understated or might go undetected. Furthermore, the use of an external worker reference population usually increases study costs.

Another approach is to use an internal reference population, consisting of some segment of the full study cohort, usually assumed to be non-exposed to the hazardous agents of concern (Gilbert, 1982). This approach may not eliminate bias from the Healthy Worker Effect, but will usually reduce it (Pearce et al., 1986). An additional advantage of using an internal reference population is that similarity of data quality is anticipated for all groups compared. In contrast, there are often disparities in the amounts and quality of data between the study cohort and an external reference population. The principal difficulty of choosing an internal reference population is that it may not be possible to identify a "non-exposed" group, and thus observed exposure–response relationships may be diminished spuriously.

Previously, we discussed subcohort analysis, where subcohorts are defined on the basis of employment duration, time since first exposure, and so on, and rates from an external reference population provide expected numbers. Use of an internal reference group is typical of analyses that are primarily directed at exploring associations of disease rates with certain work areas, tasks, or exposure levels within the workplace. Strategies of analysis focused on etiologic questions are considered next.

4.2. Subcohort Analysis

The second level of cohort data analysis is a comparative examination of disease rates between subcohorts defined on the basis of their exposure experience. This analysis, of course, requires that job and/or exposure level data are available or can be reconstructed for the cohort.

Classification with Respect to Job Categories

Exposure data in occupational epidemiology can be depicted in a variety of ways. The crudest characterization is simply ever versus never employed in the industry, and the relevant analysis consists of comparisons of disease rates between the cohort and an external reference population. This analysis can be accomplished with the SMR approach, as described earlier.

Table 5-9. Respiratory disease mortality in various job categories of metal trades occupations

Job category	Respiratory cancer		Nonmalignant respiratory disease	
	Obs	SMR	Obs	SMR
Welders	53	1.31	40	1.25
Shipfitters	12	0.57	28	1.44
Helpers	20	1.28	19	1.01
Riggers	15	0.92	14	0.85
Mechanics	7	0.92	5	0.74
Burners	11	1.28	16	2.21
Boilermakers	15	1.57	15	1.63
Others	14	1.98	9	1.28
Total	147	1.17	146	1.25

Source: Beaumont and Weiss (1980).

Characterization of workers into groups defined on the basis of process division in the plant or similarity of jobs and tasks is an objective scheme that is especially valuable when exposure intensity data are limited or nonexistent (see Chapter 2).

Example 5.4

The simplest way to apply a process division or job grouping scheme in an occupational cohort study is to categorize each worker into only one grouping. Table 5-9 gives an example of mutually exclusive categorization with data adapted from Beaumont and Weiss' (1980) cohort mortality study of metals tradesmen. Workers sometimes changed job categories, usually from a "helper" to a skilled job category. Because such workers often performed skilled work before their job designations were officially changed, the investigators assigned them to the skilled job categories. The findings reveal evidence of disease clustering in various trades, yet the role of specific causative agents is undetermined.

A simple classification system of the sort illustrated in Example 5.4 requires that all of the person-years for each worker and any cases (deaths) be assigned to only one job category. Several options are available for mutually exclusive job categorization. A worker can be classified according to (1) the first job, (2) the last job, (3) the job held longest, or (4) the presumed "most hazardous" job. Options 1 and 2 are the least desirable, although inadequate job history data may necessitate one or the other. Options 1 and 2 will be wasteful of job history and exposure information for workers who have assumed more than one job in the plant. Option 3 is the most common method of worker categorization because the longest-held job is most representative of a worker's occupational experience. Option 4 requires investigator judgment about the types and concentrations of exposures in various jobs, based either on specific knowledge of the industrial processes and job activities or on heuristic evidence of toxic reactions among workers in various jobs in the plant, for example, seemingly frequent reports of illness or injury from one job type or work area. Option 4 becomes an ordinal ranking scheme (see the following discussion) when judgment regarding exposure potential is thought to be reliable. On balance, then, categorizing workers into their longest-held jobs is the most defensible strategy for a mutually exclusive exposure classification scheme.

A simple mutually exclusive classification system is attractive from the standpoint of ease of computation. However, there are problems associated with this approach. For example, in the study by Beaumont and Weiss (1980) (Example 5.4), the investigators noted that their method of assigning all the person-years and expected deaths to the category including the last job held (option 2) "introduced a small bias, in that person-years and expected deaths for the helper experience were sometimes allocated to a skilled category. The result was slightly conservative [underestimated] mortality ratios for the skilled groups and slightly inflated ratios for the helper category." Such bias can be substantial in more complex situations of job mobility.

Bias of this type can be reduced by beginning counting of person-years and case occurrences for a particular job category only at the point in time that a worker enters that job category. In Example 5.4, this method would avoid underestimating effect estimates (e.g., SMRs) for the skilled groups but would not rectify the problem of inflated mortality ratios for the helper categories because they would still not include the person-time for helpers who moved to skilled jobs. Furthermore, this method is wasteful of information because some person-years may be excluded from the analysis.

Similar problems can occur for other job assignment options (e.g., categorizing workers into the longest-held job). These problems are compounded if workers change jobs frequently or if workers spend equal amounts of time in two or more jobs (see Example 5.5). Thus, any analysis that does not take into account movement between job categories may produce misleading results.

The solution is to make full use of all the person-time information available. This is usually done in the context of an analysis involving

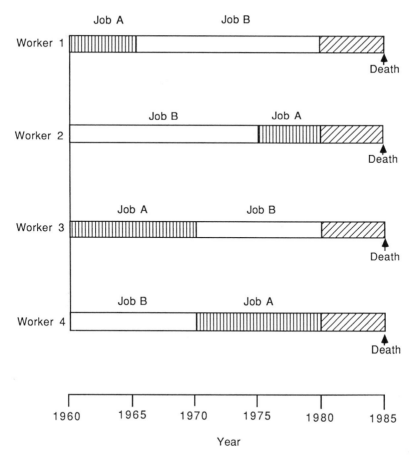

Figure 5-5. Job category assignments for four hypothetical workers.

internal comparisons, but it can also be used with SMR comparisons against an external reference population. Essentially, *a separate analysis is carried out for each job category.* The simplest such analysis is a comparison of the disease rates of workers who have ever worked in a particular job category with those of workers who have never worked in that category. Each analysis thus involves all the person-time experience and cases (or deaths) in the study.

Example 5.5

Figure 5-5 depicts the employment experience of four hypothetical workers who moved between only two jobs, A and B. To simplify the problem, we can assume that all four were hired in 1960 at age 40 years, terminated employment in 1980, and died of the disease of interest in 1985. If one were to adopt a decision algorithm such that each worker is assigned to the job category containing the job held longest, then workers 3 and 4 would present an unresolvable problem; worker 1 would be classified into category B, as would worker 2 because both had worked for 15 of their 20 years of employment in job B, even though the temporal sequencing of employment in these jobs is reversed for the two.

Considering further the four workers in Figure 5–5, we can see that workers 1 and 2 will be indistinguishable if a mutually exclusive, longest-duration job categorization is used, yet differences in their temporal patterns of exposures in job B will be obscured. The procedure that will account for these age and calendar year differences, as well as for time spent in other jobs (in this example, job A), is to carry out a separate analysis for each job category, with each analysis including all the person-time and deaths in the study. For example, the analysis for job B would consist of comparing the mortality among persons who *ever* worked in job B with that of persons who *never* worked in job B. Thus, for workers 2 and 4, all 25 years of follow-up and the subsequent death would be allocated to the "ever" category for job B. On the other hand, the first five years of follow-up for worker 1 would be allocated to the "never" category (because up to that point he had never worked in job B). The subsequent 20 years of follow-up (and the death) for worker 1 would be assigned to the "ever" category for job B. Hence, all the person-years and deaths in the study would be allocated to one of two categories (ever/never) for job B. The mortality experience of these two categories could then be compared with one of the effect measure estimates described earlier in this chapter.

More generally, it is preferable to examine the effect of duration of employment in each job category rather than a simple ever/never comparison. When employment duration is incorporated into a job category analysis, person-years are distributed, by age and calendar year and other confounders, into employment duration strata within job categories. The cases or deaths are then assigned to each job category of employment, as before, but within a job category, cases are placed in the longest achieved duration stratum. In Example 5.5, when evaluating job A, the first five person-years for worker 3 would be allocated to the zero to four years' duration of employment stratum, and the next 20 years and the death to the five to nine years duration stratum. Next, we would evaluate worker 3's employment in job B. The years 1960–74 would be assigned to the zero to four years' employment duration stratum for job B, and the next 10 years (and the death) would be assigned to the five to nine years' duration stratum. Thus, the approach described here involves conducting multiple analyses, one for each job category, and no arbitrary assumptions are made about the relative hazards of various job categories.

When only a few job categories are to be considered, it may be possible to perform a separate analysis for each, while controlling for duration in the others (e.g., the job A analysis might be stratified on duration of employment in job B, as well as on age, calendar

Table 5-10. Standardized rate ratios (SRRs) for lung cancer mortality among phosphate industry workers, according to employment duration in job categories

| Job category | Length of employment (yr) | | | | | |
| | $<1^a$ | | 1–9 | | ≥ 10 | |
	Obs	SRR	Obs	SRR	Obs	SRR
Mining and separation	74	1.00	27	1.54	15	0.76
Rock processing	92	1.00	17	1.75	7	0.95
H_2SO_4 and H_3PO_4 manufacturing	105	1.00	8	1.34	3	0.87
Fertilizer manufacturing	111	1.00	5	0.78	0	0
Skilled crafts	94	1.00	10	0.85	12	1.83
Plant services	86	1.00	20	1.28	10	1.98
Administration	92	1.00	15	1.07	9	0.62

Source: Checkoway et al. (1985a).

[a]Reference category, includes 0.

year, and other confounders). However, this can become unwieldly when there are more than two or three job categories, especially when the categories are not mutually exclusive, as occurs when categorization is made with respect to specific exposures that overlap jobs. In this situation, the initial analyses should consider each job category separately, such that each analysis includes all person-years and events in the study. Simultaneous assessment of the effects of multiple job categories can then be made selectively by focusing on the job categories that are related to disease.

Example 5.6

Table 5–10 displays data on lung cancer mortality from the cohort study of phosphate industry workers (Checkoway et al., 1985a). A total of 116 lung cancer deaths occurred during the 30 years of follow-up, and workers were classified into non-overlapping job categories. It should be noted that each line of the table represents a separate analysis, and therefore includes all 116 lung cancer deaths in the study. The columns denote increasing employment duration strata within job categories. Each worker contributes person-years into each employment duration stratum in which he worked. Within a job category, person-years accumulation for the <1, 1–9, and ≥10-year duration strata begin, respectively, at the date of entry into the cohort, the date at which one year of cumulative employment in the the job category was achieved, and the date at which ten years cumulative employment in the job category occurred. All person-years were further stratified according to age and calendar year in this example. Increasing lung cancer mortality gradients with employment duration were found for two job categories: Skilled Crafts and Plant Services.

Another general strategy for conducting subcohort analysis is to compare disease rates between subcohorts defined on the basis of employment in job categories that are ranked with respect to expo-

Table 5-11. Standardized Rate Ratios (SRRs) for lung cancer mortality among white male phosphate industry workers, according to employment duration in jobs grouped with respect to exposure potential

Jobs grouped by exposure to:	Length of employment (yr)					
	<1[a]		1–9		≥10	
	Obs	SRR	Obs	SRR	Obs	SRR
Alpha radiation	85	1.00	22	1.82	6	1.08
Phosphoric acid and soluble phosphates	99	1.00	14	1.04	3	0.49
Sulfuric acid	103	1.00	10	1.25	3	0.66
Soluble fluorine compounds	99	1.00	13	1.13	4	0.73
Mineral dust	92	1.00	19	1.64	5	1.05
Fertilizer dust	104	1.00	10	1.04	2	0.60

Source: Checkoway et al. (1985a).

[a]Reference category, includes 0.

sure intensity for the agent(s) of interest. *Ordinal rankings* can be made either on the basis of informed judgment or with reference to exposure measurements. Ordinarily, if there are sufficient exposure data to permit estimation of individual workers' exposures, then one would attempt to reconstruct a quantitative profile for each worker (see the following discussion). However, there are times when the industrial hygiene or health physics data are incomplete and only permit an ordinal ranking of jobs and work areas.

The simplest, and often most reliable, ranking system is a dichotomous yes–no rating of jobs with respect to exposure potential. Under such a scheme, jobs are grouped according to the probability of exposure.

Example 5.7

Table 5–11 shows lung cancer mortality data from the previously discussed study of phosphate industry workers (Checkoway et al., 1985a). The results are expressed as SRRs for employment duration in various job categories grouped on a dichotomous basis with respect to exposures to a number of suspected hazardous agents. The job groupings are not mutually exclusive because many jobs entail exposures to more than one substance. When job categories overlap in this way, as frequently happens, it may be difficult to distinguish effects of individual agents. In this study no regularly increasing gradient of lung cancer mortality was found for any of the agents considered. In comparison with the lung cancer mortality data in Table 5–10, these data are less informative.

A somewhat more refined scheme involves polychotomous ordinal rankings, such as "low," "moderate," and "high." Rankings of

Table 5–12. Lung cancer mortality among amosite asbestos factory workers, according to ordinally ranked jobs

Highest exposure category	Obs	SMR
Background	10	1.06
Low	12	1.34
Medium	41	2.25
Heavy	8	4.25

Source: Acheson et al. (1984).

this type require more thorough exposure data than the simple dichotomous scheme.

Example 5.8

Data from Acheson et al.'s (1984) historical cohort study of amosite asbestos factory workers illustrate the application of a polychotomous ordinal ranking of jobs (Table 5–12). There is a striking lung cancer mortality gradient with increasing exposure rank, although it should be mentioned that workers were assigned into the highest exposure categories in which they worked. Thus, the points made previously about improper assignment of person-years and possible confounding from job mobility patterns may apply in this study. Nonetheless, the impressive trend demonstrated is unlikely to be an artifact of such bias.

Ordinal ranking can be further combined with a duration-of-exposure dimension. Thus, we would classify workers into strata of employment duration within ordinally ranked job categories. This method approximates a cumulative exposure categorization scheme as the exposure intensity and employment duration estimates become more precise.

Example 5.9

Newhouse et al. (1985) conducted a historical cohort mortality study of asbestos products manufacturing workers. The industrial hygiene data that were available permitted an ordinal classification of jobs into "low–moderate" and "severe" exposure categories. Workers were then classified into employment duration strata within these exposure designations. The data on lung cancer mortality presented in Table 5–13 reveal a pronounced effect of severe exposures for the greater than two-year duration stratum; this effect is more accentuated among female than male workers.

When quantified exposure data are available for all or most workers, either by means of linkage of job and work area data to employment history information or, more rarely, from personal monitor-

Table 5–13. Lung cancer mortality among asbestos products factory workers, followed 30 years or longer, according to duration of employment in ordinally ranked jobs

Exposure category and duration	Obs	SMR
Men		
Low–moderate, ≤2 years	10	2.2
Low–moderate, >2 years	6	2.1
Severe, ≤2 years	17	2.3
Severe, >2 years	16	4.8
Women		
Low–moderate	0	0
Severe, ≤2 years	10	5.4
Severe, >2 years	10	14.7

Source: Newhouse et al. (1985).

ing, it will be possible to define subcohorts on the basis of maximum exposure intensity or with respect to cumulative exposure levels. Maximum intensity can be considered either relative to each worker's experience or with reference to some predetermined level, such as the Threshold Limit Value (Copes et al., 1985). In effect, exposure intensity data form the basis of a more precise ranking scheme than ordinal assignment, although the methods of analysis are similar. Care should be given to the attribution of person-years when stratifying on maximum intensity because similar peak intensities occurring at different ages may have decidedly different health consequences.

Some diseases are strongly related to *cumulative exposure* (CE), where CE is simply the summed products of exposure intensities and their associated durations (Chapter 2). Typical examples of CE in occupational epidemiology are million particles of dust per cubic foot × years, fibers per cc × years, and parts per million × years for chemical exposures.

Example 5.10

An example of subcohort analysis of disease rates by CE levels is demonstrated with data on asbestosis mortality among chrysotile asbestos textile workers (Dement et al., 1983b) in Table 5–14. In this study (which is described in greater detail later in this chapter), directly age- and calendar year–adjusted mortality rates were computed for subcohorts classified into fibers per cc × days CE categories. The age and calendar year distributions of person-years of the entire cohort served as the reference category. The person-years were distributed into all achieved CE categories, and deaths were assigned to the highest category reached. These data evidence a striking trend of asbestosis mortality with increasing CE levels, small numbers notwithstanding.

Table 5-14. Cumulative exposure–response relationship for asbestosis mortality among chrysotile asbestos textile plant workers

Cumulative exposure category (fibers/cc × days)	Obs	Deaths per 1,000 person-years
<1,000	2	0.32
1,000–9,999	1	0.18
10,000–39,999	6	1.98
40,000–100,000	6	5.99
>100,000	2	15.87

Source: Dement et al. (1983b).

In an analysis of disease rates in relation to CE there is no ambiguity as to where a case or death should be assigned—the highest achieved CE level (as in Example 5.10). This situation is certainly simpler and more intuitively appealing than the multiple counting procedures involved in job category subcohort analysis. Use of CE as an exposure index has the obvious advantage of a simplified analysis and relatively straightforward interpretation of results, yet strict reliance on CE as the sole exposure variable may be wasteful of information. Because CE incorporates intensity and duration of exposure, only effects attributable to the absolute amount of exposure will be apparent in a conventional analysis of CE and disease rates. The relative importance of the components of CE, intensity and duration, and temporal sequencing of a varying intensity schedule may go unnoticed.

As an illustration, consider the hypothetical data on disease rates in Table 5–15. Inspection of the rates reveals a strong effect of intensity but no effect of duration of exposure. The bottom half of this table shows rates according to CE levels. If we were to restrict

Table 5-15. Hypothetical example of disease rates according to exposure intensity, duration, and cumulative exposure

Intensity level	Duration of exposure (yr)		
	10	20	25
4	3[a]	3	3
5	6	6	6
10	12	12	12

	Cumulative exposure								
	40	50	80	(100	100	100)[b]	125	200	250
Disease rate	3[a]	6	3	(3	6	12)	6	12	12

[a]Rate per 1,000.

[b]Three combinations of intensity and duration give cumulative exposures of 100.

Table 5-16. Relative risks (SMRs) for respiratory cancer according to duration of employment and dust concentration in asbestos cement manufacturing

Average dust concentration (mppcf)[a]	Duration of employment (yr)		
	<2	2–10	>10
<5	1.00[b]	1.30	0.76
5–20	1.00	0.51	3.30
>20	1.34	1.71	4.54

Source: Weill et al. (1979).

[a]Millions of particles per cubic foot.

[b]Reference category.

our attention to the association of disease with CE and ignore the intensity- and duration-specific disease rates, then the difference in effect of these two component parameters would go undetected. Moreover, in this example the observed CE–response curve, which suggests a positive, though irregular, trend will be greatly influenced by the disease rate for the CE = 100 category, which can vary from 3 to 12, depending on the joint distribution of intensity and duration.

Example 5.11

Data from the historical cohort study by Weill et al. (1979) of respiratory cancer among workers in the asbestos cement industry (Table 5–16) provide a good example of an examination of the independent and joint effects of exposure intensity and duration. By independent, we mean the effect of one factor in the absence, or in this instance, at the lowest level(s), of another factor(s). These data indicate no pronounced effects for either intensity or duration, as can be seen from the leftmost column and top row of the table, respectively. However, there is a marked effect of CE that can be discerned from the trends in the rightmost column and bottom row.

The temporal pattern of exposures may also have a bearing on disease rates. To illustrate, consider the four hypothetical worker exposure profiles depicted in Figure 5–6. In each instance, CE is equal to 100 units, but the intensity schedule varies between workers. The exposures for these four workers will have equivalent effects only when the following conditions are met: (1) there is no threshold intensity greater than the lowest value (in this example, 5); (2) similar exposure intensities at different ages have equivalent consequences; and (3) prolonged, uninterrupted exposure is not required for disease induction. In other words, CE will be the expo-

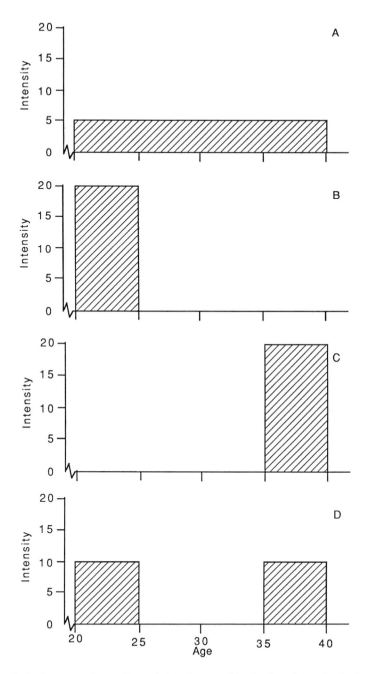

Figure 5–6. Exposure intensity and duration profiles for four hypothetical workers receiving equivalent cumulative exposures of 100 units.

sure variable of sole interest when the probability of disease induction (and/or severity) depends on the total amount of exposure received, irrespective of the rate of delivery of exposure.

Variability of exposure effects between the configurations in Figure 5–6 could arise if any of the preceding three criteria are not satisfied. For example, if cancer induction requires prolonged, uninterrupted exposure, then configuration A would confer the greatest risk, provided that there is no threshold above the given constant intensity. Early or late carcinogenic effects for exposures above some threshold intensity (e.g., 5) would preferentially result from configurations B and C, respectively, whereas configuration D might pose the greatest risk to workers exposed to a carcinogen that causes both early- and late-stage changes but requires above-threshold intensities. If, on the other hand, we consider a disease whose severity is influenced profoundly by exposure intensity, then configurations B, C, and D might be more hazardous than A, and distinctions between these three would depend on whether disease severity is amplified by above-threshold exposures early or later in life (Axelson, 1985).

The foregoing discussion is offered to highlight some of the potential problems associated with a conventional subcohort analysis that is restricted to CE. The arguments illustrated in Figure 5–6 are based on simplified hypothetical situations. In most occupational cohort studies, exposure patterns are considerably more complex than this; thus, CE may be the best method for summarizing exposure data for a subcohort analysis. Also, disentangling peak intensity, duration, and CE effects will often be complicated by a high degree of correlation between these variables. For example, workers with the highest CE values are also those most likely to have experienced the most intense or prolonged peak exposures. One approach to assess the effects of these exposure factors is to attempt stratification on two of the three variables while examining the effects of the other. Thus, we might try to stratify on peak intensity and CE in an analysis of exposure duration. Such stratification may not be successful, although inspection of graphical displays of cases' and noncases' exposure profiles over time may assist in understanding the relationship between the exposure variables and disease.

4.3. Missing Exposure Data

Unavailability of work history or exposure data is a hindrance to subcohort analysis in many occupational cohort studies. This situation may arise for several reasons. Data for workers employed during the earliest years of plant operations may have been discarded or lost over the years, or exposure data may have been collected only for workers thought to be most heavily exposed to presumed toxins. The treatment of missing data in subcohort analyses will depend on the types and amounts of data that are missing. Some available data may be of such poor quality that they are useless, and thus are effectively missing.

We can consider two types of missing exposure data. The first is work history information from which job assignment data for cohort members are compiled. Missing data on jobs for some workers will necessitate the creation of an "unknown" job category. That is, although there is documentation that certain workers were probably employed during particular time periods, there is insufficient information to permit assignment into specific jobs or work areas of the plant. Moreover, assignment into quantitative exposure categories will be impossible when exposure levels are determined by linking environmental measurements with jobs, tasks, or work locations. Subcohort analysis will then require that the "unknown" category be treated as a separate designation, with cases (deaths) and person-years assigned in the same manner as for the identifiable job categories.

Example 5.12

Approximately 6 percent of workers in a historical cohort study of nuclear industry workers had inadequate work history information for assignment into specific job categories (Checkoway et al., 1985c), thus requiring the creation of an "unknown" category. Table 5–17 shows cancer mortality data (SRRs) for the cohort of 8,371 male workers, classified according to employment duration in 12 separate job categories, including Unknown. The results of this subcohort analysis do not indicate any consistent patterns with respect to job assignment, although the elevated SRRs for the 1–9 and ≥10-year duration strata for the Unknown category are provocative. Comparisons between workers assigned to this category and the remaining cohort members did not reveal any differences in periods of employment or radiation doses, however.

Alternative strategies, such as deleting the "unknowns" from subcohort analyses or pooling them with other job categories of lesser concern (e.g., those assumed to be non-exposed) into an "other" category, are inappropriate and may introduce bias. Deleting the "unknowns" is wasteful of information, whereas the latter approach involves the unwarranted assumption that the "unknowns" share common exposure profiles with workers in identifiable jobs.

Missing data on quantitative exposures can occur for two main reasons. First, the data may simply be missing. For example, if per-

Table 5-17. Cancer mortality (all sites combined) among nuclear workers, according to employment duration in job categories

	Duration of employment (yr)					
	$<1^a$		1–9		≥ 10	
Job category	Obs	SRR	Obs	SRR	Obs	SRR
Radioisotopes	191	1.00	2	0.88	0	0
Chemical operations	198	1.00	0	0	0	0
Monitoring	188	1.00	4	0.92	1	0.38
Biology	192	1.00	1	0.66	0	0
Chemistry	182	1.00	6	0.40	5	0.50
Physics	183	1.00	7	1.27	3	1.06
Engineering	170	1.00	14	0.95	9	1.26
Administration	178	1.00	14	1.25	1	0.22
Maintenance	124	1.00	47	2.02	22	1.06
Shipping and receiving	189	1.00	1	0.13	3	1.65
Other	161	1.00	23	1.74	9	1.04
Unknown	176	1.00	11	2.33	6	1.14

Source: Checkoway et al. (1985c).

[a]Reference category, includes people who never worked in a particular job category.

sonal exposure monitoring in a plant began some years after the facility opened, then there will be no data for workers employed prior to the onset of monitoring. Second, some workers may have been eligible for monitoring but were not entered into the monitoring program because they were considered unlikely to receive significant exposures. In the first case, there is no justifiable alternative to deleting workers with missing exposure data from an exposure–response subcohort analysis. The second situation of unmonitored workers presents several options (as discussed earlier in Chapter 2). These include (1) exclusion from subcohort analysis, (2) assignment of the cohort's average or median exposure levels for the relevant time periods for which data are missing, and (3) assignment of exposure levels of zero if there is ample evidence that monitoring actually was restricted to exposed workers.

There seldom is one clearly superior choice for handling missing exposure data. Consequently, it is often advisable to conduct subcohort analyses using each of several reasonable options to determine the extent to which exposure–response relationships vary under different approaches of treating missing data.

4.4. Disease Induction and Latency Analysis

For all diseases or injuries there are requisite time lags between exposure to etiologic factors and clinical manifestation. In the extreme case of an acute episode, such as an electrocution following exposure to high voltage or eye irritation from a noxious gas, the time lag is effectively nil because the response is virtually instantaneous. However, many occupationally related diseases are delayed effects of exposure, where the time lag may range from hours or days (e.g., pulmonary edema) to decades (e.g., cancer).

Latency is the term often applied to the time interval between exposure and disease manifestation or recognition. The concept of disease latency continues to be a topic of discussion among epidemiologists who have offered various definitions. Rothman (1981) provides a clear operative definition of latency as the period from disease initiation to manifestation. This definition is consistent with the idea that there is some period of time when the disease exists in a "hidden" state in an individual.

A related concept is *induction time,* which can be defined as the period from first exposure to an agent or collection of agents to disease initiation (Rothman, 1981). There is no feasible way to determine the exact point in time following exposure onset when any disease has been induced in a person. Even if we had at our disposal the technological means of determining precisely when, say, the final malignant cell transformation occurred that progressed to a cancer, adopting such a procedure for an individual worker or for a cohort of workers would not be practical.

Figure 5–7 illustrates the relationship between induction and

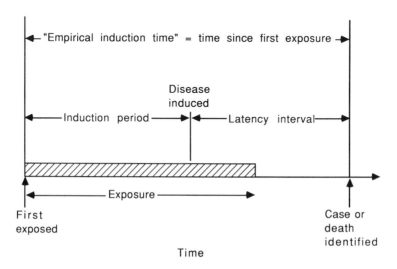

Figure 5-7. Disease induction and latency intervals.

Table 5–18. Some common methods to address disease induction and latency intervals

1. Restrict study population to retirees
2. Begin follow-up after some minimum time period
3. Truncate exposures at some arbitrary time point and include only cases occurring thereafter
4. Lag exposures

latency intervals. The induction time, although depicted here as a fixed interval, will of course vary, depending on the nature of the exposure and disease, as well as on individual responses to exposure. Many occupational exposures can be considered to be chronic, extending over periods of years or decades, but may also be intermittent within the period of exposure. Intermittent exposures, although relevant for induction of some diseases, will not be discussed here so as to simplify matters. Thus, although we cannot usually estimate induction time, we can determine the interval from exposure onset to disease manifestation or recognition. Rothman (1981) refers to this interval, which is the sum of induction and latency times, as the *empirical induction time.*

Several methods for taking into account latency and induction have been developed for occupational cohort studies (Table 5–18). The first is to restrict the study population to retirees (Enterline, 1976; Collins and Redmond, 1976). However, including only retirees in a cohort study excludes persons who developed disease and died while still employed; hence, this strategy is potentially wasteful of information. Also, retirees' exposure patterns may be atypical of the experience of many members of the complete cohort. For example, short-term workers in some occupations are assigned to the most heavily exposed jobs and may terminate early for just that reason.

A second approach is to begin follow-up after some minimum elapsed time period. Thus, cases (deaths) and person-years of observation occurring during that interval are not included in the analysis. This strategy should not be confused with the requirement for beginning person-year counting after the time when the minimum employment duration cohort inclusion criterion has been attained.

Example 5.13

The data in Table 5–19 from a historical cohort mortality study among workers at a polyvinyl chloride polymerization factory (Waxweiler et al., 1976) illustrate the method of starting follow-up after a specified time interval following cohort incep-

Table 5–19. Cancer mortality among workers exposed to vinyl chloride, according to latency period

Cancer cause of death	10-year latency		15-year latency	
	Obs	SMR	Obs	SMR
All cancers	35	1.49	31	1.84
Brain and CNS	3	3.29	3	4.98
Respiratory	12	1.56	11	1.94
Biliary and liver	7	11.55	7	16.06
Lymphopoietic	4	1.59	3	1.76

Source: Waxweiler et al. (1976).

tion. SMRs were computed after deleting the first 10 or 15 years after entry into the cohort. This technique incorporates an implicit assumption that any deaths that occurred before the specified interval (10 or 15 years) were probably unrelated to workplace exposures. It would also have been desirable had the authors presented findings for a zero-year interval. Nonetheless, the increased SMRs for the 15-year, compared to the 10-year, interval appear consistent with an occupational etiology for these cancers.

A third approach that has been used for investigating exposure–response relationships is to truncate exposures at either a fixed age or a fixed time interval since first exposure and to begin person-year and case (death) tabulation thereafter. This method attempts to avoid including "irrelevant" exposures, but its particular shortcoming is the arbitrariness of the truncation boundary for age or time since exposure onset.

Example 5.14

McDonald and colleagues (1980) used an exposure truncation technique to account for induction time in their study of the association between cumulative exposure to asbestos dust and cause-specific mortality among a cohort of miners and millers. In this study, only exposures received before age 45 years were counted, and follow-up began at that age. The results (SMRs) are given in Table 5–20. Positive gradients were seen for each of the diseases listed, especially for lung cancer and pneumoconiosis mortality.

A fourth technique for avoiding exposure and follow-up overlap is to *lag exposures* by some assumed latency interval (y), such that a worker's current person-year at risk is assigned to the exposure level (either intensity, duration, or, most commonly, cumulative exposure) achieved y years earlier. Consider an example using CE as the exposure index. If by age 40 years a worker had accumulated 25 CE units, and by age 50 years his CE was 45 units, then under an

Table 5–20. Cause-specific mortality among asbestos miners in relation to exposures to dust accumulated to age 45

| | Cumulative exposure (mppcf × years) | | | | | |
| | <30 | | 30–299 | | ≥300 | |
Cause of death	Obs	SMR	Obs	SMR	Obs	SMR
All causes	1,668	1.02	1,138	1.04	642	1.30
Pneumoconiosis	5	2.98	12	10.81	27	54.00
Lung cancer	91	0.93	81	1.18	70	2.25
Esophagus and stomach cancer	68	1.22	42	1.14	26	1.58
Colon and rectum cancer	34	0.62	28	0.77	18	1.11

Source: McDonald et al. (1980).

assumed latency interval of ten years, his person-year at risk for age 50 years would be assigned to the 25 CE unit level.

Example 5.15

An example of exposure lagging is provided in Table 5–21, which contains data from Gilbert and Marks' (1979) analysis of multiple myeloma mortality in relation to cumulative radiation doses received by workers at the Hanford Works nuclear plant. Data are shown for analyses incorporating two- and ten-year lag intervals. The mortality trends, although irregular, persist when a ten-year lag is imposed.

Exposure lagging has the particular advantage of including the entire enumerated cohort and all members' complete exposure histories, unlike the other methods described earlier, which sacrifice information by either subject exclusion or exposure truncation. We have described exposure lagging for situations where exposure data can be expressed quantitatively. It is also possible to apply lagging in an analysis of duration of employment, either considered in the industry at large or in specific job categories. The latter can become computationally cumbersome when there is a considerable degree of mobility between job categories, however.

Table 5–21. Multiple myeloma mortality among nuclear workers, according to cumulative radiation doses, lagged 2 and 10 years

| | Dose category (rem) | | | | | | | |
| | 0–<2 | | 2–<5 | | 5–15 | | >15 | |
Lag interval	Obs	SMR	Obs	SMR	Obs	SMR	Obs	SMR
2 years	3	0.7	0	0	0	0	3	6.0
10 years	3	0.6	0	0	2	4.0	1	10.0

Source: Gilbert and Marks (1979).

Of the latency analysis methods reviewed here, exposure lagging is the superior approach because it provides maximum use of the data. It is possible to vary the assumed latency period by trying different lag periods and contrasting the results. The other methods previously described do not involve clear and consistent assumptions about the empirical induction time. For example, truncating exposures after 20 years means that two workers exposed at the same intensity for 20 years and 50 years respectively, are classified into the same exposure category. Lagging exposures by ten years for these two workers would place them (appropriately) in different exposure categories.

5. PLANNING A COHORT STUDY

Decisions as to which occupational cohorts warrant epidemiologic study should be made primarily on the bases of public health and scientific concerns. The occupational groups that are exposed to either known or suspected toxins are the obvious targets for study. However, such decisions are seldom straightforward because one needs to anticipate the likely study results and their interpretation before embarking on a full-scale cohort study (Steenland et al., 1987). The questions that arise most commonly are (1) Is the study cohort sufficiently large to yield statistically reliable data? (2) Will the cohort have an adequate length of follow-up for studying delayed effects, some of which may be rare diseases? and (3) Are the exposure data suitable for assessing exposure–response relationships?

The first two questions can be viewed from a purely statistical perspective as issues of study size requirements (see Chapter 4). We are of the opinion that study size, or statistical power, considerations should be given less weight in decision making than concerns about worker health or scientific interest. Nonetheless, statistical instability cannot be dismissed out of hand because the decision as to whether a cohort should be studied is seldom clearcut, and statistical power can provide some guidance.

Specification of minimum induction or latency times requires some judgment. Obviously, if we are planning to investigate cancer mortality in an occupational cohort, where the vast majority of workers had been hired recently (say, within the preceding five to ten years), then the likelihood of an informative study would be small. However, there may still be an interest on the part of the workers or management to enumerate the cohort, retrospectively and prospectively, with the intention of conducting an ongoing cancer surveillance program.

Likewise, there would be a motivation for following a very small group of workers who had experienced a dramatic or unique exposure episode, such as an industrial accident entailing exposures to high levels of recognized toxins.

The adequacy of exposure data is a critical determinant of a study's value. In planning studies of cohorts exposed to agents previously documented as health hazards, one would like to have exposure data at least as complete and accurate as those in the least detailed of the previous studies. For example, another cohort study of cancer mortality among radiation-exposed workers with no quantified dose data is of questionable usefulness, given the vast body of data on this topic. On the other hand, unique, previously unstudied workplace environments provide ample reason for initiating a cohort study, even when data on specific exposures cannot be obtained.

6. EXAMPLE OF A COHORT STUDY: ASBESTOS TEXTILE PLANT WORKERS

The example presented in this section is a historical cohort study of the mortality experience of workers at an asbestos textile manufacturing plant. This study, conducted by Dement and colleagues (1983a,b), was sponsored by the U.S. National Institute for Occupational Safety and Health (NIOSH). This is an especially valuable study for review because it illustrates a number of the study design and data analysis issues that have been discussed in this chapter. We will also use the data from this study to illustrate methods applicable to case–control studies in Chapter 6 and to demonstrate advanced statistical and exposure modeling procedures in Chapters 8 and 9. The findings that we will present are the result of our reanalyses of the data that were provided to us by NIOSH and Dr. Dement. Minor discrepancies that may appear between ours and the published data are attributable to different analytic techniques and computer algorithms used for the analyses.

6.1. Description of the Plant and Study Cohort

The plant, located in Charleston, South Carolina, began production of asbestos products in 1896. Asbestos textiles used for fireproof fabrics and automotive parts (e.g., brake linings) were the main products manufactured.

Personnel employment data needed to reconstruct the cohort were available only for the years 1940 and later (although there are exposure data collected since 1930). Thus, workers who terminated employment prior to 1940 did not enter into the cohort. The cohort was defined as white males who were employed for at least one month in textile operations at any time between January 1, 1940, and December 31, 1965. Mortality follow-up was performed for the years 1940 to 1975 inclusive. The one-month minimum employment restriction was imposed to permit an evaluation of the mortality patterns of workers who were exposed to asbestos for a reasonable length of time. The restriction on hire date was made to ensure that all workers would have had at least ten years of follow-up beyond the date of hire (first exposure). Thus, this is a dynamic cohort insofar as workers hired after the date of cohort inception (January 1, 1940) were included.

6.2. Vital Status Tracing and Cause-of-Death Determination

The investigators used several sources to perform vital status follow-up on the cohort. These included the Social Security Administration, the Internal Revenue Service (which used to provide information on persons who made income tax payments for specific years), state motor vehicle bureaus, and postal correction services. For persons not traced by these methods, searches were conducted among listings of city residence (Polk) directories, voter registration lists, and funeral home records. Death certificates were obtained from state vital statistics offices.

The results of the tracing are shown in Table 5–22. Vital status was determined for all but 2.1 percent of the cohort, and cause-of-death information was obtained for 94.5 percent of identified

Table 5–22. Vital status and cause of death among 1,261 white male asbestos textile workers: 1940–75

Vital status	Number	Percent
Alive	927	73.5
Dead	308	24.4
(with death certificate)	(291)	(94.5)
(without death certificate)	(17)	(5.5)
Unknown	26	2.1
Total	1,261	100

Table 5–23. Characteristics of the cohort of 1,261 white male asbestos textile workers

Total person-years of observation	32,362.0
Mean length of follow-up (years)	25.7
Mean age at entry into cohort (years)	25.6
Mean year of entry into cohort	1,946.8
Mean age at death (years)	53.5

deaths. Nearly 25 percent of the cohort had died during the follow-up interval. This is a somewhat high overall percentage of deaths but is attributable primarily to the long follow-up period (36 years) and, as we will see, to a pronounced occupational mortality hazard.

Some additional descriptive information on the cohort is presented in Table 5–23. The cohort contributed 32,362 person-years of observation, with a mean duration of follow-up of 25.7 years. The latter figure is important insofar as it indicates that there was a sufficiently long period of observation for the study of cancer and pneumoconiosis mortality, which were of major a priori interest. Also shown in Table 5–23 are the mean age at entry into the cohort (25.6 years), the mean year of entry (1946.8), and the mean age at death (53.5 years). A table such as this provides valuable information about the cohort's demographic and work experience history. For example, the relatively young age at entry suggests that the mortality patterns seen are unlikely to be attributable to previous employment in other occupations, although a proper verification of that assumption would require obtaining the additional relevant data.

6.3. Results

Overall Patterns of Cause-Specific Mortality

SMRs were computed relative to prevailing rates for U.S. white males for the years 1940–75 (Table 5–24). In our calculations, workers with unknown vital status contributed person-years of observation up to the date of last employment. In the original analysis Dement et al. (1983b) considered the unknowns to be alive as of the end of the study (December 31, 1975). The difference in handling the unknowns causes only trivial discrepancies in the results.

The SMR for all causes is elevated (1.50), although the SMR for arteriosclerotic heart disease (0.76) is consistent with a Healthy Worker Effect. The major contributors to the overall excessive mor-

Table 5–24. Cause-specific SMRs for white male asbestos textile workers: 1940–75

Cause of death	Obs	Exp[a]	SMR
All causes	308	205.33	1.50
All cancers	59	36.20	1.63
Digestive system	13	10.00	1.30
Trachea, lung, bronchus	35	10.90	3.21
All other cancers	11	15.28	0.72
Arteriosclerotic heart disease	49	64.47	0.76
Nonmalignant respiratory disease	28	9.77	2.87
Pneumonia	4	3.97	1.01
Emphysema	0	2.25	0
Asthma	0	0.50	0
Other respiratory disease	24	3.05	7.87
Digestive system diseases	8	11.84	0.68
Genitourinary system diseases	6	3.42	1.75
All accidents	34	25.42	1.34
Motor vehicle accidents	11	12.35	0.89
Suicide	5	7.12	0.70

[a]Based on rates for U.S. white males, 1940–75.

tality among the cohort are lung cancer (SMR = 3.21); nonmalignant respiratory diseases, principally asbestosis (SMR = 2.87); and accidents (SMR = 1.34).

Lung Cancer Mortality

We can focus our attention on lung cancer mortality because of its frequently demonstrated association with asbestos and because the number of deaths (35) is large enough for some stratified analyses.

Table 5–25 gives SMRs, again relative to rates for U.S. white males, cross-classified according to age at risk and year of death. What is particularly noticeable about these data is that the SMRs in the body of the table are based on very small numbers, and therefore tend to be unstable. As we mentioned earlier, small numbers frequently pose a problem in a stratified analysis where stratification is done for more than one factor. Thus, the most reliable results from these data are those given in the margins ("Total" column and row). The lung cancer excesses were most pronounced among workers during the sixth and seventh decades of life. Inspection of the trend over time reveals the greatest excesses during the 1940s and 1950s, although these findings are especially influenced by lung cancer deaths that occurred among persons aged 50–59 years during 1940–49 (1) and 1950–59 (8). On balance, there appears to be a fairly consistent lung cancer mortality excess that had not abated by the end of follow-up.

Table 5–25. Observed and expected lung cancer mortality according to age and year of death among white male asbestos textile workers: 1940–75

| Age | Year of death | | | | Total |
	1940–49	1950–59	1960–69	1970–75	
<40	(0/0.03)[a]	(0/0.13)	(0/0.15)	(0/0.05)	(0/0.35)
	0[b]	0	0	0	0
40–49	(0/0.11)	(1/0.54)	(3/1.49)	(2/1.44)	(6/3.58)
	0	1.87	2.02	1.39	1.68
50–59	(1/0.103)	(8/0.56)	(5/1.75)	(1/2.11)	(16/4.52)
	19.42	14.39	2.86	0.47	3.54
60–69	(0/0.03)	(1/0.25)	(2/1.12)	(8/1.64)	(11/3.05)
	0	4.02	1.78	4.88	3.61
70–79	(0/0)	(0/0.001)	(2/0.04)	(0/0.50)	(2/0.73)
	—	0	55.56	0	2.74
≥80	(0/0)	(0/0)	(0/0.004)	(0/0.06)	(0/0.06)
	—	—	0	0	0
Total	(2/0.308)	(10/1.36)	(12/4.17)	(11/5.06)	(35/10.90)
	6.49	7.35	2.88	2.17	3.21

[a]Obs/Exp.

[b]SMR, based on rates for U.S. white males 1940–75.

The lung cancer SMRs with respect to year of hire and age at hire (Table 5–26) are consistent with an effect that requires a long induction and latency period; the SMRs are highest for persons hired before 1940 at ages younger than 40 years. A detailed review of the SMRs within the table reveals especially pronounced excesses for

Table 5–26. Observed and expected lung cancer mortality according to age and year of hire among white male asbestos textile workers: 1940–75

| Age at hire | Year of hire | | | | | Total |
	1920–29	1930–39	1940–49	1950–59	1960–65	
<20	(2/0.16)[a]	(3/0.51)	(1/1.08)	(0/0.09)	(0/0.35)	(6/1.84)
	12.20[b]	(5.88)	(0.93)	0	0	3.26
20–29	(1/0.15)	(6/1.15)	(2/2.30)	(2/0.22)	(0/0.01)	(11/3.83)
	6.71	5.22	0.87	8.93	0	2.87
30–39	(0/0.002)	(7/0.78)	(7/1.86)	(0/0.38)	(0/0.02)	(14/3.04)
	0	9.02	3.77	0	0	4.61
40–49	(0/0.005)	(3/0.20)	(1/1.17)	(0/0.41)	(0/0.02)	(4/1.81)
	0	15.00	0.85	0	0	2.22
≥50	(0/0)	(0/0.05)	(0/0.24)	(0/0.09)	(0/0)	(0/0.38)
	—	0	0	0	—	0
Total	(3/0.32)	(19/2.68)	(11/6.65)	(2/1.20)	(0/0.05)	(35/10.90)
	9.38	7.08	1.65	1.67	0	3.21

[a]Obs/Exp.

[b]SMR, based on rates for U.S. white males 1940–75.

Table 5–27. Observed and expected lung cancer mortality according to length of follow-up and duration of employment among white male asbestos textile workers: 1940–75

Duration of employment (yr)	Length of follow-up (yr)					
	0–4	5–9	10–19	20–29	≥30	Total
0–4	(0/0.16)[a]	(0/0.26)	(3/1.36)	(5/3.08)	(6/2.00)	(14/6.80)
	0[b]	0	2.21	1.62	3.00	2.04
5–9		(0/0.11)	(0/0.14)	(0/0.32)	(1/0.29)	(1/0.89)
		0	0	0	3.41	1.13
10–19			(3/0.53)	(0/0.20)	(2/0.27)	(5/1.44)
			11.32	0	7.35	3.48
20–29				(6/1.01)	(6/0.33)	(12/1.33)
				5.92	18.18	9.06
≥30					(3/0.82)	(3/0.82)
					3.66	3.66
Total	(0/0.16)	(0/0.37)	(6/2.03)	(11/4.61)	(18/3.73)	(35/10.9)
	0	0	2.96	2.39	4.82	3.21

[a]Obs/Exp.
[b]SMR, based on rates for U.S. white males 1940–75.

workers hired at ages younger than 30 years during the 1920s and 1930s (i.e., workers with the longest durations of follow-up).

The effects of duration of employment and follow-up are presented in Table 5–27. The noteworthy findings are the absence of any lung cancer deaths during the first ten years of observation and the increasing, albeit somewhat irregular, pattern with duration of employment. The results with regard to duration of follow-up support the conclusions drawn from the preceding table.

The past exposure profiles of cohort members were estimated by means of linking the workers' job history information from personnel records with environmental measurement data for specific work areas and tasks within the textile plant. Exposure data were available for the years 1930–75 and could be expressed in units of fibers (longer than 5 μm) per cc of air (fibers/cc). Cumulative exposures were estimated for all workers in the cohort as the summed products of air concentrations of asbestos and time (in days) spent in various jobs (Dement et al., 1983a). The exposure reconstruction thus permitted an analysis of lung cancer mortality in relation to cumulative exposure level.

Three types of analysis were used to evaluate trends of lung cancer mortality with cumulative exposure levels (fibers/cc $\times$ days). The first was an SMR analysis, where observed and expected numbers of deaths were computed for each cumulative exposure level (Table 5–28). The expected numbers were derived by applying the

Table 5–28. Standardized mortality ratios (SMRs) for lung cancer according to cumulative asbestos exposure levels and latency

Cumulative exposure (1,000 fibers/ cc × days)	Latency (yr)								
	0			5			15		
	Obs	Exp[a]	SMR	Obs	Exp	SMR	Obs	Exp	SMR
<1	5	3.76 (0.43, 3.10)[b]	1.33	5	3.86 (0.42, 3.02)	1.30	7	4.62 (0.61, 3.12)	1.51
1–9	10	3.72 (1.29, 4.94)	2.69	10	3.78 (1.27, 4.87)	2.65	13	3.68 (1.88, 6.04)	3.53
10–39	7	2.19 (1.28, 6.59)	3.20	10	2.25 (2.13, 8.17)	4.45	9	2.08 (1.97, 8.21)	4.33
40–99	11	1.10 (4.99, 17.89)	10.00	9	0.90 (4.56, 18.98)	10.02	6	0.42 (5.25, 31.32)	14.39
≥100	2	0.13 (1.68, 53.89)	14.93	1	0.12 (0.11, 45.98)	8.27	0	0.10 (0, 36.68)	0

[a]Based on rates for U.S. white males, 1940–75.
[b]95 percent confidence interval for SMR.

rates in the U.S. population to the numbers of person-years of observation in each of the exposure categories, with adjustment made for age and calendar year on a quinquennial basis. Separate analyses were performed using exposure lag intervals of 0, 5, and 15 years.

As can be seen from Table 5–28, there is a strong gradient of increasing lung cancer mortality with increasing exposure level, which occurs irrespective of the lag interval assumed. (The SMR for the highest exposure category under a 15-year lag interval is 0 because no lung cancer deaths achieved this level of cumulative exposure 15 years prior to death.)

The second method of data analysis involved SRR calculations, where the lowest cumulative exposure category (<1,000 fibers/cc × days) served as the reference (Table 5–29). The pattern of results from the SRR analysis is quite similar to that obtained from the SMR analysis (Table 5–28), which suggests that confounding by age or calendar year did not distort the SMR comparisons. One noteworthy feature of these tables is that there is an excess of lung cancer mortality at all levels of cumulative exposure; the SMR for the lowest exposure category is between 1.30 and 1.51, depending on

Table 5-29. Standardized rate ratios (SRRs) for lung cancer according to cumulative asbestos exposure levels and latency

Cumulative exposure (1,000 fibers/ cc × days)	Latency (yr)					
	0		5		15	
	Obs	SRR	Obs	SRR	Obs	SRR
<1[a]	5	1.00 (—)[b]	5	1.00 (—)	7	1.00 (—)
1–9	10	2.12 (0.61, 7.71)	10	2.29 (0.62, 8.41)	13	2.71 (0.78, 9.37)
10–39	7	1.17 (0.25, 5.41)	10	2.18 (0.51, 9.27)	9	2.77 (0.60, 12.83)
40–99	11	4.39 (1.00, 19.26)	9	4.94 (1.20, 20.28)	6	8.00 (1.79, 37.75)
≥100	2	23.83 (2.89, 196.65)	1	23.24 (1.38, 390.83)	0	0 (—)

[a]Reference category.
[b]95 percent confidence interval for SRR.

the lag interval chosen. (This excess, of course, is not discernible from the SRR results because the SRR for that category is 1.00, by definition.) The excess in the lowest exposure stratum may reflect either a greater cigarette smoking prevalence among the cohort than the national population or a genuine increased risk at low exposure levels.

Finally, Mantel–Haenszel analyses were carried out (Table 5–30).

Table 5-30. Mantel-Haenszel summary rate ratios (RR$_{M-H}$) for lung cancer mortality according to cumulative asbestos exposure levels and latency

Cumulative exposure (1,000 fibers/ cc × days)	Latency (yr)					
	0		5		15	
	Obs	RR$_{M-H}$	Obs	RR$_{M-H}$	Obs	RR$_{M-H}$
<1[a]	5	1.00 (—)[b]	5	1.00 (—)	7	1.00 (—)
1–9	10	1.81 (0.63, 5.43)	10	1.99 (0.68, 7.03)	13	2.72 (1.08, 8.02)
10–39	7	1.88 (0.82, 4.91)	10	3.13 (1.01, 14.89)	9	3.83 (1.35, 12.62)
40–99	11	8.01 (2.61, 32.02)	9	7.94 (2.47, 40.22)	6	12.96 (4.76, 42.16)
≥100	2	15.88 (3.70, 64.67)	1	9.13 (1.55, 66.23)	0	0 (—)

[a]Reference category
[b]95 percent confidence interval for RR$_{M-H}$

As expected, these results are similar to both the SMR and SRR findings.

7. SUMMARY OF ADVANTAGES AND LIMITATIONS OF OCCUPATIONAL COHORT STUDIES

In this chapter we have described methods for assembling and following occupational cohorts and for making disease rate comparisons with external and internal reference populations. These comparisons permit evaluations of the cohort's overall disease experience and associations with various jobs, work areas, and exposures within the workplace. What may not be evident from the discussion is the scope of work required to conduct an occupational cohort study successfully. These studies typically involve the efforts of epidemiologists, industrial hygienists, statisticians, computer programmers, and clerical staff. The magnitude of the effort will depend on the size of the cohort studied and on the volume and complexity of the exposure data to be assimilated. For example, vital status tracing and cause-of-death ascertainment for a cohort of 5,000 workers are seldom completed in less than one year, and a thorough reconstruction of exposures and analysis of data might require another one to two years. These comments pertain primarily to historical cohort studies. Prospective cohort studies are usually substantially more expensive and time-consuming.

However, cohort studies do have particular advantages. First, by design, they include all or as many members of the occupational (dynamic) cohort as can be identified and traced. There is a statistical precision advantage to this approach, but more important, cohort studies offer the broadest available picture of the health experience of the workforce because rates for multiple health outcomes can be examined. More intensive investigations of exposure–response associations are best done for a selected subset of diseases of a priori interest and those discovered to occur at an excessive rate in the cohort.

The second, less obvious, advantage of cohort studies is that the process of enumerating a cohort makes the investigator aware of the particular characteristics of the workforce (e.g., the ethnic, gender, and social class groups most heavily represented and the subgroups of the cohort most completely traced). As we shall see in the following chapters, other study designs that include only samples of the cohort do not offer as complete a view of the entire worker population available for study. Finally, phenomena characteristic of occupational populations, such as bias resulting from the Healthy Worker Effect, are examined most directly in cohort studies.

Glossary

adjustment of rates   Summarizing stratum-specific rates into single (summary) estimates (e.g., standardized rates).

cohort   The study population to be followed.

dynamic cohort   A study population that includes workers who were hired, terminated, or died at variable points in time.

expected number   The number of cases or deaths that would have occurred in the study cohort had rates in the reference population prevailed.

external reference group   Comparison group of persons outside of the study cohort; usually the national or regional population.

fixed cohort   A study population that includes workers hired (or employed) only at a single point in time or during some specified brief time interval.

historical cohort study   Follow-up to the present of retrospectively enumerated study population.

internal reference group   Comparison group selected from within the study cohort, usually the person-time experience and rates of the non-exposed or least exposed workers.

person-years   Time unit of follow-up; denominator of disease rate; number of persons multiplied by associated durations of follow-up.

pooled rate ratio   Weighted average of stratum-specific rate ratios.

prospective cohort study   Follow-up into the future of cohort enumerated during the present.

rate   Number of newly occurring cases or deaths divided by the person-years of observation.

rate ratio   Ratio of rates in populations compared; usually an exposed group and a non-exposed reference group.

risk   The average probability of developing (or dying from) disease during some specified time interval.

reference population   Comparison population; usually assumed non-exposed.

standardized rate   Weighted average of stratum-specific rates, where the rates can be the person-time distribution of the exposed, reference, or some other population.

standardized rate ratio   Summary rate ratio, combined across strata of a confounder(s).

subcohort   Segment of the cohort, defined on the basis of age, year of hire, duration of employment, duration of follow-up, or exposure level.

Notation

a_i Number of exposed cases (deaths) in stratum i

b_i Number of non-exposed cases (deaths) in stratum i

N_{1i} Number of person-years in the exposed group in stratum i

N_{0i} Number of person-years in the non-exposed group in stratum i
M_i Total number of cases (deaths) in stratum i
T_i Total number of person-years in stratum i
SR   Standardized rate
RR_s General expression for standardized rate ratio estimator
SMR   Standardized mortality (morbidity) ratio
SRR   Standardized rate ratio
RR_{M-H} Mantel–Haenszel summary rate ratio
Obs   Total number of cases (deaths) in the exposed group
Exp   Total number of cases (deaths) expected in the exposed group
χ^2 Mantel–Haenszel chi-square statistic (1 degree of freedom)

References

Acheson ED, Gardner MJ, Winter PD, and Bennett C (1984): Cancer in a factory using amosite asbestos. *Int J Epidemiol* 13:3–10.

Armitage P (1971): *Statistical Methods in Medical Research*. London: Blackwell Scientific Publications. Oxford Press.

Axelson O (1985): Dealing with exposure variable in occupational health epidemiology. *Scand J Soc Med* 13:147–152.

Baker SP (1975): Determinants of injury and opportunities for intervention. *Am J Epidemiol* 101:98–102.

Bailar JC, and Ederer F (1964): Significance of variance to Poisson expectations. *Biometrics* 20:639–643.

Beaumont JJ, and Weiss NS (1980): Mortality of welders, shipfitters and other metal trades workers in Boilermakers Local No. 104, AFL-CIO. *Am J Epidemiol* 112:775–786.

Berry G (1983): The analysis of mortality by the subject-years method. *Biometrics* 39:173–184.

Breslow NE (1984): Recent developments in cohort analysis. In: Blot WJ, Hirayama T, and Hoel DG (eds), *Statistical Methods in Cancer Research*. Hiroshima, Japan: Radiation Effects Research Foundation, pp. 95–197.

Breslow NE, Lubin JH, Marek P, and Langholz B (1983): Multiplicative models and cohort analysis. *J Am Stat Assoc* 78:1–12.

Case RAM, and Lea AJ (1955): Mustard gas poisoning, chronic bronchitis and lung cancer. *Br J Prev Soc Med* 9:62–72.

Checkoway H, Mathew RM, Hickey JLS, et al. (1985a): Mortality among workers in the Florida phosphate industry. II. Cause-specific mortality relationships with work areas and exposures. *J Occup Med* 27:893–896.

Checkoway H, Mathew RM, Hickey JLS, et al. (1985b): Mortality among workers in the Florida phosphate industry. I. Industry-wide cause-specific mortality patterns. *J Occup Med* 27:885–892.

Checkoway H, Mathew RM, Shy CM, et al. (1985c): Radiation, work experience and cause-specific mortality among workers at an energy research laboratory. *Br J Ind Med* 42:525–533.

Chiazze L (1976): Problems of study design and interpretation of industrial mortality experience. *J Occup Med* 18:169–170.

Claude R, and Frentzel-Beyme R (1984): A mortality study of workers employed in a German rock wool factory. *Scand J Work Environ Health* 10:151–157.

Clayton DG (1982): The analysis of prospective studies of disease aetiology. *Commun Stat* 11:2129–2155.

Cohen EN, Brown BW, Wu M, et al. (1980): Occupational disease in dentistry and chronic exposure to trace anesthetic gases. *J Am Dent Assoc* 101:21–31.

Collins JF, and Redmond CK (1976): The use of retirees to evaluate occupational hazards. *J Occup Med* 18:595–602.

Copes R, Thomas D, and Becklake MR (1985): Temporal patterns of exposure and nonmalignant pulmonary abnormality in Quebec chrysotile workers. *Arch Environ Health* 40:80–87.

Delzell E, and Monson RR (1981): Mortality among rubber workers. IV. General mortality patterns. *J Occup Med* 23:850–856.

Dement JM, Harris RL, Symons MJ, and Shy CM (1983a): Exposures and mortality among chrysotile asbestos workers. Part I. Exposures. *Am J Ind Med* 4:409–420.

Dement JM, Harris RL, Symons MJ, and Shy CM (1983b): Exposures and mortality among chrysotile asbestos workers. Part II. Mortality. *Am J Ind Med* 4:421–433.

Doll R (1955): Mortality from lung cancer in asbestos workers. *Br J Ind Med* 12:81–86.

Ederer F, Axtell LM, and Cutler SJ (1961): The relative survival rate: a statement of methodology. *Natl Cancer Inst Monogr* 6:101–121.

Elandt-Johnson RC (1975): Definition of rates: some remarks on their use and misuse. *Am J Epidemiol* 102:267–271.

Enterline PE (1976): Pitfalls in epidemiologic research: an examination of the asbestos literature. *J Occup Med* 18:150–156.

Finkelstein M, Kusiak R, and Suranyi G (1981): Mortality among workers receiving compensation for asbestosis in Ontario. *Can Med Assoc J* 125:259–262.

Flanders WD (1984): Approximate variance formulas for standardized rate ratios. *J Chronic Dis* 37:449–453.

Fox AJ, and Goldblatt PO (1982): *Longitudinal Study: Socio-demographic Differential*. London: Office of Population Census Surveys.

Gaffey WR (1976): A critique of the standardized mortality ratio. *J Occup Med* 18:157–160.

Gardner MJ (1986): Considerations in the choice of expected numbers for appropriate comparisons in occupational cohort studies. *Med Lav* 77:23–47.

Gilbert ES (1982): Some confounding factors in the study of mortality and occupational exposure. *Am J Epidemiol* 116:177–188.

Gilbert ES, and Marks S (1979): An analysis of the mortality of workers in a nuclear facility. *Radiation Res* 79:122–148.

Greenland S (1982): Interpretation and estimation of summary ratios under heterogeneity. *Stat Med* 1:217–227.

Greenland S (1984): A counter example to the test-based principle of setting confidence limits. *Am J Epidemiol* 120:4–7.

Greenland S, and Robins JM (1985): Estimation of a common effect parameter from sparse follow-up data. *Biometrics* 41:55–68.

Gustafsson L, Wall S, Larsson LG, and Skog L (1986): Mortality and cancer incidence among Swedish dock workers—a retrospective cohort study. *Scand J Work Environ Health* 12:22–26.

Hernberg S, Partenen T, Nordman C-H, and Sumari P (1970): Coronary heart disease among workers exposed to carbon disulfide. *Br J Ind Med* 27:313–325.

Hill ID (1972): Computing man-years at risk. *Br J Prev Soc Med* 26:132–134.

Jarvholm B (1987): Comparing mortality in an occupational cohort with incidence rates of the general population—bias introduced through the use of five-year age intervals. *Am J Epidemiol* 125:747–749.

Johnson ES, Fischman HR, Matanoski GM, and Diamond E (1986): Cancer mortality among white males in the meat industry. *J Occup Med* 28:23–32.

Kleinbaum DG, Kupper LL, and Morgenstern H (1982): *Epidemiologic Research: Principles and Quantitative Methods*. Belmont, CA: Lifetime Learning Publications.

Last JM (1983): *A Dictionary of Epidemiology*. Oxford: Oxford University Press.

Lynge E (1985): A follow-up study of cancer incidence among workers in the manufacture of phenoxy herbicides in Denmark. *Br J Cancer* 52:259–270.

Mantel N, and Haenszel W (1959): Statistical aspects of the analysis of data from retrospective studies of disease. *J Natl Cancer Inst* 22:719–748.

Marsh GM, and Enterline PE (1979): A method for verifying the completeness of cohorts used in occupational mortality studies. *J Occup Med* 21:665–670.

Marsh GM, and Preininger M (1980): OCMAP: a user-oriented occupational mortality analysis program. *Am Stat* 34:245–246.

McDonald JC, Liddell FDK, Gibbs GW, et al. (1980): Dust exposure and mortality in chrysotile mining, 1910–1975. *Br J Ind Med* 37:11–24.

McMichael AJ, Andjelkovich DA, and Tyroler HA (1976): Cancer mortality among rubber workers. *Ann NY Acad Sci* 271:125–137.

Miettinen OS (1972): Standardization of risk ratios. *Am J Epidemiol* 96:383–388.

Miettinen OS (1977): Re: estimability and estimation in case-referent studies (letter). *Am J Epidemiol* 105:498–502.

Mietinnen OS (1985): *Theoretical Epidemiology: Principles of Occurrence Research*. New York: John Wiley & Sons.

Miettinen OS, and Wang J-D (1981): An alternative to the proportionate mortality ratio. *Am J Epidemiol* 114:144–148.

Monson RR (1974): Analysis of relative survival and proportional mortality. *Comput Biomed Res* 7:325–332.

Monson RR (1980): *Occupational Epidemiology*. Boca Raton, FL: CRC Press.

Monson RR (1986): Observations on the healthy worker effect. *J Occup Med* 28:425–433.

Newhouse ML, Berry G, and Wagner JC (1985): Mortality of factory workers in East London, 1933–80. *Br J Ind Med* 42:4–11.

Pearce N, Checkoway H, and Shy C (1986): Time-related factors as potential confounders and effect modifiers in studies based on an occupational cohort. *Scand J Work Environ Health* 12:97–107.

Riihimakii V, Asp S, and Hernberg S (1982): Mortality of 2,4-dichlorophenoxyacetic acid and 2,4,5-trichlorophenoxyacetic acid herbicide applicators in Finland: first report of an ongoing prospective cohort study. *Scand J Work Environ Health* 8:37–42.

Rothman KJ (1981): Induction and latent periods. *Am J Epidemiol* 114:253–259.

Rothman KJ (1986): *Modern Epidemiology*. Boston, MA: Little Brown & Co.

Rothman KJ, and Boice JD (1979): *Epidemiologic Analysis with a Programmable Calculator*. NIH Publication No. 79-1649, Washington, D.C.: U.S. Department of Health.

Saracci R (1986): Ten years of epidemiologic investigations on man-made mineral fibers and health. *Scand J Work Environ Health* 12(Suppl 1): 5–11.

Shore RE, Pasternack BS, and Curnen MG (1976): Relating influenza epidemics to childhood leukemia in tumor registries without a defined population base: a critique with suggestions for improved methods. *Am J Epidemiol* 103:527–535.

Steenland K, Stayner L, and Grief A (1987): Assessing the feasibility of retrospective cohort studies. *Am J Ind Med* 12:419–430.

Symons MJ, and Taulbee JD (1981): Practical considerations for approximating relative risk by the Standardized Mortality Ratio. *J Occup Med* 23:413–416.

Vena JE, Sultz HA, Carlo GL, et al. (1987): Sources of bias in retrospective cohort mortality studies: a note on treatment of subjects lost to follow-up. *J Occup Med* 29:256–261.

Waxweiler RJ (1979): Methodologic considerations in occupational cohort mortality studies. Paper presented at the Annual Meeting of the Society for Epidemiologic Research, New Haven, CT.

Waxweiler RJ, Stringer W, Wagoner JK, and Jones J (1976): Neoplastic risk among workers exposed to vinyl chloride. *Ann NY Acad Sci* 271:40–48.

Waxweiler RJ, Beaumont JJ, Henry JA, et al. (1983): A modified life-table analysis program system for cohort studies. *J Occup Med* 25:115–124.

Weill H, Hughes J, and Waggenspack C (1979): Influence of dose and fiber type on respiratory malignancy risk in asbestos cement manufacturing. *Am Rev Respir Dis* 120:345–354.

Weiss W (1983): Heterogeneity in historical cohort studies: a source of bias in assessing lung cancer risk. *J Occup Med* 25:737–470.

Westerholm P (1980): Silicosis—observation on a case register. *Scand J Work Environ Health* 6(Suppl 2):1–86.

Wong O (1977): Further criticism of epidemiological methodology in occupational studies. *J Occup Med* 19:220–222.

World Health Organization (1967): *Manual of the International Statistical Classification of Diseases: Injuries and Causes of Death,* 8th revision. Geneva: World Health Organization.

Young JL, Percy CL, and Asire AJ (eds) (1981): *Surveillance, Epidemiology and End Results: Incidence and Mortality Data, 1973–77.* National Cancer Institute Monograph 57, NIH Publication No. 81-2330, Washington, D.C.

Yule GU (1934): On some points relating to vital statistics, more especially statistics of occupational mortality. *J R Stat Soc* 97:1–72.

Zack JA, and Suskind R (1980): The mortality experience of workers exposed to tetrachlorodibenzodioxin in a trichlorophenol process accident. *J Occup Med* 22:11–14.

6 Case–Control Studies

1. OVERVIEW

In Chapter 3 we argued that every occupational epidemiology study is based on the experience of a particular population as it moves over time. This population has been termed the *base population* and its experience over time, the *study base,* although both concepts are often loosely referred to as the *cohort.* The only conceptual difference between a full cohort study and a case–control study based on the same cohort is that the latter involves a sample of the study base rather than an analysis of the entire study base. There is usually little loss of precision in a case–control study compared to a full cohort study. Moreover, case–control studies offer considerable savings in time and expense. The case–control approach is particularly valuable if the study disease is rare or has a long induction time.

A second situation in which the case–control approach may be indicated is when an occupational cohort is difficult to enumerate (e.g., farmers). In this instance, a case–control study may be based on cases from a particular hospital, death registry, cancer registry, or other disease registry that serves a stable population. Registry-based occupational case–control studies will not be examined in depth because the general principles are the same as for other registry-based case–control studies, and these have been covered in several well-known texts (e.g., Schlesselman, 1982). Instead, the discussion will focus on case–control studies based on defined occupational cohorts.

In the following section, the basic case–control study design is presented. Issues in the selection of cases and controls are then examined, including sampling strategies, matching, sources of controls, and avoidance of bias. Sources and classification of exposure data are then discussed briefly. Methods for analyzing case–control data are then presented; these include overall (crude) analysis, stratified analysis, matched analysis, and analyses considering multiple exposure levels. (A discussion of mathematical modeling is deferred

170

until Chapter 8.) Examples from the published literature are used to illustrate issues of design and analysis. In particular, a case–control study nested in the cohort study of mortality among asbestos textile manufacturing workers, conducted by Dement et al. (1983), is discussed in some detail. Finally, the advantages and limitations of the case–control design are summarized.

2. BASIC STUDY DESIGN

A *cohort-based study,* often termed a *nested* case–control study, requires definition and enumeration of the cohort and its experience over time (see Chapter 5). The case group consists of all incident cases generated by the cohort or study base. Prevalent cases are rarely used because their inclusion may introduce bias due to differential prognosis. One exception is the study of congenital malformations, where the case group consists of cases discovered at birth (i.e., prevalent cases).

In a disease *registry-based study,* cases may be drawn from one or more registries (e.g., hospital records). Thus, the distinguishing feature of a registry-based study is that the case group is defined first; the tasks are then to ascertain the study base that generated the cases and to sample controls from this study base. By contrast, in a cohort-based study the study base is defined first.

Although case–control studies usually include one case group and one control group, there are at least two common departures from this situation. First, for purposes of efficiency, two or more case groups may be selected simultaneously, and both compared to a common control group. More frequently, more than one control group may be chosen for a single case group if each of several available control groups has different specific deficiencies, but none is clearly superior.

The purpose of selecting a control group is to estimate the "expected" exposure history of the study base that generated the cases. One obvious source of controls is a random sample of the study base, but the sample may be restricted to a subset that is more easily enumerable (if the entire study base is difficult to enumerate) or that is likely to yield exposure or confounder information more comparable with that obtained for the cases.

Table 6–1 shows the basic data layout for a single stratum of a case–control study, and Table 6–2 gives an example from a case–control study of cancer of the nasal cavity and paranasal sinuses and

Table 6–1. Data layout for a single stratum (i) of case–control study data

	Exposed	Non-exposed	Total
Cases	a_i	b_i	M_{1i}
Controls	c_i	d_i	M_{0i}
Total	N_{1i}	N_{0i}	T_i

formaldehyde exposure conducted by Hayes et al. (1986). The effect measure in case–control studies is the *odds ratio*, which estimates the risk ratio or rate ratio, depending on the method of control selection. From Table 6–2 we can see that the odds of a case being exposed are $31/60$ (= a/b), whereas the odds of a control being exposed are $34/161$ (= c/d). The exposure odds ratio is this $(31 \times 161)/(60 \times 34)$ (= ad/bc), or 2.45.

3. SELECTION OF CASES

In a cohort-based study, the first step in the selection of cases is to attempt to ascertain all cases generated by the cohort. Complete case ascertainment may not be achieved; however, the relative risk estimate (odds ratio) will not be biased by incomplete ascertainment. Bias may arise, for example, if heavily exposed workers receive more medical screening, and hence are more likely to have nonfatal diseases diagnosed (e.g., ischemic heart disease). Such bias is less likely to occur in mortality studies. Many occupational cohort studies are confined to mortality data; therefore, it may be necessary to use additional data sources if living cases are to be included.

Table 6–2. Exposure of cases and controls in a study of nasal cancer and formaldehyde exposure

	Exposed	Non-exposed	Total
Cases	31	60	91
Controls	34	161	195
Total	65	221	286

Source: Hayes et al. (1986).

Example 6.1

In a case–control study of bladder cancer in the U.S. rubber and tire industry (Checkoway et al., 1981), cases of bladder cancer were identified from two sources. The first source was death certificates obtained for the cohort mortality study (which covered the period 1964–73) on which the case–control study was based. The second was hospital records for all bladder cancers newly diagnosed during the period 1958–74 in the four major area hospitals. Cases among rubber industry workers were identified by cross-checking the hospital record listings against the lists of employees of the five companies included in the cohort.

In a registry-based study, the case group usually consists of all incident cases appearing in the registry during a specified period of time (usually no more than a few years). The case group ultimately can be restricted to particular age, gender, or ethnic groups, or with respect to other characteristics. Such restriction can be applied to improve information quality, to control confounding, or to facilitate the valid selection of controls. The "registry" could consist of a formal population-based registry, which incorporates all cases of a particular disease grouping such as cancer, heart disease, congenital malformations, or pneumoconiosis. Alternatively, cases might be drawn from an ad hoc registry based on records collected for other purposes, such as hospital admissions records, insurance claims, or disability pension records.

Example 6.2

In a case–control study of neuropsychiatric disorders among Swedish workers exposed to solvents (Axelson et al., 1976), a regional pension fund register was used as the source of subjects for the study. The Swedish social security system provides a disability pension to all disabled persons. Medical data including diagnoses are available through the register, as are data on years of employment in various occupations. In this study, all individuals considered for a disability pension because of some type of mental disorder were selected as cases. Patients with schizophrenia, manic-depressive psychosis of the circular type, and mental disease of obvious somatic origin (e.g., dementia from a traumatic brain injury, encephalitis) were excluded from the case group. The investigators found an odds ratio of 1.8 for nonspecific psychiatric disorders among workers exposed to solvents.

Diagnostic criteria are important in the selection of cases because the inclusion into the case group of diseases that are unrelated to the etiologic factor of interest will bias the odds ratio estimate toward the null value of 1.0. The added efficiency of case–control studies (relative to cohort studies) may permit the collection of additional diagnostic data. The validation of diagnostic data is especially important if some subtypes of a disease are more strongly related than others to the exposures under study. The goal should be to define a disease that is a homogeneous etiologic entity.

Example 6.3

Kauppinen et al. (1986) conducted a case–control study of respiratory cancer and chemical exposures nested within a cohort of 3,805 men who had worked for at least one year in the wood products industry. They requested histologic or cytologic specimens for the 57 cases from hospitals and laboratories, and these were evaluated by one pathologist. Necropsy and hospital protocols were studied for the 11 cases lacking histologic or cytologic samples. Two cases were rejected because of false preliminary diagnoses of cancer, and one was rejected as having chronic lymphocytic leukemia. This example illustrates that the detection of false positive cases is relatively straightforward. However, confirmation of the absence of disease in presumed noncases is usually more difficult; in this example, this would have required additional surveillance of all 3,748 "noncases" in the cohort.

---

4. SELECTION OF CONTROLS

4.1. Sampling Strategies

There are two main approaches to the selection of controls: cumulative incidence sampling and incidence density sampling.

Cumulative incidence sampling involves selecting controls from those free of the disease of interest at the end of the study period. For example, in the study by Arp et al. (1983) of lymphocytic leukemia and exposures to benzene and other solvents in the rubber industry, controls were selected from all members of the cohort who did not die from lymphocytic leukemia during the mortality follow-up period.

Figure 6–1 depicts a hypothetical cohort of eight initially disease-free persons followed for a period of 35 years. A case–control study of cancer involving cumulative incidence control sampling would include subject A as a case, and controls would be selected from the seven persons who did not develop cancer. If the study disease is rare, this procedure produces an odds ratio estimate approximately equal to the risk ratio. The deviation from the risk ratio only becomes substantial (greater than 10 percent) when the cumulative incidence over the study period is greater than 10 percent (Greenland and Thomas, 1982).

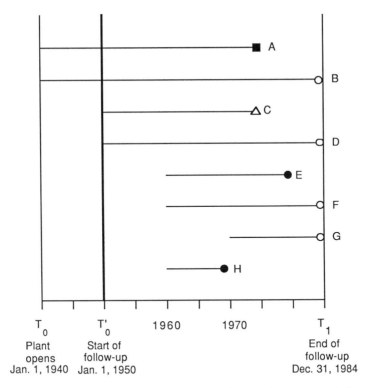

Figure 6–1. Hypothetical cohort of eight initially disease-free persons followed for 35 years (■ = cancer death, ● = other death, △ = lost to follow-up, o = alive at end of follow-up).

In the past (e.g., Arp et al., 1983), controls frequently have been sampled from persons free of the study disease at the *end* of the study period. However, Kupper et al. (1975) and Miettinen (1982) have pointed out that controls should be selected from persons free of the study disease at the *beginning* of the study period (this is usually the entire cohort), because such a sample correctly estimates the risk ratio without the need for a rare disease assumption. A sample of the entire cohort has the added advantage that it can provide controls for several simultaneous case–control studies of different diseases (Kupper et al., 1975). This approach has also been referred to as a "case–cohort" design (Prentice, 1986).

Example 6.4

Table 6–3 illustrates a hypothetical study of a cohort of 5,000 persons followed for one year. One fifth of the cohort is exposed to the risk factor of interest, and this subcohort has a doubled risk for the outcome under study. The cohort is distributed in the ratio of 1:4 between the exposed and non-exposed subcohorts. If random error is absent, a sample of the cohort (i.e., all persons free of disease at the beginning of follow-up) will equal this ratio and thus yield a correct crude risk ratio estimate of 2.00 (= (20/40)/(1000/4000)). The more traditional approach, with a rare disease assumption, is to exclude those persons who developed the disease of interest (i.e, to sample only from among persons free of disease at the end of follow-up). This produces a risk ratio estimate of 2.02 (= (20/40)/(980/3960)). The bias resulting from cumulative incidence sampling is small in this example, but a more severe bias would occur in a study of a less rare disease.

Despite its popularity, cumulative incidence sampling has a number of limitations. These are particularly pronounced in case–control studies based on dynamic cohorts, because persons may commence employment (i.e., enter the cohort) at any time during the follow-up period, and their follow-up may be terminated by deaths from other causes or from losses to follow-up. One solution is to stratify on length of follow-up and to carry out cumulative incidence sampling within each stratum. Alternatively, for each case, or group of cases, the set from which controls are sampled can be restricted to subjects who have been followed for at least as long as the case(s). For example, in Example 6.3 (Kauppinen et al., 1986), controls were matched to each case on birth year and were further required to have been alive and free from respiratory cancer at the date of diagnosis of the corresponding case. Ideally, the exposure history of each control should only be considered up to the time at which the corresponding case became a case. This modified cumulative incidence sampling is very similar to incidence density sampling described in the following discussion, but it is more cumbersome to perform.

Incidence density sampling involves selecting controls from the person-time experience that generated the cases (i.e., the study base). This usually involves selecting controls from the set of persons "at risk" at the time of onset of each case (known as the *risk set*). In a cohort-based study, incidence density sampling involves considering each case in turn, and selecting one or more controls from the set of persons who were at risk at the time that the individual was identified as a case. In clinical trials, *time* is defined as follow-up time. In cohort studies it is more appropriate to use age at risk as the time dimension (Breslow et al., 1983) because age is a strong risk factor for many diseases, and age effects should be controlled as precisely as possible (although matching can, in theory, be done on any time-related factor).

To illustrate, consider a worker who died from lung cancer at age 64 years. One or more controls would be selected from the group of all persons who were "at risk" (by being alive and members of the cohort) at age 64. This "at-risk" group thus comprises all persons who entered the cohort (started work) before age 64 and lived to at least age 64. The cumulative exposures of the controls, and their status for various confounding factors, would be evaluated at age 64, rather than at the ages they subsequently attained. Suppose, for purposes of illustration, that all eight workers depicted in Figure 6–1 were the same age at time t'_0 (1/1/50). Then controls for case A would be sampled without replacement from the set of six other persons (all except H) who were at risk (i.e., members of the cohort and free from the disease under study) at the time that A became a case. Each control's exposure should only be considered up to the time at which the corresponding case became a case. The risk set that is sampled thus may include some persons who subsequently became cases (Lubin and Gail, 1984).

Incidence density sampling can be regarded as a straightforward extension of the person-time approach used in cohort studies. For example, in a cohort study, if one person died at age 64 and 863 persons were "at risk" at age 64, then the incidence rate at age 64 would be 1 per 863 person-years. Note that the denominator may include persons who also developed the disease of interest at some later time. A case–control study with incidence density sampling essentially involves using all the numerator data (cases) and sampling from the denominator data. Incidence density sampling thus permits the estimation of the incidence rate ratio without the need for a rare disease assumption (Miettinen, 1976). Furthermore, it also estimates the risk ratio more validly than cumulative incidence sampling (Greenland and Thomas, 1982).

It should be noted that almost all registry-based studies inherently use incidence density sampling. This is because cases are usually drawn from disease registrations for a relatively short time period, and controls are drawn from the source population of the registry during the same time period. In other words, controls are selected from among persons "at risk" of developing the study disease and appearing in the registry at the times (usually in the same year) when the cases occurred. Control selection thus inherently involves incidence density matching on calendar year; matching on other factors, such as age, is also conducted in an incidence density framework.

4.2. Matching

Matching involves pairing one or more controls to each case, or a group of controls to a group of cases, with respect to one or more potential confounding factors. In incidence density sampling, controls are automatically matched to cases on the basis of some time variable, such as age at risk. However, matching may also be carried out with respect to other factors by restricting the sampled "risk set" to potential controls with the same status on the matching factor as the case. In cumulative incidence sampling, matching may be carried out by restricting potential controls to specific categories of various factors, such as age at risk, gender, ethnicity, age at hire, length of follow-up, year of birth, or year of entry into the cohort. However, each additional matching factor makes it more difficult to achieve good matches.

Example 6.5

Karasek et al. (1981) conducted a case–control study of job decision latitude, job demands, and cardiovascular disease, nested within a prospective cohort study of employed Swedish males. Each case of cardiovascular disease was identified from the death certificate and matched as closely as possible with three controls with respect to age (± 2 years), tobacco smoking habit (± 5 cigarettes per day), education, and self-reported symptoms of cardiovascular disease at the start of follow-up. They found that low decision latitude (expressed as low intellectual discretion and low personal schedule freedom) was associated with increased risk of cardiovascular disease, particularly in persons with the minimum statutory education (OR = 6.6).

There are two potential advantages of matching: practical efficiency and statistical efficiency. First, matching may be done for practical efficiency. For example, when cases are identified from hospital admission records, it may be more convenient to choose as controls patients admitted on the same days as the cases, rather than developing a roster of all patients and taking a random sample. Second, matching may be done for statistical efficiency to ensure similar distributions of confounding factors in cases and controls. For example, if most of the cases are "old" and most of the controls are "young," then fine stratification on age may result in very few controls in the older age strata and very few cases in the younger age strata. This does not bias the adjusted odds ratio, but it decreases its precision: The odds ratio estimate is less stable, and its confidence limits may be relatively wide. Hence, it may be desirable to ensure that good confounder overlap is achieved by some form of matching.

Several potential problems are associated with matching in case–control studies. First, the association of disease with the matching factor is distorted and cannot be estimated validly. Second, in case–control studies a matching factor may still be a confounder unless it is controlled in the analysis. A related problem occurs when matching is performed on a nonconfounder, particularly on a correlate of exposure that is not an independent risk factor for the disease in question. The matching process effectively turns such a factor into a confounder, which must then be controlled in the analysis, thus reducing precision and increasing analytical complexity. For example, in a case–control study of radiation doses and leukemia among nuclear industry workers, matching on work area in the plant would be counterproductive if work area and radiation exposure were associated but work area was not an independent risk factor for leukemia.

Finally, matching may be expensive and time-consuming. Finding suitable controls becomes increasingly difficult as the number of matching factors increases beyond two or three. Furthermore, the increase in precision from matching is generally modest, typically involving a 5- to 15-percent reduction in the variance of the effect estimate (Schlesselman, 1982). Therefore, although most discussions of matching stress issues of statistical efficiency, practical considerations are usually more important.

4.3. Sources of Controls

The most obvious control selection procedure involves sampling from the entire study base. There are, however, two situations where it may be desirable to restrict the sample to a subset of the study base. The first occurs in both cohort-based and registry-based studies when it is thought that controls selected from a particular subset of the study base are most likely to give exposure information comparable to that obtained for the cases. The second occurs in a registry-based study when it is not possible to identify explicitly the source population for the registry (e.g., if cases are drawn from records of an urban referral hospital with no clearly defined catchment area). Both situations usually necessitate selecting controls from among persons with other diseases who appeared in the same registry (or were generated by the same cohort) during the same time period. This selection method generally improves comparability of information between cases and controls and, unless the exposure also causes some of the control diseases, identifies a control group that reflects the exposure history of the source population for the cases.

One special instance of selecting controls from among other disease registrants occurs when controls are sampled from among other deaths in a mortality study. This approach is valid when the exposure experience of the other deaths is representative of the entire at-risk population (the study base), that is, when the study exposure does not cause mortality excesses (or deficits) from other diseases. This procedure is commonly used in studies based on national or state death registries (e.g., Blair and Thomas, 1979), but it can also be used in cohort-based case–control studies in which controls are sampled from other deaths in the cohort or from national or state death registries. This approach is related to the proportionate mortality ratio (PMR) method (Chapter 3), where the proportion of deaths from a particular disease in the exposed population is compared to that expected on the basis of a non-exposed population (Miettinen and Wang, 1981).

4.4. Issues in Control Selection

When control selection involves sampling from the entire cohort, *selection bias* is a minor concern, although selection bias may still occur if the strength of the Health Worker Effect differs according to exposure level. When controls are selected from among persons with other diseases, considerable care must be taken in specifying the diseases that form the control group. In particular, a specific disease may not correctly reflect the exposure pattern in the study base, especially if it is caused by the study exposure. One approach is to include only diseases that are thought to be unrelated to exposure (Miettinen, 1985), but this requirement may be difficult to satisfy in practice because adequate evidence for the absence of exposure effects on many diseases is frequently not available (Axelson et al., 1982). An alternative approach is to select as controls a sample of all other diseases. This approach is generally more reliable because there are few factors that markedly increase risks of numerous diverse diseases. It has become common practice to exclude diseases known to be related to exposure from the pool of potential controls; however, even this restriction does not always eliminate bias (Pearce and Checkoway, 1988).

Example 6.6

Pearce et al. (1986) conducted a case–control study of non-Hodgkin's lymphoma and exposure to agricultural chemicals in New Zealand. Interviews were conducted with 83 male cases of non-Hodgkin's lymphoma or their next of kin. The cases were identified from the New Zealand Cancer Registry during the period 1977–81. Controls were selected from among other male cancer patients registered during the same period and were matched on age (± 2 years) and year of registration. However, there was concern that selection bias could occur if other cancers were caused by agricultural chemicals. It was not possible to assess this selection bias directly. Nonetheless, it was possible to assess selection bias with regard to employment in farming, which is a surrogate for agricultural chemical exposure. The occupational distribution of the other cancer controls was compared with that expected on the basis of national census data, and the number of farmers in the control group was found to be very close to that expected (Smith et al., 1988). Furthermore, the overall cancer mortality rate in New Zealand farmers was found to be close to that for all employed persons (Pearce and Howard, 1986). These two findings suggested that using the other cancer patients as controls was unlikely to have created selection bias with respect to employment in farming. Therefore, this approach was also unlikely to have created selection bias with regard to agricultural chemical exposure. Further evidence for an absence of serious selection bias was provided by comparison with an additional control group chosen from the general population that yielded very similar findings to the comparison with other cancer controls.

In some cohort-based studies, and most registry-based studies, information about exposure, or about potential confounders such as cigarette smoking, is obtained retrospectively by interviewing cases and controls, or their relatives. In this situation there is potential for information bias to occur. In particular, it has been argued that *recall bias* may occur because patients with chronic diseases (or their relatives) may ponder about the possible causes of their disease and therefore may be more likely to recall some past exposures than healthy controls. Furthermore, *interviewer bias* may occur if interviewers are aware of subjects' health status. However, there is little evidence that such bias has occurred frequently in occupational epidemiology (Axelson, 1985). Cohort-based studies ordinarily rely on routinely tabulated records (e.g., personnel records) rather than personal interviews. Hence, recall bias and interviewer bias are often not relevant, although nondifferential information bias due to inaccuracies in available records may still be of concern.

Example 6.7

Consider a cohort-based case–control study of leukemia and exposure to benzene, in which exposure classification was based on the areas of the plant in which workers were assigned. If personnel records contain detailed work history information for all employees, then the selection of a control group is relatively straightforward. The most obvious strategy would be to sample from the entire study base, preferably using incidence density sampling. Comparability of information would not be of concern in this instance because all exposure information was collected prospectively.

If a registry-based study were conducted or if appropriate records were not available in a cohort-based study, then it might be necessary to interview cases and controls (or proxy respondents) to ascertain past exposures to benzene. In this situation, there might be concerns regarding the comparability of information between the cases and controls, particularly if a larger proportion of cases than controls were dead. One strategy would involve choosing separate control groups of living and dead controls. A sample of the entire study base (in a cohort-based study) would also yield a mix of living and dead controls, although the number of dead controls might be too small for a separate analysis. When separate analyses by vital status are possible, it is not clear which findings to accept if comparisons with the living and dead controls give different results. On the other hand, if it were known that benzene had a minimal effect on overall cancer mortality, then there would be considerable advantages to selecting a single control group of persons who had developed other forms of cancer. This approach should provide the best comparability of information between cases and controls, particularly since similar proportions of cases and controls would be deceased.

It is important to attempt to validate the classification of exposure, such as by comparing interview results with other data sources, such as employer records, or by assessing interrater agreement (Goldberg et al., 1986). Alternatively, recall bias may be assessed by comparing the main exposure findings with those of other exposures for which recall bias is equally likely but which are apparently not risk factors for the study disease.

Example 6.8

Selevan et al. (1985) conducted a case–control study of occupational exposures to antineoplastic drugs and fetal loss in nurses employed in 17 Finnish hospitals. The pregnancies occurred during the period 1973–80. Each nurse with a fetal loss was matched with three nurses who gave birth. The odds ratio for occupational exposure to antineoplastic drugs during the first trimester of pregnancy was 2.30. The authors commented that "if the outcome of pregnancy produced a bias in recall of pregnancy-related exposures . . . an elevated odds ratio would be expected for anesthetic gases, since several reports have linked this exposure to fetal loss." In this study the odds ratio for anesthetic gases was 0.96; thus, they concluded that recall bias was probably minor.

---

5. EXPOSURE DATA

Exposure data will be considered only briefly, as the key issues have been discussed in Chapters 2 and 5, and more complex analyses of exposure effects will be discussed in Chapter 9. In a cohort-based study, the types and sources of exposure data are identical to those that would have been used for a full cohort analysis (e.g., Example 6.7). Registry-based studies most commonly use personal interviews regarding occupational history (e.g., Example 6.6), although studies may also be based solely on registry records if these contain occupational information.

The classification of exposure data is conceptually identical to that in cohort studies. Each case is classified exactly as it would have been in a full cohort analysis. With incidence density matching, controls are selected from the set of all persons "at risk" at the age at which the case occurred. A control's exposure is only considered up to the age when the corresponding case occurred, and all subsequent exposure history is ignored. Thus, controls are classified into the same cumulative exposure and confounder categories as the relevant person-year would have been in a cohort analysis.

As in a cohort study, cohort-based studies may involve job category analyses. Once again, the simplest approach is to carry out separate analyses for each job category in which cases and controls are classified as to whether they have "ever" or "never" worked in a particular job category. Duration of employment in each job category may also be considered. Further refinements include assigning ordinal rankings of job categories and adjusting job category-specific effect estimates for employment in other job categories.

Registry-based studies usually involve less detailed exposure data than cohort-based studies. Often subjects are classified only according to whether they have ever worked in a particular industry, or according to duration of employment in an industry. When a particular exposure is of primary concern, detailed questioning may permit more valid exposure assessment, and the classification of subjects according to factors such as number of days exposure per year and duration of exposure (Hoar et al., 1986). Job–exposure matrices may be used for screening multiple exposures. In its simplest form, a job–exposure matrix is a table with occupational categories on one axis and exposures on the other. Occupations involving exposures to a particular substance can then be grouped. This approach can be used both in studies based on routinely collected occupational information (Coggon et al., 1984) and personal interviews (Hoar et al., 1980). A recent refinement has been the use of intensive "detective work" by chemists and hygienists to translate a job history into a set of potential exposures (Gerin et al., 1985).

Example 6.9

Siemiatycki et al. (1986) undertook a multi–cancer site, case–control study to screen hypotheses about possible associations between numerous occupational exposures and various cancer sites. For each cancer site, controls were selected from among the other cancer sites in the study. Detailed lifetime job histories were obtained from subjects by personal interview. A team of chemists and hygienists then considered the details and idiosyncrasies of each job description and assigned exposure ratings in accordance with all the available information. Several associations emerged: wood dust and lung cancer (OR = 1.5), wood dust and stomach cancer (OR = 1.5), synthetic fibers and colorectal cancer (OR = 1.8), synthetic fibers and bladder cancer (OR = 1.8), cotton dust and non-Hodgkin's lymphoma (OR = 1.9), grain dust and colon cancer (OR = 2.6), grain dust and prostate cancer (OR = 2.2), and paper dust and prostate cancer (OR = 2.0).

For both cohort-based and registry-based studies, latency analyses are conceptually identical to those in cohort studies. For example, an analysis based on a latency interval assumption of ten years involves ignoring exposures within the most recent ten years when calculating exposures of cases and controls. This corresponds to lagging the exposure data by ten years in a cohort study (see Chapter 5).

6. ANALYSIS

In this section we describe the basic methods of analysis of occupational case–control data. More comprehensive reviews are given by Breslow and Day (1980), Kleinbaum et al. (1982), and Rothman (1986). First, the standard analytic methods are outlined for a single stratum. The discussion is then extended to the control of confounding with stratified analysis and the analysis of multiple exposure levels.

6.1. Crude Analysis

The basic effect measure in a case–control study is the *odds ratio* (OR). In the one-stratum case this is

$$OR = \frac{a/b}{c/d} = \frac{ad}{bc} \tag{6.1}$$

The Mantel–Haenszel chi-square (Mantel and Haenszel, 1959) tests the null hypothesis that the odds ratio is equal to unity and takes the form

$$\chi^2_{\text{M-H}} = \frac{[a - E_0(A)]^2}{\text{Var}_0(A)} \tag{6.2}$$

where a = observed number of exposed cases

$E_0(A) = \dfrac{N_1 M_1}{T}$ = the expected number of exposed cases, assuming there is no association between exposure and disease

$\text{Var}_0(A) = \dfrac{N_1 N_0 M_1 M_0}{T^2(T-1)}$ = the variance of the number of exposed cases, assuming there is no association between exposure and disease

Miettinen's (1976) test-based method can be used to calculate a confidence interval for the Mantel–Haenszel odds ratio:

$$\underline{\text{OR}}, \overline{\text{OR}} = \text{OR}^{(1 \pm Z/\sqrt{\chi^2})} \tag{6.3}$$

where Z is the appropriate standard normal deviate (e.g., $Z = 1.96$ for 95-percent limits), and χ^2 is the Mantel–Haenszel chi-square. The advantages and limitations of the test-based method (Miettinen, 1977; Greenland, 1984; Rothman, 1986) have been discussed in Chapter 5.

An alternative approach is to calculate a direct estimate of the variance of the log odds ratio (which is approximately normally distributed in large samples). In the one-stratum case the variance of ln(OR) is approximately (Woolf, 1955):

$$\text{Var}[\ln(\text{OR})] \simeq \frac{1}{a} + \frac{1}{b} + \frac{1}{c} + \frac{1}{d} \tag{6.4}$$

The square root of the variance is the standard deviation (SD), and this yields (logit) confidence limits of

$$\exp\left[\ln(\text{OR}) \pm Z\sqrt{\text{Var}[\ln(\text{OR})]} \right] \tag{6.5}$$

Example 6.10

Consider the data given in Table 6–2 for a case–control study of cancer of the nasal cavity and paranasal sinuses and formaldehyde exposure in which 31 of 91 cases and 34 of 195 controls were exposed. The odds ratio is

$$\text{OR} = \frac{31 \times 161}{60 \times 34} = 2.45$$

$E_0(A) = 20.68$ and $\text{Var}_0(A) = 10.93$, and the Mantel–Haenszel chi-square [equation (6.2)] is

$$\chi^2_{\text{M-H}} = \frac{[31 - 20.68]^2}{10.93} = 9.74$$

The square root of the Mantel–Haenszel chi-square is 3.12; thus, the test-based 95-percent confidence interval for the odds ratio is

$$\underline{OR}, \overline{OR} = 2.45^{(1 \pm 1.96/3.12)} = 1.40, 4.30$$

Alternatively, $\ln(OR) = 0.896$, $SD(\ln(OR)) = 0.291$ [from formula (6.4)], and the 95-percent logit confidence interval is

$$\underline{OR}, \overline{OR} = \exp [0.896 \pm 1.96 \times 0.291] = 1.39, 4.33$$

6.2. Stratified Analysis

The control of confounding involves the assembly of a separate table for each level of the confounder, or for each combination of levels if more than one confounder is being controlled. Table 6–1 denotes this situation by attaching the subscript i to each entry in the table [i.e., the table represents just one stratum of the confounder(s)].

Separate odds ratios can be calculated for each stratum, but it is usually also desirable to calculate a summary odds ratio. The most commonly used method is that of Mantel and Haenszel (1959):

$$OR_{M-H} = \frac{\Sigma a_i d_i / T_i}{\Sigma b_i c_i / T_i} \tag{6.6}$$

Expression (6.5) corresponds to a weighted average of the stratum-specific odds ratio estimates, with weights of $b_i c_i / T_i$ in each stratum. [A minor modification of the weights is necessary when analyzing a so-called case–cohort study (Greenland, 1986).] The Mantel–Haenszel method gives consistent estimates of the odds ratio, even when many strata contain small numbers. Also, it can be used without modification when there are zero frequencies within the body of some stratum-specific tables, provided that the marginal totals are nonzero.

A related method for summary odds ratio estimation is the precision weighting approach. This involves calculating a weighted

Table 6–3. Number of hospitalized cases during a one-year period for a hypothetical cohort

Disease outcome	Exposed population	Non-exposed population	Total
Cases	20	40	60
Noncases	980	3,960	4,940
Total	1,000	4,000	5,000

average of the stratum-specific odds ratios, using the inverses of their variances as weights (Kleinbaum et al., 1982). However, precision weighting may yield unstable estimates when there are small numbers in some strata and yields similar estimates to the Mantel–Haenszel estimator when numbers are large.

The stratified form of the Mantel–Haenszel statistic is

$$\chi^2 = \frac{[a - E_0(A)]^2}{\mathrm{Var}_0(A)} \tag{6.7}$$

where $a = \Sigma a_i$
$E_0(A) = \Sigma N_{1i} M_{1i}/T_i$
$\mathrm{Var}_0(A) = \Sigma[(N_{1i} N_{0i} M_{1i} M_{0i})/(T_i^2)(T_i - 1)]$

Miettinen's test-based method [equation (6.3)] can be used to calculate approximate confidence limits for the adjusted odds ratio using the summary Mantel–Haenszel chi square. Direct calculation of a variance estimate for the log of the Mantel–Haenszel odds ratio is relatively complex with stratified data. Many estimators have been proposed, but the one that is easiest to compute without compromising validity (in large samples) is that proposed by Robins et al. (1986):

$$\mathrm{Var}[\ln(OR_{\mathrm{M-H}})] = \frac{\Sigma PR}{2R_+^2} + \frac{\Sigma(PS + QR)}{2R_+ S_+} + \frac{\Sigma QS}{2S_+^2} \tag{6.8}$$

where $P = (a_i + d_i)/T_i$; $Q = (b_i + c_i)/T_i$; $R = a_i d_i/T_i$; $S = b_i c_i/T_i$; $R_+ = \Sigma R$; and $S_+ = \Sigma S$. In the one-stratum case this reduces to equation (6.4).

Example 6.11

Table 6–4 shows data from a study of cancer of the nasal cavity and paranasal sinuses and formaldehyde exposures (Hayes et al., 1986), stratified on the con-

Table 6–4. Exposures of cases and controls in a study of nasal cancer and formaldehyde exposure

Exposure	Exposed	Non-exposed	Total
Low wood dust exposure			
Cases	15	48	63
Noncases	18	143	161
Total	33	191	224
High wood dust exposure			
Cases	16	12	28
Noncases	16	18	34
Total	32	30	62

Source: Hayes et al. (1986).

founding factor of wood dust exposure. The overall Mantel–Haenszel odds ratio, adjusted for wood dust exposure, is

$$OR_{M-H} = \frac{(15 \times 143/224) + (16 \times 18/62)}{(48 \times 18/224) + (12 \times 16/62)} = 2.05$$

and the Mantel–Haenszel chi-square is

$$\chi^2_{M-H} = \frac{[31 - 23.71]^2}{9.61} = 5.50$$

The square root of 5.50 is 2.35, and the test-based 95-percent confidence interval is thus

$$OR, \overline{OR} = 2.05^{(1 \pm 1.96/2.35)} = 1.13, 3.73$$

Using formula (6.7) for the variance of the log of the odds ratio yields

$$Var\,[(\ln\,(OR)] = \frac{4.575}{2 \times 7.524^2} + \frac{4.416 + 2.949}{2 \times 7.524 \times 6.954} + \frac{2.538}{2 \times 6.954^2}$$
$$= 0.137$$

which has a square root of 0.370. The log of the odds ratio is 0.718, thus yielding 95-percent confidence limits of

$$OR, \overline{OR} = \exp\,[0.718 \pm 1.96 \times 0.370] = 0.99, 4.23$$

6.3. Matched Analysis

As outlined earlier, matching on a confounder in a case–control study does not ensure control of confounding; it merely ensures similar distributions of the confounders for cases and controls. If matching has only been done on factors such as age and gender, then confounding can be controlled with a broadly stratified analysis. A broadly stratified analysis is easier to conduct, and generally is more efficient statistically, than an individually matched analysis. However, an individually matched analysis will be necessary if genuine "matched sets" exist. In the latter instance, each case and corresponding matched control(s) comprise a single stratum. The Mantel–Haenszel procedure for odds ratio estimation can be used in both situations.

Table 6–5 shows the notation for a matched pairs analysis. When only one control has been matched to each case (i.e., $M = 1$), the Mantel–Haenszel estimate is simply the ratio of the number of pairs where the case is exposed and the control is not, and the number of pairs where the control is exposed and the case is not

$$OR_{M-H} = \frac{n_{10}}{n_{01}} \tag{6.9}$$

Table 6–5. Notation for matched case–control study data

Cases		Number of exposed controls					
		0	1	...	k	...	M
Exposed	(1)^a	n_{10}	n_{11}	...	n_{1k}	...	n_{1M}
Non-exposed	(0)	n_{00}	n_{01}	...	n_{0k}	...	n_{0M}

^{a}Coding notation: 1 = exposed; 0 = non-exposed.

The Mantel–Haenszel chi-square is

$$\chi^2_{\text{M–H}} = \frac{(n_{10} - n_{01})^2}{(n_{10} + n_{01})} \tag{6.10}$$

When the allocation ratio (M) is greater than 1:1, the calculations become considerably more complex, particularly if the number of controls per case varies. The Mantel–Haenszel estimate of the odds ratio is (Rothman, 1986)

$$\text{OR}_{\text{M–H}} = \frac{\sum_K \sum_{m=1}^K \dfrac{(K + 1 - m)n_{1,m-1}}{(K + 1)}}{\sum_K \sum_{m=1}^K \dfrac{mn_{0,m}}{(K + 1)}} \tag{6.11}$$

and the test for association becomes

$$\chi^2 = \frac{\left[\sum_K \sum_{m=1}^K \left[n_{1,m-1} - \dfrac{m}{(K + 1)}(n_{1,m-1} + n_{0,m}) \right] \right]^2}{\sum_K \sum_{m=1}^K (n_{1,m-1} + n_{0,m}) \dfrac{m(K + 1 - m)}{(K + 1)^2}} \tag{6.12}$$

where K is the ratio of controls to cases, and the summations are carried out over all possible values of K from $K = 1$ to $K = M$. For example, suppose that it is decided to choose four controls per case (i.e., $M = 4$), but that there are some matched sets where it was not possible to obtain exposure information for all the cases and controls. When the individual matching is maintained, any matched sets containing either no case or no controls would have to be discarded. (This is a major disadvantage of maintaining the individual matching in the analysis). Using expressions (6.11) and (6.12), the summations would be performed four times: first for the matched sets with only one control ($K = 1$, $m = 1$); second for the matched sets with two controls ($K = 2$, $m = 1,2$); third for the matched sets with three controls ($K = 3$, $m = 1,2,3$); and finally for the matched sets with four controls ($K = 4$, $m = 1,2,3,4$). In a study with complete con-

Table 6–6. Exposure of cases and controls in a matched case–control study of soft tissue sarcoma and farming

	Controls		
	Farmers	Non-farmers	Total
Cases:			
Farmers	1	11	12
Nonfarmers	8	82	90

Source: Smith et al. (1982).

trol information, (i.e., with four controls for every case), only the latter summation would be carried out.

Either Miettinen's (1976) test-based method or Robins' (1986) method can be used to calculate the confidence interval for the odds ratio. For matched pairs data, the latter yields a variance estimate of

$$\text{Var}[\ln(\text{OR})] = \frac{1}{n_{10}} + \frac{1}{n_{01}} \qquad (6.13)$$

Example 6.12

A simple matched analysis can be illustrated with data from a registry-based case–control study (Smith et al., 1982) of soft tissue sarcoma and farming occupations (Table 6–6). The odds ratio is

$$\text{OR}_{\text{M-H}} = 11/8 = 1.375$$

and the Mantel–Haenszel chi-square is

$$\chi^2_{\text{M-H}} = \frac{(11 - 8)^2}{(11 + 8)} = 0.47$$

Test-based confidence limits are

$$\underline{\text{OR}}, \overline{\text{OR}} = 1.375^{(1 \pm 1.96/0.69)} = 0.56, 3.40$$

Expression (6.12) yields a variance estimate for ln(OR) of

$$\frac{1}{11} + \frac{1}{8} = 0.216$$

which has a square root of 0.465; ln(OR) = 0.318, yielding 95-percent confidence limits of

$$\underline{\text{OR}}, \overline{\text{OR}} = \exp[0.318 \pm 1.96 \times 0.465] = 0.55, 3.42$$

6.4. Extension to Multiple Exposure Levels

It is often desirable to extend the analysis to the consideration of three or more exposure levels. The simplest approach is to treat the data as a series of 2 × 2 tables and to calculate odds ratios for each level compared to the lowest level of exposure. However, caution is needed when using the Mantel-Haenszel procedure because the weights given to the various confounder strata will often be different for each pairwise comparison of exposure levels (i.e., the Mantel–Haenszel estimates are not mutually standardized). Therefore, the odds ratio estimates for the different levels will not be strictly comparable if the odds ratios are not uniform across strata of confounders. (This problem was discussed in Chapter 5.) The solution is to use a uniform set of weights, such as that used in an SRR analysis, in which the weights come from the lowest exposure category. In a case–control analysis, the weights are proportional to the confounder distribution of the controls in the lowest exposure category because these weights should represent the confounder distribution of the lowest exposure category in the study base (Miettinen, 1972). Like all directly weighted procedures, this approach is susceptible to instability resulting from small numbers.

An extension of the Mantel-Haenszel procedure (Mantel, 1963) provides a chi-square trend statistic with one degree of freedom. Table 6–7 shows the contingency table for stratum i. Scores (Y_j) are assigned to each exposure level (j) (e.g., the scores can be 0, 1, 2, etc., for increasing exposure levels). The chi-square with one degree of freedom is based on the deviation of $\Sigma A_j Y_j$ from its expectation, conditional on the null hypothesis, and subject to all the marginal totals being fixed:

$$\chi^2 = \frac{[\Sigma A_j Y_j - E_0(\Sigma A_j Y_j)]^2}{\mathrm{Var}_0(\Sigma A_j Y_j)} \qquad (6.14)$$

where $E_0(\Sigma A_j Y_j) = (N_1/T)\Sigma M_j Y_j$; $\mathrm{Var}_0(\Sigma A_j Y_j) = (N_1 N_0/T^2(T-1)) [T\Sigma M_j Y_j^2 - (\Sigma M_j Y_j)^2]$, and j indexes the exposure category.

When there are two or more strata of the confounder or control variable, the deviations of $\Sigma A_j Y_j$ from its expectation are summed separately across strata, and $\mathrm{Var}_0(\Sigma A_j Y_j)$ is also summed separately

Table 6-7. Notation for the Mantel–Haenszel extension test: contingency table for stratum i of a specified set of confounders

	\multicolumn{5}{c}{Study factor level (j) and score (Y_j)}				
	0	1	2	...	$k-1$	
	Y_0	Y_1	Y_2	...	Y_{k-1}	Total
Cases	A_0	A_1	A_2	...	A_{k-1}	N_1
Controls	B_0	B_1	B_2	...	B_{k-1}	N_0
Total	M_0	M_1	M_2	...	M_{k-1}	T

across strata in a manner analogous to that for the standard Mantel–Haenszel statistic. The chi-square trend statistic relies on the
assignment of scores to each exposure level and is derived from a
linear regression. This statistic is still valid in the case of a nonlinear
trend, since the derivation of both the expectation and variance of
$\Sigma A_j Y_j$ makes no assumption of linearity. For example, scores of 0,
1, 10, 100, and so on, can be assigned if there is prior evidence to
assume that the effect should be exponential rather than linear. A
major drawback of the Mantel extension procedure is that it does
not yield odds ratio estimates, but only provides a p-value. Various
other methods are available for evaluating trends across multiple
exposure levels, but the most useful of those involve mathematical
modeling (see Chapter 8).

Example 6.13

Analysis of multiple exposure levels can be illustrated with data from the study by
Hayes et al. (1986) of cancer of the nasal cavity and paranasal sinuses and formaldehyde exposure (see Table 6–8). The method is illustrated for a single stratum of
wood dust exposure, with three formaldehyde exposure levels. Comparing exposure level 1 to level 0 yields an odds ratio of 2.35 (95-percent confidence interval
1.10, 5.03), and comparing level 2 to level 0 yields an odds ratio of 2.53 (95-percent
confidence interval 1.24, 5.16). From expression (6.14), $\Sigma A_j Y_j = 96$, $E_0(\Sigma A_j Y_j) = 63.64$, and $\text{Var}_0(\Sigma A_j Y_j) = 91.47$. The Mantel extension trend chi-square (with 1
d.f.) is thus

$$\chi^2 = \frac{(96 - 63.64)^2}{91.47} = 11.45$$

---

7. EXAMPLE: NESTED CASE–CONTROL STUDY OF ASBESTOS TEXTILE PLANT WORKERS

The following example illustrates some of the methods presented
earlier. It involves a nested case–control study of lung cancer and
asbestos exposure, based on the cohort of 1,261 white male asbestos
workers from one textile manufacturing plant (Dement et al., 1983)
described in Chapter 5.

7.1. Study Design

The case group includes all 35 lung cancer deaths generated by the
cohort during the period 1940–75. All exposure information was
collected prospectively; thus, there were no potential problems with

Table 6-8. Exposure of cases and controls in a study of nasal cancer and formaldehyde exposure

Study factor level	0	1	2	Total
Score	0	2	4	
Cases	60	14	17	91
Controls	161	16	18	195
Total	221	30	35	286

Source: Hayes et al. (1986).

comparability of information between cases and controls. Hence, controls were chosen by sampling from the entire cohort. Because of the small number of cases, a 4:1 control-to-case matching ratio was used, thus yielding 140 worker controls. Controls were selected by incidence density matching on age at risk. It was not considered necessary to match on other factors.

7.2. Analysis: Dichotomous Exposure

The initial analysis used a dichotomous exposure classification. Cases and controls were classified as to whether their cumulative asbestos exposure was greater or less than 10,000 fibers/cc $\times$ days. (A latency period of zero years was assumed in this initial analysis). Table 6–9 shows the exposure distribution of cases and controls. The crude odds ratio (equation 6.1) is

$$OR = \frac{20 \times 92}{48 \times 15} = 2.56$$

The Mantel–Haenszel chi-square [equation (6.2)] is:

$$\chi^2 = \frac{(20 - 13.60)^2}{6.69} = 6.12$$

Table 6-9. Exposure of cases and controls: 1,000 fibers/cc $\times$ days[a]

	Asbestos exposure		
	<10	≥ 10	Total
Cases	15	20	35
Controls	92	48	140
Total	107	68	175

[a]Odds ratio = 2.56.

Table 6–10. Exposure distribution of cases and controls by age: 1,000 fibers/cc × days

Age group	Cases' exposure		Controls' exposure		Odds ratio
	<10	≥10	<10	≥10	
45–49	5	1	17	7	0.49
50–54	3	7	29	11	6.15
55–59	0	6	18	6	∞
60–64	1	4	13	7	7.43
65–69	4	2	11	13	0.42
70–74	2	0	4	4	0
Total	15	20	92	48	2.38[a]

[a] Adjusted odds ratio

and χ is 2.47. The approximate (test-based) 95-percent confidence interval for the odds ratio is [expression (6.3)]:

$$\underline{OR}, \overline{OR} = 2.56^{(1 \pm 1.96/2.47)} = 1.21, 5.40$$

Table 6–10 shows the exposure distribution of cases and controls stratified by age. The adjusted Mantel–Haenszel odds ratio is 2.38, and the Mantel–Haenszel chi-square is 6.08, yielding a 95-percent confidence interval of 1.19, 4.74. The data in Table 6–10 suggest that the odds ratio is not uniform across strata.

Table 6–11 gives the distribution of matched sets classified according to asbestos exposure. For example, there were 15 cases classified as "non-exposed" (cumulative exposure of less than 10,000 fibers/cc × days), each of which had four matched controls. In one of these, all four matched controls were exposed, in six of them two of the four matched controls were exposed, and so on. Using formula (6.11) and a fixed matching ratio of $K = 4$ (since all matched sets include four controls), the adjusted odds ratio is

Table 6–11. Distribution of matched sets according to asbestos exposure: 10,000 or more versus less than 10,000 fibers/cc × days

	Number of controls with 10,000 or more fibers/cc × days				
	0	1	2	3	4
Cases:					
≥10,000	3	7	9	1	0
<10,000	4	4	6	0	1

$$\mathrm{OR_{M-H}} = \frac{(4 \times 3 + 3 \times 7 + 2 \times 9 + 1 \times 1)}{(1 \times 4 + 2 \times 6 + 3 \times 0 + 4 \times 1)} = 2.60$$

The Mantel–Haenszel chi-square [formula (6.12)] is

$$\chi^2 = \frac{[(3 - 7 \times 1/5) + (7 - 13 \times 2/5) + (9 - 9 \times 3/5) + (1 - 2 \times 4/5)]^2}{[(7 \times 4/25) + (13 \times 6/25) + (9 \times 6/25) + (2 \times 4/25)]}$$

$$= 6.10$$

The corresponding test-based confidence interval is 1.23, 5.59. These findings are very similar to those of the crude and stratified analyses, suggesting that little confounding by age exists in the data. The minor differences in the crude, age-stratified, and matched analyses are due to minor variations in the grouping and weighting of strata under the three analytic approaches.

7.3. Analysis: Multiple Exposure Levels

For the analysis of multiple exposure levels cases and controls were classified into the same five cumulative exposure categories used in Chapter 5. Table 6–12 shows the exposure distribution of cases and controls, and the crude odds ratios obtained comparing each level with the lowest exposure level. The strong exposure–response trend is similar to that found in the full cohort analysis (Table 5–29).

Table 6–13 gives the cumulative exposure distributions stratified by age. Once again, pairwise comparisons have been made between each level with the lowest exposure level. The crude (Table 6–12) and adjusted (Table 6–13) odds ratios are generally similar, but there are some discrepancies at the higher exposure levels, suggesting that there is residual confounding in these categories. However, the findings for the higher exposure categories are unstable because of small numbers. Also, some age strata (e.g., 45–49 years) contain no cases or controls in the highest exposure category. Two analytic

Table 6–12. Exposure distribution of cases and controls: 1,000 fibers/cc × days

	Asbestos exposure				
	<1	1–9	10–39	40–99	≥100
Cases	5	10	7	11	2
Controls	49	43	28	16	4
Odds ratio	1.00	2.28	2.45	6.74	4.90

Table 6–13. Exposure distribution of cases and controls by age: 1,000 fibers/cc × days

Age group		Asbestos exposure				
		<1[a]	1–9	10–39	40–99	≥100
45–49	Cases	3	2	1	0	0
	Controls	8	9	7	0	0
50–54	Cases	1	2	3	3	1
	Controls	15	14	4	7	0
55–59	Cases	0	0	3	3	0
	Controls	10	8	3	3	0
60–64	Cases	0	1	0	4	1
	Controls	9	4	5	2	0
65–69	Cases	1	3	0	1	1
	Controls	5	6	6	4	3
70–74	Cases	0	2	3	0	0
	Controls	2	2	3	0	1
Total	Cases	5	10	7	11	2
	Controls	49	43	28	16	4
Adjusted odds ratio		1.00	1.95	2.46	6.27	8.78

[a]Reference category.

approaches can be adopted. One approach is simply to discard strata that contain zero marginals, since they contribute nothing to the analysis. For example, in the comparison of the highest and lowest exposure categories, the 45–49-year age stratum contains no cases or controls in the highest exposure category, and the 70–74-year age stratum contains no cases at either of the two levels being compared. Both of these strata could be excluded from the analysis. The alternative approach, adopted here, is to pool such strata with adjacent strata that do not have zero marginals (e.g., the 45–49-year and the 50–54-year age strata were pooled for the comparison of the highest and lowest exposure categories). This approach has the advantage that all the data are included in the analysis, but it is only valid when the expanded stratum width does not introduce (residual) confounding.

Table 6–14 contrasts the findings for the crude and age-adjusted analyses. The odds ratio estimates are similar, suggesting again that little confounding by age exists in the data.

7.4. Discussion

This example illustrates the efficiency of the case–control approach, which provided effect estimates, based on 175 subjects, very similar to those obtained with a full cohort analysis of 1,261 subjects

Table 6–14. Comparison of findings for crude analysis and stratified analysis

1,000 fibers/cc × days	Crude		Stratified	
	Odds ratio	95% confidence interval	Odds ratio	95% confidence interval
<1	1.00	—	1.00	—
1–9	2.28	0.73, 7.08	1.95	0.61, 6.27
10–39	2.45	0.72, 8.29	2.46	0.83, 7.25
40–99	6.74	2.20, 20.68	6.27	2.09, 18.86
≥100	4.90	0.81, 29.72	8.78	1.17, 65.97
Chi-square (trend)	8.86		9.16	

described in Chapter 5. In this instance, exposure data had already been assembled for all cohort members, and the case–control approach was also used for illustration. There is a considerable reduction in time and expense from a case–control analysis because exposure data are assembled only for the cases and controls actually chosen. However, it should be emphasized that, although the case–control approach provides generally valid overall estimates of effect, the findings may be less stable for particular subgroups.

8. SUMMARY OF ADVANTAGES AND LIMITATIONS OF CASE–CONTROL STUDIES

The major advantage of case–control studies is that they save time and expense relative to cohort studies, with little loss of precision. For example, the difference in precision between selecting four controls per case and doing a full cohort analysis (of a relatively common exposure) is generally very small (Miettinen, 1969). Registry-based case–control studies have the additional advantage of enabling the study of an exposure when an exposed cohort cannot be enumerated feasibly. This is particularly valuable for studying exposures that primarily occur in scattered small workplaces. A further commonly ascribed advantage is that a case–control study permits the evaluation of several different risk factors. In fact, cohort studies can also evaluate effects of multiple exposures, although at a greater cost. In many instances, the savings in time and cost from the case–control approach may permit the collection of additional exposure and confounder information.

Any case–control study is subject to the same biases as a full analysis of the study base. Additional problems of selection bias can occur but are usually not a major problem in cohort-based studies because the study base is fully enumerable. Information bias is generally of lesser concern if the study includes data collected prior to the occurrence of disease. Information bias is of more concern in studies involving data collected after the occurrence of disease, but this is relevant both to historical cohort studies and nested case–control studies. A further problem with the case–control design is that the medical community, and the wider public, is less familiar with it than cohort studies. Thus case–control findings may be difficult to explain. Problems related to the interpretation and acceptance of findings from case–control studies can be mitigated by stressing the inherent link between the case–control and cohort approaches.

In summary, occupational case–control studies are commonly depicted as being relatively fast and efficient, but being more susceptible to bias than cohort studies. The latter is generally true of registry-based studies. Cohort-based case–control studies have the former advantages but are no more prone to bias than cohort studies.

Glossary

odds   The ratio of the proportion of a group experiencing an event to the proportion not experiencing the event.
odds ratio   The ratio of two odds, used to estimate risk ratios or rate ratios.
relative risk   A general term to denote the rate ratio, risk ratio, or odds ratio.
response rate   The proportion of intended study subjects for whom appropriate information was obtained.
study base   The population–time experience of the base population.

Notation

a_i	Exposed cases in stratum i
b_i	Non-exposed cases in stratum i
c_i	Exposed controls in stratum i
d_i	Non-exposed controls in stratum i
$E_0(A)$	Expected number of exposed cases under the null hypothesis
N_{1i}	Number of exposed persons in stratum i
N_{0i}	Number of non-exposed persons in stratum i
M_{1i}	Number of cases in stratum i
M_{0i}	Number of controls in stratum i
OR	Odds ratio effect measure
OR_i	Odds ratio in stratum i of confounder
<u>OR</u>	Lower confidence limit for odds ratio

$\overline{OR}$	Upper conficence limit for odds ratio
T_i	Total number of persons in stratum i
$Var_0(A)$	Variance of number of exposed cases under the null hypothesis
χ^2_{M-H}	Mantel–Haenszel chi-square
N_1	Total number of cases, summed across multiple exposure levels
N_0	Total number of controls, summed across multiple exposure levels
A_j	Cases at exposure level j
B_j	Controls at exposure level j
Y_j	Score assigned to exposure level j
n_{1i}	Number of matched sets where case is exposed and i controls are exposed
n_{0i}	Number of matched sets where case is non-exposed and i controls are exposed
M	Allocation ratio of controls to cases

References

Arp EW, Wolf PH, and Checkoway H (1983): Lymphocytic leukemia and exposures to benzene and other solvents in the rubber industry. *J Occup Med* 25:598–602.

Axelson O (1985): The case-referent study—some comments on its structure, merits and limitations. *Scand J Work Environ Health* 11:207–213.

Axelson O, Hane M, and Hogstedt C (1976): A case-referent study on neuropsychiatric disorders among workers exposed to solvents. *Scand J Work Environ Health* 2:14–20.

Axelson O, Flodin U, and Hardell L (1982): A comment on the reference series with regard to multiple exposure evaluations in a case-referent study. *Scand J Work Environ Health* 8(Suppl 1):15–19.

Blair A, and Thomas TL (1979): Leukemia among Nebraska farmers: a death certificate study. *Am J Epidemiol* 110:264–273.

Breslow NE, and Day NE (1980): *Statistical Methods in Cancer Research, Volume I: The Analysis of Case–Control Studies.* Lyon, France: International Agency for Research on Cancer.

Breslow NE, Lubin JH, and Marek P (1983): Multiplicative models and cohort analysis. *J Am Stat Assoc* 78:1–12.

Checkoway H, Smith AH, McMichael AJ, et al. (1981): A case-control study of bladder cancer in the United States rubber and tyre industry. *Br J Ind Med* 38:240–246.

Coggon D, Pannett B, and Acheson ED (1984): Screening for new occupational hazards of cancer in young persons. *Ann Occup Hyg* 28:145–150.

Dement JM, Harris RL, Symons MJ, and Shy CM (1983): Exposures and mortality among chrysotile asbestos workers. Part II: Mortality. *Am J Ind Med* 4:421–433.

Gerin M, Siemiatycki J, Kemper H, et al. (1985): Obtaining occupational exposure histories in epidemiologic case-control studies. *J Occup Med* 27:420–426.

Goldberg MS, Siemiatycki J, Kemper H, et al. (1986): Inter-rater agreement in assessing occupational exposure in a case-control study. *Br J Ind Med* 43:667–676.

Greenland S (1984): A counterexample to the test-based principle of setting confidence limits. *Am J Epidemiol* 120:4–7.

Greenland S (1986): Adjustment of risk ratios in case-base studies (hybrid epidemiologic designs). *Stat Med* 5:579–584.

Greenland S, and Thomas DC (1982): On the need for the rare disease assumption in case-control studies. *Am J Epidemiol* 116:547–553.

Hayes RB, Raatgever JW, de Bruyn A, et al. (1986): Cancer of the nasal cavity and paranasal sinuses, and formaldehyde exposure. *Int J Cancer* 37:487–492.

Hoar SK, Morrison AS, Cole P, et al. (1980): An occupational exposure and linkage system for the study of occupational carcinogens. *J Occup Med* 22:722–726.

Hoar SK, Blair A, Holmes FF, et al. (1986): Agricultural herbicides use and risk of lymphoma and soft-tissue sarcoma. *J Am Med Assoc* 256:1141–1147.

Karasek R, Baker D, Marxer F, et al. (1981): Job decision, job demands, and cardiovascular disease: a prospective study of Swedish men. *Am J Public Health* 71:694–705.

Kauppinen TP, Partanen TJ, Nurminen MM, et al. (1986): Respiratory cancers and chemical exposures in the wood industry: a nested case-control study. *Br J Ind Med* 43:84–90.

Kleinbaum DG, Kupper LL, and Morgenstern H (1982): *Epidemiologic Research: Principles and Quantitative Methods*. Belmont, CA: Lifetime Learning Publications.

Kupper LL, McMichael AJ, and Spirtas R (1975): A hybrid epidemiologic study design useful in estimating relative risk. *J Am Stat Assoc* 70:524–528.

Lubin JH, and Gail MH (1984): Biased selection of controls for case-control analyses of cohort studies. *Biometrics* 40:63–75.

Mantel N (1963): Chi-square tests with one degree of freedom. Extensions of the Mantel–Haenszel procedure. *J Am Stat Assoc* 58:690–700.

Mantel N, and Haenszel W (1959): Statistical aspects of the analysis of data from retrospective studies of disease. *J Natl Cancer Inst* 22:719–748.

Miettinen OS (1972): Standardization of risk ratios. *Am J Epidemiol* 96:383–388.

Miettinen OS (1976): Estimability and estimation in case-referent studies. *Am J Epidemiol* 103:226–235.

Miettinen OS (1977): Letter to the editor, re: Estimability and estimation in case-referent studies. *Am J Epidemiol* 105:498–502.

Miettinen OS (1982): Design options in epidemiologic research: an update. *Scand J Work Environ Health* 8(Suppl 1):7–14.

Miettinen OS (1985). The "case-control" study: valid selection of subjects. *J Chronic Dis* 7:543–548.

Miettinen OS, and Wang J-D (1981): An alternative to the proportionate mortality ratio. *Am J Epidemiol* 114:144–148.

Pearce NE, and Checkoway H (1988): Case–control studies using other diseases as controls: problems of excluding exposure-related diseases. *Am J Epidemiol* 127:851–856.

Pearce NE, and Howard JK (1986): Occupation, social class and male cancer mortality in New Zealand, 1974–78. *Int J Epidemiol* 15:456–462.

Pearce NE, Smith AH, Howard JK, et al. (1986): Non-Hodgkin's lymphoma and exposure to phenoxyherbicides, chlorophenols, fencing work, and meat works employment: a case-control study. *Br J Ind Med* 43:75–83.

Prentice RL (1986): A case-cohort design for epidemiologic cohort studies and disease prevention trials. *Biometrika* 73:1–11.

Robins JM, Breslow NE, and Greenland S. (1986): Estimation of the Mantel–Haenszel variance consistent with both sparse-data and large-strata limiting models. *Biometrics* 42:311–323.

Rothman KJ (1986). *Modern Epidemiology*. Boston, MA: Little, Brown & Co.

Schlesselman JJ (1982): *Case-Control Studies: Design, Conduct, Analysis*. New York: Oxford University Press.

Selevan SG, Lindbohm M-L, Hornung RW, et al. (1985): A study of occupational exposure to antineoplastic drugs and fetal loss in nurses. *N Engl J Med* 313:1173–1178.

Siemiatycki J, Richardson L, Gerin M, et al (1986): Associations between several sites of cancer and nine organic dusts: results from an hypothesis-generating case-control study in Montreal, 1979–1983. *Am J Epidemiol* 123:235–249.

Smith AH, Fisher DO, Pearce NE, et al (1982): Do agricultural chemicals cause soft tissue sarcoma? Initial findings of a case-control study in New Zealand. *Community Health Stud* 6:114–119.

Smith AH, Pearce NE, and Callas PW (1988): Cancer case-control studies with other cancers as controls. *Int J Epidemiol* 17:298–306.

Woolf B. (1955): On estimating the relationship between blood group and disease. *Ann Hum Genet* 19:251–253.

7 Cross-Sectional Studies

1. OVERVIEW

Cross-sectional studies occupy an important place in occupational epidemiology because of their applicability to the study of nonfatal diseases, symptoms, and exposure effects on physiologic functions. This chapter reviews the basic study design features and issues of occupational cross-sectional studies. The topics to be covered include one-time and repeated survey designs, subject selection options, methods of data analysis for disease prevalence and physiologic variable comparisons, and sources of bias to which cross-sectional studies are most vulnerable. Finally, we summarize the principal advantages and shortcomings of occupational cross-sectional studies.

2. STUDY DESIGN FEATURES

There are two general designs of cross-sectional studies. The first is a survey conducted to determine the prevalence of disease or physiologic status of the worker population, or some subset thereof, at one point in time. This type of cross-sectional study can be termed a *one-time survey.* The second approach, the *repeated survey,* is an extension of the one-time survey in which subsequent health (and exposure) assessments are made on the workforce. The common element of all cross-sectional studies is that the health outcome is the number of cases of disease existing in the population at a point in time. It should be recognized that the term *disease* is used loosely here to encompass actual diseases (e.g., ischemic heart disease), symptoms (e.g., numbness in the extremities), and physiologic states (e.g., white blood cell differential counts).

Although cross-sectional studies can be regarded as variants of other epidemiologic designs, they have the distinguishing characteristic of always involving measurement of disease *prevalence* rather than incidence. Disease prevalence denotes the number of cases existing in the population. *Point prevalence* refers to the prevalence estimated at one point in time (e.g., the number of workers with chronic bronchitis determined during a survey conducted in 1988). *Period prevalence* denotes the number of cases that existed during some time interval (e.g., the number of workers with carpal tunnel syndrome during the years 1974–88). Period prevalence is seldom estimable in occupational epidemiology. Moreover, the interpretation of period prevalence is not clear because it is a mixture of the initial point prevalence and subsequent incidence rates. Thus, we shall restrict our attention to point prevalence, henceforth referred to simply as prevalence.

Prevalence is computed as the number of cases divided by the number of workers in the study. Thus, prevalence is a proportion. The term *prevalence rate* is sometimes used, although some authors (e.g., Elandt-Johnson, 1975) reserve the term *rate* for the number of new cases occurring over time. Prevalent, or existing, cases include cases that developed during different time periods but where the individuals were still alive and continued to mainfest disease at the time of the cross-sectional study. There is a direct link between disease incidence, duration of disease, and prevalence (Freeman and Hutchison, 1980).

Prevalence studies are particularly valuable for nonfatal, degenerative diseases with no clear point of onset. Medical care for such diseases (e.g., chronic bronchitis) is often not sought until disease has become relatively advanced (Kelsey et al., 1986). Disease prevalence will be greatest for diseases that occur relatively frequently in the workforce (i.e., high incidence rate) and persist for long periods of time. Disease persistence means that the disease is not rapidly fatal in its own right, does not routinely lead to fatal complications, and is not a transitory condition with only brief periods of activity. Most prevalence studies are limited to active workers, and thus will not detect diseases that result in rapid termination of employment. Osteoarthritis is an example of a condition that is prevalent in some occupations involving repetitive musculoskeletal stresses and that would therefore be suitable for a cross-sectional study. Acute myelogenous leukemia, by contrast, would be virtually impossible to investigate in a cross-sectional study.

2.1. One-Time Surveys

The most common type of cross-sectional study is the *one-time survey* in which disease prevalence in the worker population is measured

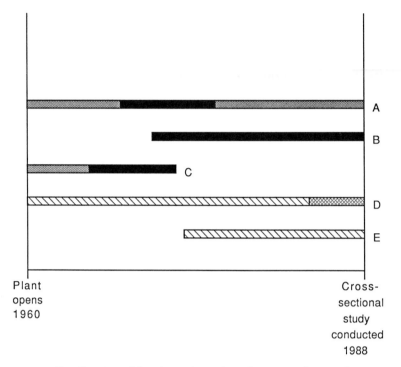

Figure 7–1. Classification of five hypothetical workers according to disease and exposure status in a one-time cross-sectional study (▨ = non-exposed and no disease, ▨ = non-exposed and disease, ▨ = exposed and no disease, ■ = exposed and disease).

at one point in time. Figure 7–1 shows how five hypothetical workers would be classified in a cross-sectional study conducted in 1988. Workers A, B, and C are in the "exposed" category, whereas workers D and E are "non-exposed." In a cross-sectional study, all the workers except C would be included because worker C had previously left employment. Among the exposed, worker B would be classified as a case, but worker A would not, because his disease was not present at the time of the study. Among the non-exposed, worker D would be a case. Thus, a simple comparison of exposed and non-exposed would suggest equal prevalences, despite the fact that the incidence of disease was greater among the exposed. We discuss biases of this type later in the chapter.

Example 7.1

Sjogren and Ulfarvson (1985) conducted a cross-sectional study of the prevalence of respiratory disease symptoms among welders exposed to aluminum, stainless

Table 7-1. Chronic bronchitis among welders and non-exposed workers

	Welders			Non-exposed		
Type of welding	Total	No. with bronchitis	%	Total	No. with bronchitis	%
Gas-shielded on aluminum	59	4	6.8	64	2	3.1
Coated electrodes on stainless steel	44	4	9.1	46	2	4.3
Railroad track	149	7	4.7	70	1	1.4

Source: Sjogren and Ulfvarson (1985).

steel, or chromium. The study included 59 aluminum welders, 44 stainless steel welders, and 149 railroad track welders exposed to chromium compounds as exposed groups, and 180 non-exposed workers with similar distributions of age and smoking habits. The comparison group consists of nonwelding industrial workers from the same companies as the welders. Table 7-1 shows the prevalence of reported chronic bronchitis by exposure category. The prevalence of chronic bronchitis is elevated among the welders in each category.

2.2. Repeated Surveys

Repeated surveys, sometimes called panel studies, are series of cross-sectional studies performed over time, usually on the same group of workers. The objective of a repeated survey is to evaluate change in health status in relation to change in exposure. The design of a repeated survey is depicted in Figure 7–2. Because a repeated survey involves follow-up of worker groups, it can be considered as a special case of prospective cohort study. Repeated surveys are especially useful for the study of physiologic variables, such as pulmo-

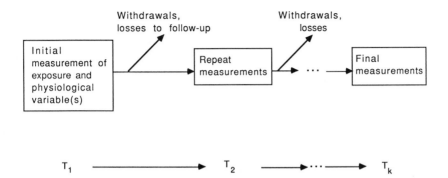

Figure 7–2. Design of repeated survey of physiological variable change.

Table 7–2. Pulmonary function decline among firefighters in relation to number of fires fought

Number of fires	Forced vital capacity (mL)	Forced expiratory volume 1 sec (mL)
1–40	−51	−49
41–99	−78	−71
≥100	−135	−109

Source: Peters et al. (1974).

nary function or blood pressure, for which changes over several years may indicate early stages of disease processes.

Example 7.2

In a repeated survey of pulmonary function declines among firefighters, Peters and associates (1974) made measurements at two points in time, 1970–71 and 1971–72. The changes in forced vital capacity (FVC) and forced expiratory volume in 1 second (FEV_1) were examined with respect to the numbers of fires fought during the year between the two measurements. As shown in Table 7–2, there are marked trends in ventilatory decline that coincide with the extent of firefighting activity during the interval between measurements.

When physiologic change is the study outcome, the best approach is to include the same subjects in a repeated survey. However, some repeated surveys include new enrollees or may even be performed on completely new groups of workers. In the latter instance, the original cross-sectional study is replicated. One might choose to replicate a cross-sectional study on a different group(s) of workers if the study objective were to estimate disease prevalence or physiologic function under changed exposure circumstances. For example, if in 1960 we had studied the prevalence of hypertension among workers exposed to high levels of a cardiovascular toxin and exposures had been reduced subsequently, then it might be desirable to conduct a new prevalence survey in 1988 on a different group of workers. Hypertension, if not treated, is a persistent condition; thus, including workers from the original survey would prevent us from determining the effects of lowered exposures.

When the health outcome is not thought to be persistent, including the same subjects in a repeated survey generally is more valid than selecting new subjects, because most confounding can be eliminated if individuals' measurements in the two (or more) surveys can be linked. Studying the same subjects repeatedly may also be advantageous in terms of statistical efficiency because there usually is less variability in measurements within individuals than between groups (Berry, 1974).

3. SOURCES OF HEALTH AND EXPOSURE DATA

3.1. Health Outcome Data

A major advantage of cross-sectional studies is that a broad spectrum of health outcomes can be studied. These span the range from clinical diseases (e.g., myocardial infarction) that might also be included in cohort or case–control studies to subtle physiologic changes (e.g., liver enzyme levels) that can only be detected by specialized laboratory techniques. Consequently, there are diverse sources of and methods used to obtain health outcome information (Table 7–3). Typical sources include physical examinations, radiographic surveys, laboratory reports, medical records, insurance claims, and questionnaires administered to workers. Data from more than one of these sources are included in many cross-sectional studies, particularly when there are multiple health outcomes of interest or when the major health outcome requires confirmatory data from several sources to establish diagnoses. Silicosis, for which complementary evidence from radiographs, physical examinations, and pulmonary function testing is needed to establish an unequivocal diagnosis, is one such example.

3.2. Exposure Data

The sources of exposure data useful for cross-sectional studies depend on the nature of the health outcome under investigation. For example, in a study of the concurrent relationship between lead

Table 7–3. Sources of health data in occupational cross-sectional studies

Source	Example
1. Physical examinations	Dermatitis
2. Radiographic surveys	X-ray survey for pulmonary fibrosis
3. Laboratory reports	Serum lipids
4. Medical records	Hypertension history
5. Insurance claims	Back injuries
6. Questionnaires	Respiratory disease symptoms

Table 7–4. Sources of exposure data in occupational cross-sectional studies

1. Industrial hygiene measurements
2. Job histories
3. Biological samples
4. Questionnaires administered to workers and supervisors

exposure and kidney function, air and perhaps urinary concentrations of lead are the relevant exposure factors. By contrast, we might be interested in knowing not only the "current" exposure of the workers but also their cumulative exposures to lead. Accordingly, we would supplement current exposure data with an index of lifetime working lead exposure derived from a compilation of past work history information.

Some of the most useful sources of exposure data are current and past industrial hygiene measurements, job histories, biological samples of compounds or their metabolites, and questionnaires administered to workers or their supervisors (Table 7–4). When possible, it is desirable to attempt to corroborate exposure measurements or reports from more than one source.

4. SUBJECT SELECTION OPTIONS

There are several options for selecting workers for inclusion in a cross-sectional study. The ideal approach is to study all active and retired workers who have ever worked in the plant or industry, but this is rarely practical. The most complete and feasible approach usually is to include all active workers in the plant or industry. Other, more restrictive strategies are to include subsets of workers chosen on the basis of exposure characteristics or, less frequently, to select workers with respect to health experience. The advantages and drawbacks of the various selection options are considered in the following discussion.

4.1. Plant- or Industrywide Studies

Including all workers actively working in a plant or industry is analogous to conducting a cohort study on the entire workforce. This approach is justified when health data are recorded routinely for all workers, such as from preemployment and subsequent examinations. A plant- or industrywide survey generally is improved when exposure data are also obtained and tabulated for all employees (e.g., radiation dosimetry in a nuclear plant). However, except in small workforces of fewer than, say, 100 workers, this approach can become prohibitively expensive, especially when elaborate and costly diagnostic or laboratory procedures are required.

Another justification for including all workers, even when health data are not readily available, is when the industry under study involves exposures to known hazards. The cross-sectional study then becomes potentially of immediate benefit to workers by serving as a means of disease screening and referral for treatment for identified cases.

Example 7.3

Samet et al. (1984) conducted a cross-sectional study of respiratory disease and spirometry among uranium miners from the Colorado Plateau who had achieved a minimum of ten years experience. Previous research (Archer et al., 1973) had indicated that dust and radiation exposures might be causally related to emphysema among underground uranium miners. The study by Samet and co-workers included 192 workers from an eligible pool of 238 male miners (nonparticipants were either ill, on vacation, or refused participation). Questionnaires eliciting symptom reports and pulmonary function tests were administered to the workers. The symptom results for workers, classified according to years worked in mining, are summarized in Table 7–5. These data, which were adjusted for smoking habits, demonstrate symptom excesses among the longest-tenured ($\geq$20 years) workers. The most pronounced prevalence gradient was detected for dyspnea.

As with cohort studies, sometimes it may be advisable to restrict the subjects in a cross-sectional study to workers with a minimum employment duration if there is reason to believe that exposure effects require minimum induction or latency times. Excluding short-term workers with possibly atypical sociodemographic char-

Table 7–5. Prevalence of respiratory symptoms according to years of underground uranium mining

Symptom	<10 yr ($N = 47$)	10–19 yr ($N = 70$)	$\geq$20 yr ($N = 70$)
Chronic cough	19.9[a]	14.1	22.7
Chronic phlegm	32.5	31.9	36.6
Persistent wheeze	19.7	26.1	34.0
Dyspnea	5.3	9.6	23.7

[a]Prevalence per 100 workers, standardized by smoking habits.
Source: Samet et al. (1984).

acteristics is another reason for imposing a minimum employment duration criterion in some studies. In the study described in Example 7.3, the investigators chose a ten-year minimum employment in mining inclusion criterion because it was presumed that the respiratory effects considered required prolonged exposures.

4.2. Selection on Exposure Status

Most often, workers are selected for cross-sectional studies on the basis of their exposure status. That is, workers with particular exposure profiles within a plant or industry are targeted for study. In Example 7.1 we saw that welders were chosen specifically because of their exposures and were compared with other workers assumed non-exposed to welding fumes. Isolation of exposure groups of particular interest, including non-exposed workers, can be more cost- and time-efficient than studying an entire workforce. Alternatively, subsets of exposed workers can be selected from a plant-wide survey for more intensive medical investigation. In the latter instance the overall survey would serve as a disease screening mechanism.

Example 7.4

The investigators in Example 7.1 (Sjogren and Ulfvarson, 1985) stratified the railroad welders with respect to exposure levels of chromium and total particulates. Comparisons of respiratory symptoms (cough, phlegm, and irritation) prevalence between the exposure groups and the non-exposed workers reveal an association with higher levels of chromium, but not with total particulates (Table 7–6).

The design of a cross-sectional study, wherein samples of subjects are selected on the basis of exposure level from a larger pool of

Table 7–6. Respiratory symptom prevalence among railroad track welders in relation to exposures to chromium and total particulates

Exposure group	Total number	No. with symptoms	Percent
Non-exposed	70	3	4.3
Chromium			
$<20\ \mu g/m^3$	41	11	26.8
$\geq 20\ \mu g/m^3$	8	4	50.0
Total particulates			
$<5\ mg/m^3$	25	8	32.0
$\geq 5\ mg/m^3$	24	7	29.2

Source: Sjogren and Ulfvarson (1985).

Table 7-7. Mean hand-grip strength among forestry workers, according to total hours of chain saw operation

Total hours chain saw operation	Number	Mean grip strength (kg)
Reference group[a]	36	52.5
0–2,499	28	46.5
2,500–4,999	40	43.6
5,000–7,499	25	41.8
≥7,500	41	40.1

Source: Miyashita et al. (1983).

[a]Forestry workers not operating chain saws.

workers, is an efficient strategy in that it facilitates evaluating exposure–response gradients, especially when workers from the entire range of exposures are sampled.

Example 7.5

Miyashita et al. (1983) selected 134 forestry workers who routinely use chain saws from a pool of some 2,000 forestry workers. A comparison group of 36 forestry workers not exposed to vibrations was also selected. Both the exposed and non-exposed workers were men aged 40–59 years. The exposed workers were classified into categories of cumulative chain saw operation experience, and various musculoskeletal responses were compared between the groups. The results for hand grip strength (Table 7–7) evidence a marked decrement with increasing cumulative hours of operating chain saws.

Examples 7.4 and 7.5 also illustrate two methods of exposure classification. In the study of welders (see Example 7.4), exposure classification was made according to levels measured at the time of the study, whereas in the study of forestry workers (see Example 7.5), cumulative exposure was used to categorize workers. In general, current exposures are more pertinent than cumulative exposure in studies of short-term sequelae, and cumulative exposures are more appropriate for delayed or progressive effects.

4.3. Selection on Disease Status

Subject selection for a cross-sectional study can also be made with respect to disease status. Here the study is a case–control design that is limited to prevalent cases. In this situation, cases of disease among the workforce are compared with noncases with respect to exposure. For example, we might compare the exposure profiles of

Table 7–8. Types of comparison groups in occupational cross-sectional studies

Reference source	Example
1. National surveys of general population	National Health and Nutritional Examination Survey in United States
2. Published normative values for physiologic variables	Prediction equations for pulmonary function, by age, gender, height, and smoking status
3. Other non-exposed industry workers	Meat packing plant workers in a study of lead toxicity among battery plant workers
4. Internal reference groups	Workers with the lowest exposures in the plant under study

a group of workers with peripheral neuropathy with a comparison group of other workers free of the disease. As in a typical case–control study, matching on confounders could be applied.

4.4. Comparison Populations

Considering only the most typical cross-sectional design, wherein subject selection is based on exposure status, there are several selection options for comparison populations (Table 7–8). As with cohort studies, we can classify the comparison groups as either external or internal populations.

External Comparisons

Data from general population prevalence surveys can form the basis for comparisons of disease prevalence or physiologic variable distributions with the study population. For example, the National Health and Nutrition Examination Surveys conducted on samples of the U.S. population (National Center for Health Statistics, 1973) have generated a considerable amount of data on cardiovascular diseases, blood pressure, diabetes, and other conditions. Comparisons against a general population can be made for the entire workforce or for subsets of workers designated according to exposure levels. Disease prevalence comparisons with a general population may be biased by the Healthy Worker Effect in much the same way that mortality comparisons with an external comparison population frequently are biased in cohort studies. In fact, the same diseases that usually occur less frequently in industrial cohorts in mortality studies (e.g., chronic respiratory diseases) are also less common among worker populations in prevalence studies (Sterling and Weinkam, 1985). The Healthy Worker Effect may even be stronger in prevalence studies because they typically include only actively employed workers.

Another source of external comparison data is published laboratory values for physiologic variables. Examples include pulmonary function values, blood cell counts and differential white cell distributions, serum lipid values, and various blood chemistries. These data are used to represent "normative" values, providing either normal ranges or, in some instances, predicted values for individuals based on gender, ethnicity, anthropometric variables, or smoking habits.

Example 7.6

In a study of pulmonary function loss among firefighters exposed to high concentrations of toluene diisocyanate (TDI) at one particular incident, Axford et al. (1976) compared temporal changes in FEV_1 and FVC among 35 firefighters with predicted changes determined from published values for men of the same age and ethnic group (Cotes, 1975). Their findings are presented in Table 7–9. During the first six months the firefighters experienced greater than predicted declines of both FEV_1 and FVC; however, during the subsequent 37 months the firefighters' lung function declines were slightly less than expected. These results suggest that the effects of acute exposure to TDI are greatest during the first six months following exposure.

One should be cautious about relying on published normative data for comparisons when the sources of the reference data are not specified explicitly. Often there is no way of knowing the characteristics of the population from which such data were generated. Some of the sources of these data include healthy volunteers (frequently, medical students), blood donors, and patients receiving routine medical examinations. Surveys conducted on randomly selected

Table 7–9. Average annual loss in FEV_1 and FVC among firefighters during 43-month period following acute exposure to toluene di-isocyanate

Period	Average loss per year (L)	
	FEV_1	FVC
First 6 months	0.066	0.216
Next 37 months	0.014	−0.029 (gain)
Entire period	0.019	0.010
Expected loss for normal men	0.031	0.021

Source: Axford et al. (1976).

groups from the general population are a better source of external reference values than those previously described.

Workers from another industry also can be chosen as an external comparison group. The most desirable strategy is to select the comparison group from an industry that employs workers with sociodemographic characteristics similar to those of the exposed group but free from the exposure of interest and from other exposures that can cause the health outcomes under study. For example, if we are studying neurobehavioral effects among workers exposed to organic solvents in a paint manufacturing plant, then a suitable external comparison group might be workers in some other factory who were not exposed to solvents or neurotoxic metals (e.g., lead battery plant workers would be eliminated from consideration).

Example 7.7

Sarto and co-workers (1984) conducted a cytogenetic survey among 22 workers from a benzene manufacturing plant. As a comparison group, the investigators selected an equal number of workers from among 100 volunteers at a nearby metallurgical factory where there were no known clastogenic exposures. The exposed and non-exposed workers were matched individually with respect to age, gender, smoking habits, and residential area. The exposed workers were divided into two groups. The first consisted of nine manufacturing workers exposed to average benzene concentrations less than 2 ppm; the second group included 13 other workers (laboratory, maintenance personnel, and plant foremen) exposed to average benzene concentrations of about 5 ppm. There are no consistent differences in sister chromatid exchange levels between exposed and non-exposed workers, although the exposed groups had higher average numbers of cells with structural chromosomal aberrations (Table 7–10).

Table 7–10. Mean number of sister chromatid exchanges (SCE) per metaphase and percent metaphases with structural chromosomal aberrations (SCA) among workers exposed to benzene

Group	Number	SCE per metaphase	Percent metaphases with SCA
Plant workers[a]	9	11.0	1.7
Reference group	9	10.1	0.5
Other workers[b]	13	8.1	1.4
Reference group	13	9.2	0.8

Source: Sarto et al (1984).

[a]Benzene manufacturing workers.

[b]Laboratory workers, workers involved in benzene tank filling, empyting, and rinsing, and plant foremen.

Internal Comparisons

Internal comparison groups chosen from among the workforce included in a cross-sectional study are used primarily to examine prevalence gradients according to exposure levels. The methods for subdividing the study population in a cross-sectional study are the same as those described in Chapter 5 for cohort studies, and therefore will not be reiterated. The principal difference between subcohort analysis and subgroup analysis in cross-sectional studies is that, in the most general case, subcohort analysis requires attribution of person-time into each attained exposure stratum, whereas in cross-sectional studies the exposure subgroups are treated as fixed categories (as exposure is only assessed at one point in time), thus simplifying the analysis considerably.

We have already seen examples of internal comparisons in the studies by Sjogren and Ulfvarson (1985) of welders (see Example 7.4) and Miyashita et al. (1983) of chain saw operators (see Example 7.5). In the latter study the comparison was with other forestry workers without chain saw exposure, although we might also consider the workers with 0–2,500 cumulative person-hours of chain saw work as another internal reference category (see Table 7–7).

Usually, it is most desirable to select internal comparison groups because prevalence comparisons with non-exposed workers tend to be less influenced by the Healthy Worker Effect, other sources of selection bias, and confounding. Small numbers of non-exposed workers may necessitate the use of an external comparison, however.

5. METHODS OF DATA ANALYSIS

In this section we describe methods for the analysis of cross-sectional study data. Methods for comparing disease prevalence are outlined first. Next, we consider the analytic techniques useful for comparing distributions of physiologic variables, including changes over time that would be measured in a repeated survey.

5.1. Comparisons of Prevalence

Table 7–11 displays the basic data layout for a cross-sectional study comparing disease prevalence between exposure groups. This data

Table 7–11. Data layout for ith stratum of a cross-sectional study

	Exposed	Non-exposed	Total
Disease	a_i	b_i	M_{1i}
No disease	c_i	d_i	M_{0i}
Total	N_{1i}	N_{0i}	T_i

format represents the fourfold table for the *i*th stratum of some confounder (e.g., age).

If we denote the prevalence of a particular disease in the study population by *P*, then it can be shown (Rothman, 1986) that the prevalence odds is equal to the incidence rate (*I*) times average disease duration (*D*) when the incidence rate is constant over time:

$$\frac{P}{(1 - P)} = ID \qquad (7.1)$$

Thus, the prevalence odds [expression (7.1)] is the basic outcome measure in a cross-sectional study because it is directly proportional to the disease incidence that is of intrinsic interest. Hence, the *prevalence odds ratio*, which is the ratio of the prevalence odds in the exposed to the prevalence odds in the non-exposed, is the basic effect measure in a cross-sectional study. This means that the methods for estimating odds ratios in case–control studies (see Chapter 6) can also be applied in cross-sectional studies. In particular, prevalence odds ratios can be calculated using the Mantel–Haenszel method (Mantel and Haenszel, 1959) as given in expression (6.6). Also, test-based confidence intervals (Miettinen, 1976) [expression (6.3)], which uses the Mantel–Haenszel chi-square [formula (6.2)], can be used. An alternative method for confidence interval estimation, given by Robins et al. (1986) [expression (6.8)], can be used instead of the test-based method. Since these procedures have been discussed in Chapter 6, we concentrate here on methods involving prevalence itself, which approximates the prevalence odds when the disease is rare.

The prevalences among the exposed (P_1) and non-exposed (P_0) are, respectively,

$$P_1 = a/N_1 \qquad (7.2)$$

and

$$P_0 = b/N_0 \qquad (7.3)$$

Prevalence comparisons can take the form of difference or ratio measures. The *prevalence difference* (PD) is simply expression (7.2) − expression (7.3), or

$$PD = P_1 - P_0 \tag{7.4}$$

The *prevalence ratio* (PR) is the quotient of the two prevalences:

$$PR = \frac{P_1}{P_0} \tag{7.5}$$

To illustrate the calculations for this simplest case, consider the data on chronic bronchitis prevalence among welders (Sjogren and Ulfvarson, 1985) from Table 7–1. Among aluminum welders the prevalence is 4/59, or 6.78 cases per 100 workers, and the prevalence among the non-exposed workers from the same industry is 2/64, or 3.13 per 100. Thus, the prevalence difference is $6.78 - 3.13 = 3.65$, and the prevalence ratio is $6.78/3.13 = 2.17$.

Summary Measures of Effect

It is usually of interest to compute a single prevalence difference or ratio across strata of a confounder so as to simplify the presentation of results. One procedure for combining prevalence differences across strata to obtain a summary measure is to compute a weighted average of the differences, where the weights are the inverses of the variances of the stratum-specific prevalence differences. An approximation of the variance of a prevalence difference (Rothman, 1986) is given as

$$Var(PD_i) \cong \frac{a_i c_i}{(N_{1i})^3} + \frac{b_i d_i}{(N_{0i})^3} \tag{7.6}$$

where the notation follows that of Table 7–11. The *summary prevalence difference* (SPD) then becomes

$$SPD = \frac{\sum_i W_i PD_i}{\sum_i W_i} \tag{7.7}$$

where the W_i are the inverses of the variances of the stratum-specific PD_i. The confidence interval for an inverse variance-weighted prevalence difference (Kleinbaum et al., 1982) is given as

$$\underline{SPD}, \overline{SPD} = SPD \pm Z / \left(\sqrt{\sum_i W_i} \right) \tag{7.8}$$

where the W_i are the stratum-specific inverses of the variances; and Z is the standard normal deviate (e.g., $Z = 1.96$ for 95-percent confidence interval).

One can compute a Mantel–Haenszel estimate of the SPR (Greenland and Robins, 1985) according to the following expression:

$$\text{SPR}_{\text{M}-\text{H}} = \frac{\sum_i a_i N_{0i}/T_i}{\sum_i b_i N_{1i}/T_i} \tag{7.9}$$

Confidence intervals for $\text{SPR}_{\text{M}-\text{H}}$ can be obtained by computing the variance of $\ln(\text{SPR}_{\text{M}-\text{H}})$ and exponentiation. An approximate formula for the variance of $\ln(\text{SPR}_{\text{M}-\text{H}})$ (Greenland and Robins, 1985) is

$$\text{Var}[\ln(\text{SPR}_{\text{M}-\text{H}})] = \frac{\sum_i (M_{1i}N_{1i}N_{0i} - a_i b_i T_i)/T_i^2}{\left(\sum_i a_i N_{0i}/T_i\right)\left(\sum_i b_i N_{1i}/T_i\right)} \tag{7.10}$$

The confidence interval for $\text{SPR}_{\text{M}-\text{H}}$ is then

$$\underline{\text{SPR}}_{\text{M}-\text{H}}, \overline{\text{SPR}}_{\text{M}-\text{H}} = \exp\left[\ln(\text{SPR}_{\text{M}-\text{H}}) \pm Z\sqrt{\text{Var}[\ln(\text{SPR}_{\text{M}-\text{H}})]}\right] \tag{7.11}$$

Example 7.8

The hypothetical data in Table 7–12 can be used to illustrate the computations involved in summary estimates of the prevalence difference and prevalence ratio. Data for only two age strata (<40 and ≥ 40 years) are presented to simplify the calculations. For the <40 years age stratum, the prevalence among the exposed

Table 7–12. Hypothetical example of cross-sectional data stratified according to age

Age group	Exposed	Non-exposed	Total
<40			
Disease	6	2	8
No disease	34	28	62
Total	40	30	70
≥ 40			
Disease	15	10	25
No disease	50	90	140
Total	65	100	165

and non-exposed are, respectively, 0.15 (= 6/40) and 0.07 (= 2/30), yielding a prevalence difference of 0.08 and a prevalence ratio of 2.1. For the older (≥ 40 years) stratum, the corresponding prevalences are 0.23 (= 15/65) for the exposed and 0.10 (= 10/100) for the non-exposed. Thus, among the older workers the prevalence difference is 0.13 and the prevalence ratio is 2.3.

We can compute the SPD using expressions (7.6) and (7.7). From expression (7.6), the variance for the <40 years stratum is $(6)(34)/(40)^3 + (2)(28)/(30)^3 = 0.0053$, and the variance for the ≥ 40 years stratum is $(15)(50)/(65)^3 + (10)(90)/(100)^3 = 0.0036$. Using the inverses of these variances as weights, SPD = $((1/0.0053)(0.08) + (1/0.0036)(0.13))/((1/0.0053) + (1/0.0036)) = 0.110$, which, as expected, is intermediate between the two stratum-specific prevalence differences. Applying expression (7.8) yields a 95-percent confidence interval of $\underline{SPD}$ = 0.019 and $\overline{SPD}$ = 0.201. The Mantel–Haenszel estimate for SPR [from expression (7.9)] is 2.29, and the Mantel–Haenszel chi-square [expression (6.2)] is 6.32. From expressions (7.10) and (7.11), the 95-percent confidence interval for SPR_{M-H} is 1.18, 4.64.

When there are more than two or three confounders, the stratified analysis methods described here may be difficult to apply because of small numbers in some strata. In this situation, mathematical modeling may be used (see Chapter 8). The best approach is to model the prevalence odds using logistic regression, as is done for case–control data.

5.2. Comparisons of Physiologic Variable Distributions

In some cross-sectional studies the health outcomes are continuously distributed physiologic variables rather than simply the presence or absence of disease or symptoms. Appropriate statistical analysis procedures are described in standard textbooks on regression analysis (Snedecor and Cochran, 1967; Kleinbaum and Kupper, 1978; Draper and Smith, 1981). The reader is referred to these texts to gain a comprehensive understanding of specific techniques and their underlying mathematical properties. The following section summarizes some practical methods for the analysis of data that are obtained in occupational cross-sectional studies of physiologic variability.

One-Time Survey Data

In the simplest situation one would compare distributions of physiologic variables (e.g., pulmonary function) between exposed workers and a comparison group. One common, and useful, first approach is to compare mean values between the groups. If a statistical test is desired, then Student's t-test for unmatched or matched data, depending on whether exposed workers and the comparison group have been matched, can be computed. The extension of the t-test to multiple exposure categories is analysis of variance (Draper and Smith, 1981), where an overall test of significance (F-test) is performed between the means of all the groups.

The t-test and analysis of variance F-test are only strictly suitable for normally distributed data. Some physiologic variables are not normally distributed, but a logarithmic transformation of the data may make the data more normally distributed.

The general method for examining the relationship between exposure and continuous health outcome variables is *multiple linear regression* analysis. The regression model takes the form

$$Y = B_0 + B_1X_1 + B_2X_2 + \cdot \cdot \cdot + B_kX_k + e \tag{7.12}$$

where Y represents the outcome variable, the X_i are the exposure and confounding variables, the B_i are their coefficients, and e is the random error term. B_0 is an intercept term that is merely the average value for the outcome variable for the entire group that would be seen if none of the exposure variables nor any of the confounders had any effect. The coefficients indicate the amount of change in the outcome variable *per unit change* of the exposure or confounder. Thus, the regression model estimates the effects of each independent variable (X_i) adjusted for the effects of all other variables in the model.

The simplest form of expression (7.12) is $Y = B_0 + B_1X$, in which X can take values of either 1 for exposed and 0 for non-exposed. (We have omitted the error term here.) If X is treated as a continuous variable (e.g., ppm of trichloroethylene), then the interpretation of B_1 is the incremental change to the outcome variable per unit of exposure (in this case, per ppm of trichloroethylene). As we have seen, it is sometimes only possible to assign ordinal exposure rankings. If, for example, we were comparing health outcome values between four exposure groups, then we would need three X variables (X_1, X_2, and X_3), each assuming values of 0 or 1 for exposed or non-exposed to a particular level. So, if we had four categories of trichloroethylene—<1.0, 1.0–2.4, 2.5–4.9, and ≥ 5 ppm—we would construct three exposure terms in the regression model as X_1, X_2, and X_3. Thus, a worker in the lowest category would be assigned values 0 for all three X terms, a worker in the second category (1.0–2.4 ppm) would be assigned a value of 1 for X_1 and 0 for each of the other X terms, and so forth. The coefficient for any one of the

Table 7-13. Multiple regression coefficients for pulmonary function variables in relation to cigarette smoking and years of uranium mining

	Independent variable	
Pulmonary function variable[a]	Current smoking[b]	Years underground mining
Forced expiratory volume in 1 sec	− 7.75	− 0.46
Maximal midexpiratory flow	− 10.85	− 0.93

Source: Samet et al. (1984).

[a]Percent of predicted value for healthy men.

[b]"1" for current smokers, "0" for all others.

X terms would then indicate the mean difference between that level and the lowest exposure level.

Example 7.9

In their study of respiratory disease among uranium miners, Samet et al. (1984) obtained spirometry measurements and correlated the results with years of uranium mining and cigarette smoking. A multiple regression analysis was used in which years of mining was treated as a continuous variable and smoking was categorized into a binary variable ($X = 1$ for current smokers and 0 otherwise). The results for two spirometry variables, FEV_1 and maximal mid-expiratory flow (MMEF), are shown in Table 7–13. Both lung function variables are expressed as percentages of predicted values derived from published standard equations for healthy men (Knudson et al., 1976). The coefficients for current smoking for both spirometry measures are larger in absolute value than the corresponding coefficients for exposure. The interpretation of the coefficient for years mining on FEV_1 is that there is a decrement of 0.46 percent of the predicted value for each year; thus, ten years of mining would be associated with a decrement of 4.6 percent of predicted.

Repeated-Survey Data Analysis

The most straightforward type of repeated survey is when health data are obtained from the same subjects at two points in time. This design is most applicable to the measurement of physiologic variables (continuous data). It is also possible to obtain repeated binary data (e.g., respiratory symptoms), but this is seldom done in occupational epidemiology. Therefore, we will focus the discussion on repeated surveys of physiologic variables.

Ordinarily, the repeated survey design assesses change in physiologic function over time, as illustrated by Example 7.2 concerning lung function in firefighters (Peters et al., 1974). The comparisons between two points in time require paired measurements in which the difference is computed for each individual. The paired design, wherein each subject serves as his own comparison, has the advantage of controlling for confounding from personal factors (e.g., smoking habit). Furthermore, differences in physiologic variables may be normally distributed even when the variables themselves are not. For example, platelet counts may be log normally distributed in a sample of workers, yet the difference between values measured at two points in time would be expected to approximate a normal distribution more closely. An exception to this generalization occurs when the variable changes over time in a predictable direction, irrespective of exposure status. Pulmonary function, for example, declines with age; thus, paired differences in pulmonary function measurements taken at two points in time may not be more normally distributed than values determined at one time.

A repeated measures survey may only include one exposed group yet still provide valid change estimates, provided that the outcome variable is not expected to change in a known direction. However, if it is known that the variable may change over time, irrespective of exposure (e.g., age or seasonal effects), then it is better to have a true comparison group from whom repeated measurements are also obtained at the same times as the exposed group. This is analogous to choosing a placebo group in a controlled therapeutic clinical trial. When only one exposed group is evaluated repeatedly, it must be assumed that the expected change of the outcome variable is zero. In general, a better estimate of the expected mean change can be obtained from the mean change occurring among the comparison group. Published data on physiologic variables may be used to generate predicted values when it is not possible to identify a suitable comparison group, in which case the changes can be expressed as percentages of predicted.

It is well recognized that when repeated measurements are made for physiologic variables, second and subsequent measurements for persons with initially extreme values tend to converge toward the group average. This phenomenon is known as *regression to the mean* (Davis, 1976). Regression to the mean only poses a problem for data interpretation in repeated surveys when subjects with extreme values are preferentially selected for repeated measurement. (This is often done in disease screening and treatment referral programs, such as blood pressure surveys.) Bias from regression to the mean is effectively eliminated when repeated measurements are made irrespective of initial values.

A repeated survey incorporating measurements made at more than two points in time requires more complicated computations that can be achieved using regression analysis. In principle, this analysis involves computing a regression slope for time on the outcome variable for each worker, obtaining an average slope for the group, and comparing this summary result with that of the reference group (Draper and Smith, 1981; Donner, 1984).

6. SOURCES OF BIAS IN CROSS-SECTIONAL STUDIES

In this section we discuss some of the biases that are most likely to pose problems in cross-sectional studies. In particular, we focus on the two main limitations of cross-sectional studies: the temporal relationship of exposure to disease and problems of studying prevalence rather than incidence.

6.1. Temporal Relationship of Exposure to Disease

Perhaps the strongest objection to cross-sectional studies has been the view that, relative to cohort and case–control studies, cross-sectional studies offer weak evidence for causality because one cannot be confident that the exposure preceded the disease. This objection has been raised in reference to the typical one-time survey design. The repeated-survey approach is really a form of cohort study, and thus has not been criticized on the issue of temporality.

The difficulty of examining causal associations in cross-sectional studies is illustrated in situations where it has been difficult to determine whether the exposure caused the disease or whether the association is spurious. A famous example of this is the study of the prevalence of cardiovascular disease among London bus drivers and conductors (Morris et al., 1953). The bus drivers, who were less physically active on the job than the conductors, had a higher prevalence of heart disease. However, the drivers' cardiovascular disease risk factors (e.g., obesity) and perhaps symptom manifestations were probably influential in their seeking jobs as drivers rather than as conductors, who have to maintain a greater level of physical exertion. Bias of this type is always of concern in cross-sectional studies that ascertain exposures simultaneously with disease. On the other hand, it is less important if prior exposure history can be obtained. Nonetheless, current exposure information may still be useful if there is reason to believe that current exposure is a reliable surrogate for past exposure. This situation would occur in an industry where there is little or no job mobility and exposure intensities or relative rankings had remained fairly constant over time.

6.2. Studying Disease Prevalence

The second major source of bias in cross-sectional studies is that they measure prevalence rather than incidence. Insofar as prevalence depends on both incidence and duration of disease, it is not always clear whether observed effects on prevalence pertain to incidence, duration, or both. For example, suppose that exposures in section A of a plant cause fatal coronary heart disease, whereas exposures in section B cause nonfatal coronary disease. A cross-sectional study might reveal a higher prevalence of coronary disease among workers in section B, even if the combined incidence of coronary heart disease (fatal and nonfatal) were the same in both sections of the plant. This type of bias can be avoided by conducting a full cohort study, which would involve a far greater cost than a cross-sectional study. Alternatively, the potential for such bias in a cross-sectional study may be reduced by restricting the study to nonfatal yet persistent health conditions.

6.3. Selection Bias

In Sections 6.1 and 6.2 we have reviewed the main sources of bias that are specific to cross-sectional studies. Other types of bias are not unique to cross-sectional studies but are considered here briefly. Selection bias is discussed first.

Figure 7–3 depicts a simple, hypothetical example of a cross-sectional study comparing disease prevalence in exposed and non-exposed workers. If the study were conducted in 1980 (t_1), then the prevalence among the exposed would be 0.3 (= 30/100) and the prevalence among the non-exposed would be 0.10 (= 10/100), giving a prevalence difference of 0.20 and a prevalence ratio of 3.0. Assume that the exposure is causally related to disease, as reflected by the 1980 results, that the disease is a persistent condition (i.e., does not resolve on removal from exposure), and that the disease becomes severe enough to force 20 percent of affected workers to leave employment from the industry altogether. Now, if the study had been conducted in 1985 (t_2) instead of 1980, and the events indicated for the intervening years had occurred, then an entirely different picture arises. Specifically, 20 percent of diseased workers

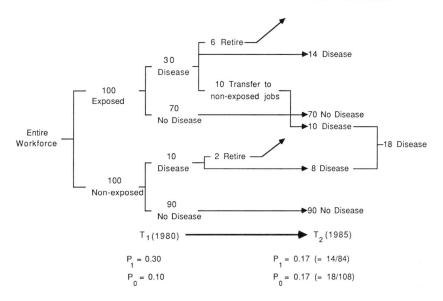

Figure 7–3. Hypothetical example of selection bias in a cross-sectional study.

in both the exposed and non-exposed had left employment, ten cases from the exposed transferred to the non-exposed jobs, possibly because their conditions were exacerbated by continued exposure, and no new cases occurred in either group. (This last assumption is a contrivance used to simplify the example.) Thus, in 1985 there would be no difference in the prevalences of the exposed and non-exposed workers; the prevalence among the exposed and non-exposed, respectively, would be $0.17 (= 14/84)$ and $0.17 (= 18/108)$. The difference in results for these two cross-sectional studies arises because there is selective migration among the diseased workers out of the exposed to the non-exposed jobs, with the net effect being an underestimated exposure effect at the second survey. It could be argued that a cross-sectional study performed at any single point in time is likely to suffer from selection bias of the type illustrated in Figure 7–3. This could go undetected unless the investigator attempts to obtain both past and current exposure data.

From the foregoing it should be apparent that subject selection in cross-sectional studies can pose major validity problems. Careful characterization of workers' current and prior exposures to occupational and nonoccupational factors can help to minimize bias resulting from workers having changed job categories within the industry but cannot remove bias due to workers having terminated employment. Also, studies of actively employed workers usually suffer from the Healthy Worker Effect when comparisons are made against an external reference population.

The most prominent shortcoming of many cross-sectional studies is that they include only actively employed workers. Limiting the study to active workers, although usually dictated by feasibility constraints, may produce misleading results when the disease of interest is a delayed exposure effect that becomes more severe with the passage of time, even after exposure ceases, or when early disease symptoms cause workers to terminate employment. As an example, cross-sectional studies of the prevalence of silicosis are ordinarily conducted on active workers (Rice et al., 1986); thus, the prevalence and severity of the disease are likely to be underestimated. Continued surveillance of workers with occupational diseases is one approach to obtain more complete data; however, maintaining contact with terminated workers and monitoring their health status tends to be a costly endeavor. Occupational disease registers [e.g., Westerholm's (1980) register of silicotics] are valuable in this regard.

Self-selection into a cross-sectional study can also be a source of bias if workers have special motivations for agreeing or refusing to participate. Workers who are concerned about their health because of disease symptoms or intense exposures may be more likely than other workers to participate. Alternatively, workers who suspect that they are experiencing job-related morbidity may be fearful of participating if the detection of disease will force them to retire or transfer to less desirable jobs. As a check on self-selection bias, one should try to obtain data on demographic and occupational variables for workers who do and do not agree to participate in the study. Comparisons between participants and nonparticipants may reveal possible selection biases. Subtle motivational influences on participation are likely to be undetectable, however.

6.4. Information Bias

As in other study designs, exposure and/or disease misclassification can occur when the source of one or both is limited to reports provided by the workers included in the study. Obtaining exposure or health data from what are hoped to be objective sources (e.g., urine bioassays for exposure, laboratory tests for health outcome data) and verifying data with alternative sources are advisable when practical. Over- or underreporting of disease symptoms or exposures on questionnaires can be checked to some extent by including irrelevant questions. The pattern of responses to the "bogus" questions gives an indication of a worker's proclivity to exaggerate or under-state his or her responses.

7. PLANNING A CROSS-SECTIONAL STUDY

7.1. Data Requirements

The decision to initiate a cross-sectional study, rather than another type of epidemiologic design, is guided by the health outcome of interest. As we have stated earlier, some health conditions can only be studied using a cross-sectional design or a repeated-survey approach. Nonfatal conditions that are relatively common (i.e., at least 5-percent prevalence) and relatively persistent states are the most suitable.

There can be several motivations for conducting cross-sectional studies. First, there may be an interest on the part of management or workers to conduct periodic or routine health and exposure monitoring. In this case, a cross-sectional study may not necessarily address questions of disease etiology, but may serve as a surveillance program for excessive exposures and disease prevalence. Of course, there will be a need for careful consideration of the types and amounts of data that should be collected. In spite of the availability of computer storage and data retrieval systems, indiscriminate col-lection of data can yield diminishing returns if data systems become overloaded with information that may never be used. A selective data collection scheme should be adopted in a surveillance program, so that data collection and storage are restricted to the most rele-vant items. For example, if we are planning to implement a medical and exposure monitoring system for workers in an automotive bat-tery factory, then primary consideration should be given to the exposures of greatest potential harm (e.g., lead, cadmium, acid mists) and the most strongly suspected health outcomes (e.g., pul-monary impairment, kidney dysfunction). Data on other health and exposure factors can be collected as resources permit. This selective approach permits subsequent cross-sectional studies to be con-ducted in a cost- and time-efficient manner.

A second reason to conduct a cross-sectional study is to investi-gate health problems suggested by workers' reports of discomfort or morbidity. One should make special efforts to ensure that studies performed in response to symptom or disease "outbreaks" are designed and executed in an unbiased manner. This means that sub-ject selection should be extended beyond inclusion of just the workers who report adverse exposure or health conditions or volunteers with particular motivations. Also, suitable comparison subjects should be obtained whenever possible.

The third reason to conduct a cross-sectional study is to address questions of disease etiology. Previous epidemiologic or toxicologic research may indicate deleterious consequences of exposure. Thus, a cross-sectional study on a group of exposed workers may be an attractive and logical next step. The informativeness of the study will be determined by the presence of exposure gradients in the workplace or the availability of appropriate external comparison groups, the ability to characterize exposures, and the availability of sensitive indicators of change in health status.

7.2. Subject Selection

We have stressed the value of including workers with the highest exposures as well as a non-exposed comparison group in a cross-sectional study. Worker participation is also an important consideration when planning a study. Obviously, a study that involves invasive medical maneuvers or lengthy questionnaires stands less chance of worker acceptance than a clearly focused study that does not create discomfort or inconvenience to workers. Ethical concerns also come into play. Although all epidemiologic studies should assure confidentiality of sensitive information, maintaining confidentiality is especially significant in cross-sectional studies because they usually involve more intensive medical examination and personal data collection than other study designs. Workers should also be apprised at the outset of the purposes of the study. If the health measurement to be made has no clear clinical implication, then this should be so stated. For instance, sister chromatid exchange levels are useful for detecting exposures to some mutagens, but an increased level in a worker's lymphocytes does not necessarily predict an elevated cancer risk (Vainio, 1985). Studies that are purely of research interest should be presented as such, even at the risk of reducing subject participation.

8. SUMMARY OF ADVANTAGES AND LIMITATIONS OF OCCUPATIONAL CROSS-SECTIONAL STUDIES

The principal advantage of cross-sectional studies is that they are the most suitable epidemiologic means for studying nonfatal diseases and effects on physiologic variables. Additionally, repeated surveys, in which health and exposure data are determined for the same workers at various times, offer possibilities for assessing short- and long-term physiologic changes.

Another important advantage of cross-sectional studies is that they permit collection of data on confounders directly from workers, rather than from proxy respondents, as often occurs in case–control studies. Data on confounding variables, especially nonoccupational risk factors, are seldom available in cohort mortality studies. Finally, cross-sectional studies can be incorporated into ongoing surveillance programs, thus permitting screening for impaired health or excessive exposure.

The general perception of the main weakness of cross-sectional studies is that this design is less appropriate for investigating causal associations than cohort or case–control studies. One reason for this view is that cross-sectional studies measure disease prevalence, which is affected by determinants of incidence and disease duration. Thus, inferences drawn from cross-sectional studies involve additional assumptions to those required in other epidemiologic designs that measure incidence. Other limitations are not the result of an intrinsic defect in the cross-sectional design; rather, they occur because of incomplete exposure data or the failure to include all of the workers who theoretically should be studied. Specifically, some cross-sectional studies are restricted to correlating health and exposure data where both are obtained at the time of the study. Proper accounting of past exposures in the design and analysis should mitigate the problem of incomplete data.

The principal shortcoming of most cross-sectional studies is that they are confined to actively employed workers. Consequently, disease prevalence or severity is underestimated, especially for diseases that continue to progress after exposure cessation. Moreover, many cross-sectional studies are subject to a Healthy Worker Effect bias, again because they are limited to actively employed workers. These problems arise because of the difficulties associated with tracing and examining terminated workers, some of whom may be at greatest risk for disease.

Repeated surveys can provide more conclusive evidence for causal associations with exposures than one-time surveys, but the gains in information need to be balanced against added costs and logistical problems.

Glossary

one-time survey   Cross-sectional study conducted at one point in time.
prevalence   Number of cases in a population at one point in time (point prevalence) or during some specified time interval (period prevalence).

prevalence difference   Prevalence among exposed workers minus prevalence among non-exposed comparison group.

prevalence odds   The proportion of persons with disease divided by the proportion without disease.

prevalence odds ratio   The prevalence odds in the exposed divided by the prevalence odds in the non-exposed.

prevalence ratio   Prevalence among exposed workers divided by the prevalence among non-exposed workers.

repeated survey   Study where health (and sometimes exposure) data are measured at multiple points in time, usually on the same group of workers.

Notation

D Average duration of disease
I Incidence rate
N_{0i} Number of non-exposed subjects in the ith stratum
N_{1i} Number of exposed subjects in the ith stratum
P_0 Prevalence among the non-exposed
P_1 Prevalence among the exposed
PD_i Prevalence difference in the ith stratum
PR_i Prevalence ratio in the ith stratum
SPD   Standardized prevalence difference (e.g., inverse variance weighted average of stratum-specific PD_i).
SPR   Standardized prevalence ratio (e.g., Mantel–Haenszel weighted average of PR_i).

References

Archer VE, Wagoner JK, and Lundin F (1973): Uranium mining and cigarette smoking effects on man. *J Occup Med* 15: 204–11.

Axford AT, McKerrow CB, Parry-Jones A, and LeQuesne PM (1976): Accidental exposure to isocyanate fumes in a group of firemen. *Br J Ind Med* 33:65–71.

Berry G (1974): Longitudinal observations: their usefulness and limitations with special reference to the forced expiratory volume. *Bull Eur Physiopathol Respir10:643–655.*

Cotes JE (1975): *Lung Function Assessment and Application in Medicine*, 3rd ed. Oxford: Blackwell Scientific Publications.

Davis CE (1976): The effect of regression to the mean in epidemiologic and clinical studies. *Am J Epidemiol* 104:493–498.

Donner A (1984): Linear regression analysis with repeated measurements. *J Chron Dis* 37:441–448.

Draper NR, and Smith H (1981): *Applied Regression Analysis*. New York: John Wiley & Sons.

Elandt-Johnson RC (1975): Definition of rates: some remarks on their use and misuse. *Am J Epidemiol* 102:267–271.

Freeman J, and Hutchison GB (1980): Prevalence, incidence and duration. *Am J Epidemiol* 112:707–723.

Greenland S, and Robins JM (1985): Estimation of a common effect parameter from sparse follow-up data. *Biometrics* 41:55–68.

Kelsey JL, Thompson WD, and Evans AS (1986): *Methods in Observational Epidemiology.* New York: Oxford University Press.

Kleinbaum DG, and Kupper LL (1978): *Applied Regression Analysis and Other Multivariable Techniques.* Scituate, MA: Duxbury Press.

Kleinbaum DG, Kupper LL, and Morgenstern H (1982): *Epidemiologic Research: Principles and Quantitative Methods.* Belmont, CA: Lifetime Learning Publications.

Knudson RJ, Slatin RC, Lebowitz MD, and Burrows B (1976): The maximal expiratory flow-volume curve: normal standards, variability and effects of age. *Am Rev Respir Dis* 113:587–600.

Mantel N, and Haenszel W (1959): Statistical aspects of the analysis of data from retrospective studies of disease. *J Natl Cancer Inst* 22:719–748.

Miettinen OS (1976): Estimability and estimation in case-referent studies. *Am J Epidemiol* 103:226–235.

Miyashita K, Shomi S, Itoh N, et al. (1983): Epidemiological study of vibration syndrome in response to total hand-tool operating time. *Br J Ind Med* 40:92–98.

Morris JN, Heady JA, Raffle AB, et al. (1953): Coronary heart disease and physical activity at work. *Lancet* 2:1053–1057.

National Center for Health Statistics (1973): *Plan and Operation of the Health and Nutrition Examination Survey, United States 1971–1973.* Washington, D.C. Series 1, No. 109.

Peters JM, Theriault GP, Fine LJ, and Wegman DH (1974): Chronic effect of fire fighting on pulmonary function. *N Engl J Med* 291:1320–1322.

Rice CH, Harris RL, Checkoway H, and Symons MJ (1986): Dose-response for silicosis from a case-control study of North Carolina Dusty Trades workers. In: Goldsmith DF, Winn DM, and Shy CM (eds.) *Silica, Silicosis and Cancer: Controversy in Occupational Medicine.* New York: Praeger Scientific Publications.

Robins JM, Breslow NE, and Greenland S (1986): Estimation of the Mantel–Haenszel variance consistent with both sparse data and large strata limiting models. *Biometrics* 42:311–323.

Rothman KJ (1986): *Modern Epidemiology.* Boston, MA: Little, Brown & Co.

Samet JM, Young RA, Morgan MV, et al. (1984): Prevalence survey of respiratory abnormalities in New Mexico uranium miners. *Health Phys* 46:361–370.

Sarto F, Cominato I, Pinton AM, et al. (1984): A cytogenetic study on workers exposed to low concentrations of benzene. *Carcinogenesis* 6:827–832.

Sjogren B, and Ulfvarson U (1985): Respiratory symptoms and pulmonary function among welders working with aluminum, stainless steel and railroad tracks. *Scand J Work Environ Health* 11:27–32.

Snedecor GW, and Cochran WG (1967): *Statistical Methods,* 6th ed., Ames: Iowa State University Press.

Sterling TD, and Weinkam JJ (1985): The "healthy worker effect" on morbidity rates. *J Occup Med* 27:477–482.

Vainio H (1985): Current trends in the biological monitoring of exposure to carcinogens. *Scand J Work Environ Health* 11:1–6.

Westerholm P (1980): Silicosis: observations on a case register. *Scand J Work Environ Health* 6(Suppl 2):34–36.

8 Advanced Statistical Analysis

1. OVERVIEW

The analytic methods presented in Chapters 5–7 are adequate for many occupational epidemiology studies, particularly those in which a simple exposed versus non-exposed classification is used. However, stratified analyses may not be feasible if there are multiple exposure categories or more than two or three confounders. This chapter presents an overview of the mathematical models useful for analyzing occupational cohort data. Readers requiring a more formal and detailed statistical presentation are referred to standard texts (e.g., Breslow and Day, 1980, 1987; Kalbfleisch and Prentice, 1980). Emphasis is placed on analyses involving time-related factors. We begin by presenting an overview of the importance of considering the temporal relationship of exposure and disease. The general form of the exponential model is introduced for the situation where there are two levels of one main exposure variable and the only potential confounder is age. The specific forms of Poisson regression, the Cox proportional hazards model, and logistic regression are then defined and related to the corresponding stratified methods presented in earlier chapters. Various aspects of model definition are then considered, including variable specification, estimation of joint effects, and regression diagnostics. These models are illustrated with data from the asbestos textile workers study by Dement et al. (1983). Finally, the advantages and limitations of mathematical modeling are summarized.

2. IMPORTANCE OF TIME-RELATED ANALYSIS

The term *time-related factors* refers to important determinants of disease risk that vary as a person ages (Thomas, 1983). In many occupational studies, one important time-related factor is cumulative exposure that can change as a worker accumulates exposure over

232

time. In Chapter 5 we noted the problems of analyses that do not take the time pattern of exposure into account (e.g., when all the person-time of a worker is allocated to the highest cumulative exposure category attained). By incorrect attribution of person-years, the fixed analysis results in a dampened exposure–response curve (Enterline, 1976).

It is also important that confounders be analyzed in a time-related manner (Pearce et al., 1986). The time-related confounders that have been most frequently considered include age at risk, calendar year, and length of follow-up. These all change as a worker is followed over time. Age at hire is often considered together with these factors, although it is a fixed rather than a time-related factor. Duration of employment can also be a confounder in occupational studies, although its inclusion in the model is of debatable value (see Chapter 4). Employment duration is often used as a surrogate for cumulative exposure when exposure intensity data are not available. When such data are available, duration of employment often is highly correlated with cumulative exposure. Thus, inclusion of both variables in the model is redundant.

3. GENERAL LINEAR MODELS

The general analytical approach considered here involves modeling some function of disease occurrence as a linear combination of various risk factors. The model takes the general form

$$f(Y) = b_0 + b_1 X_1 + b_2 X_2 + \cdots + b_j X_j + e \qquad (8.1)$$

where Y can represent the risk, rate, or odds of disease in persons with characteristics $X_1, X_2, \ldots, X_j$ and e is the random error term, representing an assumed random departure from the value of $f(Y)$. For convenience, e is omitted from subsequent equations. One option is to let $f(Y) = Y$ (i.e., to use the actual measure of disease as the dependent variable). However, this approach is rarely used because the risk, rate, or odds of disease cannot be less than zero, and the disease risk cannot be greater than one.

Models of the type depicted in equation (8.1) theoretically can give values much larger than 1.0 or much smaller than zero. Hence, the model is usually restricted to estimating the rate or odds of disease, and a logarithmic transformation is used so that the dependent variable in the model is $\ln(Y)$. This transformation yields a function that has a theoretical range of minus infinity to plus infinity. The family of models employing a logarithmic transformation is particularly suited to ratio, or multiplicative, measures of effect (Breslow et al., 1983; Whittemore, 1985). We concentrate on this family of models, since it is the one most commonly used in occupational epidemiology. It should also be noted that there are often good reasons for using difference (additive) measures of effect (see Chapter 4).

3.1. The Exponential Model

The transformed model can be written in the form

$$Y = \exp(b_0 + b_1 X_1 + b_2 X_2 + \cdots + b_j X_j) \tag{8.2}$$

Note that if all the X_i's are zero then $Y = \exp(b_0)$. Thus, $\exp(b_0)$ estimates the rate or odds of disease in persons with zero values for each of the X_i's. (This situation is denoted as Y_0.) Thus, the model can be formulated as

$$\frac{Y}{Y_0} = \exp(b_1 X_1 + b_2 X_2 + \cdots + b_j X_j) \tag{8.3}$$

We will first examine the simple situation where exposure is dichotomous and represented by X_1 ($X_1 = 1$ if exposed, $X_1 = 0$ if non-exposed), and the only confounder is age, which is stratified into two levels and represented by X_2 (e.g., $X_2 = 1$ if age ≥ 55 years; $X_2 = 0$ if age < 55 years). Thus, when age is included in the analysis, the model for the exposed subgroup ($X_1 = 1$) is

$$\frac{Y_E}{Y_0} = \exp(b_1 + b_2) \tag{8.4}$$

and the model for the non-exposed group ($X_1 = 0$) is

$$\frac{Y_{\bar{E}}}{Y_0} = \exp(b_2) \tag{8.5}$$

Dividing equation (8.5) into equation (8.4) yields the rate ratio (R) or odds ratio of disease in exposed persons relative to non-exposed persons:

$$R = \exp(b_1) \tag{8.6}$$

The general term *relative risk* is used to denote such ratio effect measures.

Just as one variable was needed to denote a factor with two levels, $k - 1$ variables are needed to denote a factor with k levels. The reference (non-exposed) category is assigned scores of zero for each of the $k - 1$ indicator variables. The coefficient for a particular exposure category, when exponentiated, estimates the relative risk for the category compared to the reference category. The model does not distinguish between the main exposure(s) and confounders; they are all modeled as "risk factors," and the coefficient for any factor estimates its effect, controlling for all other factors in the model. Hence, creating variables to specify multiple levels of confounders is similar to that for the main exposure.

3.2. Maximum Likelihood Estimation

The simple model presented here is analogous to the familiar methods for stratified data described in Chapter 5, in which stratum-specific estimates are combined as a weighted average, such as the standardized rate ratio (Miettinen, 1972) or the Mantel–Haenszel summary odds ratio (Mantel and Haenszel, 1959). However, in this instance a summary relative risk estimate is obtained by the method of *maximum likelihood*. (Maximum likelihood methods can also be used in a stratified analysis, but the computations are complex.) This method is based on the *likelihood function,* which represents the probability of observing the data as a function of the unknown parameters $(b_0, b_1, \ldots, b_j)$. Initial estimates of the unknown parameters (usually, $b_i = 0$ for each i) are made, and these are inserted into the likelihood function to derive new estimates that increase the value of the likelihood function. (For practical reasons the logarithm of the likelihood function is generally used, but this does not change the parameter estimates.) This process is repeated until the values of b_i ($i = 1 \ldots j$) are found that maximize the likelihood function. These are the *maximum likelihood estimates* of the parameters.

In most situations maximum likelihood estimates can only be obtained with a computer. They do not involve any directly weighted average of the stratum-specific effect estimates (like the Mantel–Haenszel estimator), but they are similar to weighted averages in the sense that more weight is effectively given to larger strata. Maximum likelihood estimation also yields standard errors for the parameters that can be used to calculate confidence intervals. For example, if the exposure variable coefficient (b_1) is 0.693, then the relative risk estimate is $\exp(0.693) = 2.0$. If the coefficient has a standard error of 0.124, then the 90-percent confidence interval is

$$\underline{R}, \overline{R} = \exp(0.693 \pm 1.645 \times 0.124)$$

where 1.645 is the appropriate standard normal deviate for 90-percent confidence intervals.

The maximized value of the logarithm of the likelihood can also be used to obtain the *log likelihood statistic,* also known as the *deviance,* by subtracting twice the maximized log likelihood from zero. The log likelihood does not itself have a well-defined distribution, but differences in the log likelihoods for different models may be interpreted as chi-square values (Breslow and Day, 1980). Such likelihood inference usually involves a nested hierarchy of models. For example, if one model contains age and another contains age and cumulative exposure, then the contribution of cumulative exposure to the model can be assessed by comparing the log likelihood statistics for the two models. This is known as the *likelihood ratio test.*

Maximum likelihood estimation can be performed with most standard statistical packages (Wallenstein and Bodian, 1987). Packages commonly used for analyzing occupational epidemiology studies include GLIM (Baker and Nelder, 1978) and various Statistical Analysis System (SAS) programs (Harrell 1983a, 1983b).

3.3. Other Models

The exponential models discussed here are the most frequently used in occupational epidemiology, but many alternatives are available. A simple linear regression is frequently used when the outcome is represented by a continuous variable (e.g., in cross-sectional studies). More generally, Thomas (1981), Guerrero and Johnson (1982), and Breslow and Storer (1985) have proposed families of models that include the linear (additive) and exponential (multiplicative) models as special cases. For example, the model of Guerrero and Johnson takes the form

$$\log R = \begin{cases} \dfrac{\log[1 + \lambda(b_1 X_1 + b_2 X_2 + \cdots)]}{\lambda}, & \lambda \neq 0 \\ b_1 X_1 + b_2 X_2 + \cdots, & \lambda = 0 \end{cases} \tag{8.7}$$

where R is the relative risk and λ is the mixture parameter that determines the assumption regarding joint effects of exposures and confounders. When $\lambda = 0$ the model corresponds to multiplicative relative risk [the exponential model in equation (8.3)]. When $\lambda = 1$ the model corresponds to additive relative risk [equation (8.1) when $f(Y) = Y$]. The model is applied separately for a range of values of λ to estimate the value of λ that best reflects the pattern of joint effects in the data. Although these models are generally fitted using GLIM (Baker and Nelder, 1978), they can also be fitted using other standard programs (Wallenstein and Bodian, 1987).

Table 8-1. Separate and joint relative risks
of two factors

| | | Factor 2 | |
		No	Yes
	No	1.0	3.0
Factor 1		(R_{00})	(R_{01})
	Yes	2.0	4.1
		(R_{10})	(R_{11})

These models are of considerable theoretical interest and have the advantage of not requiring specific interaction terms for estimating joint effects. However, this is usually only a minor advantage (particularly if the assessment of interaction is not an analytic goal). Also there are several problems with these families of models. First, the models generate a global assessment of joint effect (i.e., they assess the overall combined effects of all factors in the model rather than just the specific factors of interest). Furthermore, the Breslow–Storer and Guerrero–Johnson approaches combine models that differ both in the form of dose–response model (linear versus exponential) and the form of joint effects (e.g., additive or multiplicative). This makes the parameter λ difficult to interpret for continuous variables, but it is not a problem for categorical variables. By contrast, Thomas' (1981) model does allow for the separation of the form of dose–response model and the form of joint effects. A second problem with these models is that the findings can be difficult to interpret without interpolating back to a categorical table of separate and joint effects (such as Table 8–1). Finally, the models of Thomas (1981) and Breslow and Storer (1985) may produce quite different results (and interpretations) as a result of minor changes in the coding of the variables (Moolgavkar and Venzon, 1987). For these reasons, it is generally easier to use the simpler exponential (or additive) models described here and to include one or more interaction terms if it is desired to estimate the joint effects of two or more factors.

4. SPECIFIC APPLICATIONS

4.1. Poisson Regression

Figure 8–1 illustrates eight hypothetical workers in an occupational cohort. It differs from those depicted in Chapter 5 in that an age

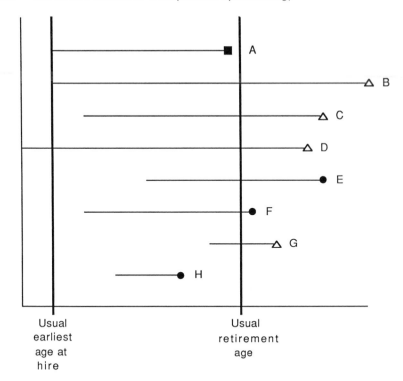

Figure 8–1. Follow-up outcomes of eight hypothetical workers (■ = cancer death, ● = other death, △ = lost to follow-up).

axis, rather than a calendar year axis, has been used to facilitate the calculation of age-specific incidence rates. Thus, each worker is depicted according to age at hire, age at termination, and age at death. If the person-years are accumulated and grouped into age strata, then an age-standardized rate ratio (SRR) can be obtained as

$$\text{SRR} = \frac{\sum \lambda_{1i} N_{0i}}{\sum \lambda_{0i} N_{0i}} \tag{8.8}$$

where λ_{1i} and λ_{0i} are the incidence rates in the exposed and non-exposed groups, respectively, and N_{0i} is the number of person-years in the non-exposed subgroup of age stratum i.

Poisson regression is an extension of this simple analysis. Assume that the rate ratio (R) is constant across strata. Then $\lambda_{1i} = R\lambda_{01}$ in each stratum i, and the standardized rate ratio (SRR) can be formulated as

$$\text{SRR} = \frac{\sum R\lambda_{0i} N_{0i}}{\sum \lambda_{0i} N_{0i}} = R \tag{8.9}$$

It can be shown (Frome and Checkoway, 1985) that it is this quantity (R) that is estimated in Poisson regression when the model fits the data well. The observed number of deaths in each exposure–age stratum is limited by the number of persons in the cohort, whereas a true Poisson variate can theoretically assume very large values. In the ideal situation where follow-up is complete, the total number of deaths is fixed, since all cohort members eventually die. The uncertainty (i.e., random variation) lies in the number of person-years that each subject will contribute before death. However, the appropriate likelihood function is proportional to that obtained by treating the person-years as fixed and the observed deaths as a Poisson variate. This latter approach is used for statistical convenience (Berry et al., 1983; Whittemore, 1985). The model has the general form

$$\frac{\lambda}{\lambda_0} = \exp(b_1 X_1 + b_2 X_2 + \cdots + b_j X_j) \tag{8.10}$$

where λ is the incidence rate for persons with specified values of X_1, $X_2, \ldots, X_j$ and the baseline incidence rate is λ_0. Standard statistical packages (e.g., GLIM) use unconditional maximum likelihood methods for Poisson regression. These yield identical estimates to those that would have been obtained using the more computationally complex conditional likelihood estimators, which assume that the number of cases in each stratum is fixed (Anderson, 1970; Greenland and Robins, 1985). Hence, unlike unconditional logistic regression (see the following discussion), the rate ratio estimates obtained by Poisson regression are not affected by small numbers in particular strata.

Poisson regression can also be formulated as an extension of SMR analyses (Breslow et al., 1983). In this instance the model takes the form

$$\frac{\text{Obs}}{\text{Exp}} = \exp(b_1 X_1 + b_2 X_2 + \cdots + b_j X_j) \tag{8.11}$$

where Obs is the observed number of events and Exp is the expected number, based on some set of standard rates such as national mortality or incidence rates. However, this approach can be cumbersome computationally and may suffer from the noncomparability of SMRs, which lack a common standard (see Chapter 5). Even when the SMRs are comparable, regression analyses of this type may be biased because the outcome variable is age-adjusted, whereas the predictor variables are not (Rosenbaum and Rubin, 1984). Hence, we do not discuss this approach further.

4.2. The Proportional Hazards Model

Consider Figure 8–1 again and suppose that age is considered to be a strong confounder. In order to obtain the greatest possible control over confounding by age, it might be considered desirable to stratify very finely on age, using months or weeks rather than years. Then each age stratum would contain at most one event: either a case of the disease of interest, a death from some other cause, or a withdrawal due to loss to follow-up. Many strata would contain no cases and thus would contribute no information to the analysis (since the rate ratio is not calculable if no cases occur). Thus, if there were 35 cases, then the analysis would involve 35 age strata, each containing just one case and the person-time experience from which it arose. Since all other persons "at risk" survived through the narrow age interval during which the corresponding case occurred, the analysis involves comparing the exposure history of the case with those of all persons who were "at risk" of becoming a case at the age at which the case developed. As in the person-time approach, each worker is classified according to his or her exposure history at that particular age. Hence, the exposure history of a worker who became a case at age 54 years and six months would be compared to those of all workers who were "at risk" at age 54 years and six months, and the comparison would not consider exposures received at subsequent ages.

This is the type of comparison made in the most common variant of the *proportional hazards model* (Cox, 1972). Thus, it can be noted that the Poisson regression model converges to the proportional hazards model as the age strata are made infinitely small. The term *proportional hazards model* is sometimes confined to models in which the baseline incidence rate has a specific functional form. However, the most commonly used estimation procedure is that based on Cox's (1975) partial likelihood function in which the baseline incidence rate is treated as an unknown "nuisance" parameter. The model has the general form

$$\frac{\lambda(t)}{\lambda_0(t)} = \exp(b_1 X_1 + b_2 X_2 + \cdots + b_j X_j) \tag{8.12}$$

where t represents age; $\lambda(t)$ is the incidence rate at age t in persons with specified values of $X_1, X_2, \ldots, X_j$; and $\lambda_0(t)$ is the unknown baseline incidence rate at age t. The major difference between this model and Poisson regression [expression (8.9)] is that Poisson regression commonly involves only a few strata, whereas the proportional hazards model creates a stratum for each case. These age strata are not explicitly included as terms in the proportional hazards model. Instead, age is the "time" variable that is used to define the set of persons "at risk" at the time (age) that each case became a case. The underlying relationship of the incidence rate with age is thus treated as an unknown nuisance function, and the rate ratio is assumed to be independent of age [i.e., it is assumed that each risk factor multiplies the (unknown) underlying age-specific rate].

This presentation of Cox's model differs from some others (e.g., Kalbfleisch and Prentice, 1980) in two main respects. First, Cox's model has been presented as an extension of Poisson regression rather than as a special case of survival analysis. In fact, Cox's estimation procedure can be viewed from either perspective, but in occupational studies it is more straightforward to view it as an extension of simple incidence rate analysis. Second, because of its original derivation from studies of survival of patients in clinical trials, survival time (length of follow-up) is often used as the time variable. However, Breslow et al. (1983) have argued that it is more appropriate to use age as the time variable in cohort studies because death rates rise rapidly with age, and age effects should be controlled as precisely as possible. By contrast, length of follow-up is generally highly correlated with duration of exposure and hence with cumulative exposure. This recommendation has been followed here.

4.3. Logistic Regression

The observation that the proportional hazards model requires creating a separate stratum for each case suggests that the model can be conceptualized as a specific form of stratified analysis, analogous to case–control analysis of matched data. In fact, the procedure for defining the risk sets involved in each proportional hazards comparison is identical to that of incidence density matching in case–control studies (Prentice and Breslow, 1978), where, for each case, controls are selected at random from the set of all persons "at risk" at the time (age) at which the case occurred. This readily suggests a related model, known as *logistic regression,* where Y is the odds of a person being a case ($= P/(1 - P)$, where P is the proportion of persons who are cases, and the effect measure of interest is the odds ratio. Logistic regression is thus the modeling analogue of the Mantel–Haenszel procedure (Mantel and Haenszel, 1959).

The logistic regression model takes the form

$$\frac{P_1/(1 - P_1)}{P_0/(1 - P_0)} = \exp(b_1X_1 + b_2X_2 + \cdots + b_jX_j) \qquad (8.13)$$

where P_0 is the proportion of non-exposed persons who are cases and P_1 is the proportion of exposed persons who are cases. It should be noted that several texts present expression (8.13) in the alternative form

$$P(X) = \frac{\exp(b_0 + b_1X_1 + b_2X_2 + \cdots + b_jX_j)}{1 + \exp(b_0 + b_1X_1 + b_2X_2 + \cdots + b_jX_j)} \qquad (8.14)$$

where $P(X)$ is the proportion of persons with characteristics X ($=X_1, X_2, \ldots$) who are cases.

When controls are sampled from the risk sets for each case and this matching is retained in the analysis, the *conditional* logistic likelihood function is identical to that for the proportional hazards model (Kalbfleisch and Prentice, 1980). This function is based on the likelihood of the observed data, *given* the marginal totals in each stratum. It can be used to analyze the entire risk set for each case and gives identical results to the proportional hazards model. However, logistic regression is more commonly used when a case–control study has been designed by sampling from these risk sets. When matching has been conducted on a number of factors and genuine "pairs" exist (e.g., twins), a fully matched analysis, using conditional logistic regression, is appropriate. However, when matching has only been performed on general factors such as age and gender, an individually matched analysis and a stratified analysis yield equally valid findings, but the latter provides a more precise effect estimate (McKinlay, 1977; Thomas and Greenland, 1983). The conditional estimation procedure can still be used, but it is computationally difficult and often is very expensive to perform when individual strata include large numbers of cases and noncases. Hence, the *unconditional* estimation procedure is generally used when the strata are large.

Logistic regression is most commonly used in case–control studies, but it originally was developed for cohort studies involving cumulative incidence comparisons (Cornfield, 1962). Persons are classified as to whether they experienced the event of interest, but the time of the event is not considered. Additionally, each worker is classified according to his or her final cumulative exposure, and final values of confounders, such as age and length of follow-up.

In a cohort analysis, logistic regression should only be used for the study of rare diseases in fixed cohorts, in which each worker has the same potential follow-up time and there are no time-related factors. However, as noted in Chapter 5, most occupational populations are dynamic, and the analysis should take that into account. Even in studies of rare diseases in fixed cohorts, the logistic model may yield effect estimates that are too large if the follow-up period is relatively long (Abbott, 1985). This problem can be minimized by dividing the follow-up period into discrete intervals and employing Cox's (1972) discrete time proportional hazards model. This approach can be applied using standard logistic regression programs (Breslow, 1986) and is closely related to the form of Mantel–Haenszel analysis known as the log-rank test (Mantel, 1966).

5. DEFINING THE MODEL

5.1. Introduction

General approaches to data analysis—including the control of confounding, effect modification, and induction and latency analyses—have been discussed in previous chapters in the context of stratified analysis. The same considerations apply when using mathematical modeling. However, the added complexity and analytical power of mathematical modeling raises additional issues that may need to be considered when defining the model. These include variable specification, estimation of joint effects, and regression diagnostics.

5.2. Exposure

It is generally preferable to use a categorical definition of the main exposure variable (Rothman, 1986), although in some instances it is also possible to use each individual's actual exposure value. The latter approach is not directly possible in inherently categorical (grouped) data models (e.g., Poisson regression), but conversions of categorical data to quasi-continuous data can be achieved by assigning scores to each exposure group. Exposure is then represented by a single variable, and exponentiating the coefficient for this variable gives an estimate of the relative risk for one unit of exposure.

However, there are potential problems with using continuous exposure variables. The continuous model assumes that exposure is exponentially related to disease risk (Greenland, 1979). Thus, each additional unit of exposure *multiplies* the relative risk by a constant value. For example, suppose that the coefficient for a particular factor is 0.693. Exponentiating this term yields a relative risk of 2.0 for one unit of exposure, whereas a person with two units of exposure ($X_1 = 2$) has an estimated relative risk of $\exp(2 \times 0.693) = 4.0 \, (= 2.0^2)$ compared to a person with no exposure. Such an exponential exposure–response relationship is rarely observed in epidemiologic data. Hence, it is generally preferable to use a categorical exposure classification, since this involves no assumptions about the shape of the exposure–response relationship and enables the detection of relationships that do not fit an exponential pattern.

An objection that is often raised against the categorical approach is that continuous exposure information is lost, and several terms are required in the model rather than just one. Accordingly, it is often argued that this approach has less statistical power than a continuous approach. Statistical power is lost, relative to the continuous approach, *if* the exposure–response relationship follows a smooth monotonic pattern throughout the exposure range. Nevertheless, statistical power is only a secondary consideration in epidemiologic studies. The main goal is to obtain valid estimates of the actual exposure–response relationship. This objective is generally achieved in a most straightforward manner with a categorical analysis.

5.3. Exposure–Response Estimation

Once the categorical analysis of overall effects has been conducted, it is possible to supplement this with a continuous analysis if this seems warranted. For example, if the exposure–response curve appears to be exponential (on the basis of prior knowledge and the observed data), then a continuous analysis can be conducted with the exponential model. If the exposure–response curve appears to be linear, then the findings of the categorical analysis can be used in a simple linear regression of the form (Rothman, 1986):

$$R = 1 + aX \tag{8.15}$$

where R is the estimated relative risk for a particular exposure category and X is the mean cumulative exposure of the persons, or person-time, contributing to that category. (In a case–control study the mean exposure of the controls in a particular category should be used.)

It is appropriate to use the mean cumulative exposure level because a linear exposure–response relationship is being assumed.

The regression model is constrained to have an intercept of 1.0, so that the model estimates the excess relative risk per unit exposure. Each relative risk estimate is weighted by the inverse of its variance, which can be estimated by

$$\text{Var}(R) = (R^2)(\text{SE}(b))^2 \tag{8.16}$$

where $\text{SE}(b)$ is the standard error of the b-coefficient estimated from the exponential model and $R = \exp(b)$ (Rothman, 1986). For example, suppose a particular cumulative asbestos exposure category has a mean of 3,400 fibers/cc $\times$ days and that the coefficient for this category is 0.693, with standard error of 0.332. Then the estimated relative risk is $\exp(0.693) = 2.0$, and its inverse variance is $1/(2.0 \times 0.332)^2 = 2.268$. Hence, $R = 2.0$ and $X = 3,400$, and this data point would be weighted by a factor of 2.268 in the linear regression analysis.

It should be noted that the linear relative risk model presented here is not the same as an additive model. The latter assumes that all factors in the model are additive and have linear exposure–response relationships. The model considered here assumes that all factors are multiplicative (e.g., that the rate ratio for exposure is constant across age groups) but that the main exposure has a linear exposure–response relationship.

5.4. Confounding

As for the main exposure, it is generally desirable to use a set of categorical variables to denote levels of confounders. It is most appropriate to use continuous confounder variables when the relationship with disease is known to be approximately exponential. For example, an exponential relationship with age does appear to hold approximately for certain diseases (e.g., solid tumors). However, one should first carry out a categorical analysis and confirm that the data do show an exponential relationship (or at least one that is monotonically increasing) before using continuous variables. In general, it is still preferable to use a categorical approach, but a continuous variable may be required if there are problems with small numbers. It is usually desirable to adjust for all potential confounders when estimating the exposure effect. However, if there is a strong correlation between some risk factors, then the model will be unstable because of multicollinearity (see Section 5.6). In this situation it may be necessary to eliminate some potential confounders from the model.

5.5. Joint Effects

Estimating the joint effect(s) of two or more factors is often an important analytic goal. If two factors are strictly independent (i.e., there are no cases of disease that are caused only by the joint effect of the two factors), then their joint effect will not exceed additivity (Miettinen, 1982). In other situations, joint effects can range from less than additive to greater than multiplicative. Thus, one needs to be careful about the assumptions involved in an analysis relying on a particular model. In particular, the exponential models considered here assume that all risk factors have multiplicative effects. However, it is still possible to calculate the separate and joint effect(s) of two or more factors and assess the findings on an additive scale.

To illustrate, consider that X_1 and X_2 are dichotomous variables representing two workplace exposures. An interaction term (X_3) may be defined as $X_3 = (X_1)(X_2)$. If a person is exposed to both factors, then $X_3 = 1$; otherwise $X_3 = 0$. The model is thus

$$\frac{Y}{Y_0} = \exp(b_1 X_1 + b_2 X_2 + b_3 X_3) \tag{8.17}$$

The exponential model assumes that the relative risk for factor 1 does not depend on the presence or absence of factor 2. If this assumption is correct, then there is no statistical interaction of the two factors (i.e., $b_3 = 0$). If the relative risk for factor 1 is greater in persons exposed to factor 2 (i.e., the combined effect of the two factors is greater than the product of their independent effects), then b_3 will be greater than zero. If the relative risk for factor 1 is smaller in persons exposed to factor 2 (i.e., the combined effect of the two factors is less than the product of their independent effects), then b_3 will be less than zero.

To estimate the separate and joint effects of the two factors, let R_{10} be the relative risk for factor 1 alone and R_{01} be the relative risk for factor 2 alone. Then if $b_1 = 0.693$ (i.e., $R_{10} = \exp(0.693) = 2$) and $b_2 = 1.099$ (i.e., $R_{01} = \exp(1.099) = 3.0$), then the model assumes that the joint effect of the two factors is $2.0 \times 3.0 = 6.0$. Suppose the data actually deviate from this model, however, and b_3 is estimated as -0.377. Then $\exp(-0.377) = 0.69$. The joint effect of factors 1 and 2 is estimated by summing all relevant coefficients. In this case they are b_1, b_2, and b_3, since a person exposed to both factors has values of 1 for X_1, X_2, and X_3, whereas a person exposed to neither factor has values of 0 for all three variables. Thus, the relevant term is $0.693 + 1.099 - 0.377 = 1.415$, which when exponentiated yields an estimate of $R_{11} = 4.12$ ($= 2.0 \times 3.0 \times 0.69$). We can thus derive the information given in Table 8–1. Under additivity, the joint effect of X_1 and X_2 (R_{11}) would be $1.0 + (2.0 - 1.0) + (3.0 - 1.0) = 4.0$. The observed joint effect is 4.1, suggesting that the effects of the two factors are approximately additive. This supports the suggestion that the two factors operate independently in the causation of the study disease, although the data could also be consistent with a wide range of other models.

Confidence intervals for R_{10} and R_{01} can be calculated using the standard errors for their coefficients (b_1 and b_2). Since the coefficient for R_{11} is obtained by summing the coefficients b_1, b_2, and b_3, its variance (the square of its standard error) is given by

$$\mathrm{Var}(b_1 + b_2 + b_3) = \mathrm{Var}(b_1) + \mathrm{Var}(b_2) + \mathrm{Var}(b_3) \quad (8.18)$$
$$+ 2[\mathrm{Cov}(X_1,X_2) + \mathrm{Cov}(X_1,X_3) + \mathrm{Cov}(X_2,X_3)]$$

where $\mathrm{Cov}(X_i,X_j)$ is the covariance of factors X_i and X_j. (These data are readily available from standard packaged programs.) Thus, if $\mathrm{Var}(b_1) = 0.014$, $\mathrm{Var}(b_2) = 0.618$, $\mathrm{Var}(b_3) = 0.042$, $\mathrm{Cov}(X_1,X_2) = 0.450$, $\mathrm{Cov}(X_1,X_3) = -0.178$, and $\mathrm{Cov}(X_2,X_3) = -0.189$, then

$$\mathrm{Var}(b_1 + b_2 + b_3) = 0.014 + 0.618 + 0.042$$
$$+ 2[0.450 - 0.178 - 0.189]$$
$$= 0.840$$

and hence, $\mathrm{SE}(b_1 + b_2 + b_3) = 0.917$ (the square root of 0.840). The 90-percent confidence interval for R_{11} is thus

$$\underline{R},\overline{R} = \exp(1.50 \pm 1.645 \times 0.917) = 1.00, 20.38$$

5.6. Regression Diagnostics

The exponential models examined here were first developed for analyzing experimental data, usually involving relatively "balanced" designs. Maximum likelihood methods have good statistical properties in such ideal settings but may be unduly sensitive to imbalances in epidemiologic data (Prebigon, 1981). Regression diagnostic techniques have been developed to ascertain whether certain problems are occurring. We will discuss briefly three relevant issues: multicollinearity, influential data points, and goodness of fit.

Multicollinearity occurs when a variable is nearly a linear combination of other variables in the model. In particular, if there is a strong correlation between a confounder(s) and the main exposure, then the exposure effect estimate will be unstable, and its standard error will be large. For example, cumulative exposure is often strongly correlated with duration of employment in occupational studies. The attempt to include both factors in the same model may thus lead to unstable effect estimates with large standard errors. Multicollinearity is of particular concern when an interaction term is included in the model, since it will be correlated with each of the two or more component factors.

Although methods for assessing the presence of multicollinearity are well developed for linear regression (Belsey et al., 1980), less work has been done on assessing multicollinearity in exponential models. Collinearity involving only two factors can be assessed by examining the matrix of multiple correlation coefficients (that can be generated by most packaged programs). If a confounder (e.g., duration of employment) is strongly correlated with the main exposure variable (e.g., if the correlation is greater than 0.8), then multicollinearity problems may occur. These may be minimized by increasing the size of the study (although this is rarely feasible) or by "centering" continuous variables about the mean.

Another alternative is to delete the confounder(s) from the model. The most desirable situation is when the factor(s) causing multicollinearity problems is not a strong confounder and hence can be deleted from the model without seriously affecting the validity of the exposure effect estimate. If deleting a confounder(s) leaves the main effect estimate virtually unchanged, but greatly reduces its standard error, this suggests that the "smaller" model provides more precise estimates of the main effect without compromising validity. However, it is less clear how to proceed when a strong confounder(s) is a source of multicollinearity, since the increase in precision due to deleting such a confounder(s) may be offset by an increase in bias due to inadequate control of confounding (Robins and Greenland, 1986).

Influential data points are data points that profoundly influence the maximum likelihood estimate. For example, if a worker with very heavy exposure lives to an age of 100 years without developing the study disease, then including or excluding this worker from an analysis involving a continuous cumulative exposure variable may result in markedly different effect estimates. Such longevity may be merely a chance phenomenon, in which case one would not want it to influence the effect estimates unduly. This problem is largely avoided if only categorical variables are used, particularly if fine categorization is used to isolate extreme data points in separate categories, where they will automatically be discarded if no comparison data are available (Rothman, 1986). Influential data points are of more concern in analyses using continuous variables. One assessment procedure involves deleting each data point in turn to ascertain whether the coefficient estimates are affected considerably by whether a particular data point is included. Such methods can also be used in exponential models (Pregibon, 1981; Storer and Crowley, 1985) but are not, as yet, routinely done.

Most tests for *goodness of fit* involve grouping the data and comparing the observed number of cases in each group with that predicted by the model (usually with a chi-square statistic). Since Poisson regression involves grouped data (see the following discussion), goodness of fit tests are relatively straightforward. In particular, it is possible to calculate the deviance of the maximized likelihood for a particular model from that of an unconstrained model (with one parameter for each possible combination of risk factors). This deviance follows a chi-square distribution when the predicted values in each cell of a categorical analysis are reasonably large (at least three). Thus, the deviance can be used to assess goodness of fit. Similar methods are available for other exponential models, but the data must first be grouped by the investigator. One common procedure is to group the data into deciles of risk (as predicted by the model) and to compare the number of observed and expected cases in each decile (Lemeshow and Hosmer, 1982).

Although the value of goodness of fit tests is clear in the statistical context, where prediction is often a primary goal, their value is not so clear in more purely etiologic studies. It may be reassuring to know that a model fits well, but a poor-fitting model may still give valid effect estimates. The lack of fit indicates that there is some strong risk factor, or an interaction between risk factors already included in the model, which has not been adequately controlled. However, a poor fit does not indicate whether the uncontrolled factor is associated with exposure, and hence is a confounder. For example, Frome and Checkoway (1985) give an example of skin cancer incidence (Scotto et al., 1974), where the inclusion of age in a model reduces the goodness of fit chi-square from 2,569.7 with 14 d.f. to 8.2 with 7 d.f., thus clearly improving the fit of the model. However, in this example, age is only a weak confounder, and the rate ratio for exposure (the city of residence) only changes from 2.23 to 2.10 when age effects are controlled. Thus, although a poor fit may raise concerns about uncontrolled confounding, it does not show that it is actually occurring.

6. EXAMPLE: STUDY OF ASBESTOS TEXTILE WORKERS

6.1. Introduction

The following example illustrates some of the principles discussed earlier. It involves the study of lung cancer in 1,261 white male workers from one asbestos textile manufacturing plant (Dement et al., 1983) described in Chapters 5 and 6. The analysis has been confined to the following factors: cumulative exposure in thousands of fibers/cc × days, age, calendar year, and length of follow-up. Duration of employment could have been included as a potential confounder, but a preliminary analysis revealed that this factor was not a confounder and that its inclusion in the model created instability resulting from collinearity with cumulative exposure. Age at hire (first exposure) was not included in the model because it is a linear function of age at risk and length of follow-up, which were already included. However, age at hire is an important potential effect modifier; this possibility is explored in Chapter 10.

6.2. Computational Methods

Poisson regression was used as the primary analytic method because it involved the lowest cost and provided the greatest flexibility and simplicity of use. Table 8–2 lists the variables included in the analysis. Table 8–3 shows the records for a hypothetical worker for whom follow-up started on January 1, 1954 (at age 26.1 years), and finished on January 1, 1964. At the midpoint of the first year of follow-up the value of calendar year was 1954.5, age at risk was 26.6 years, duration of employment was 0.5 years, and follow-up time was 0.5 years. The worker accumulated 0.1 units of exposure

Table 8–2. Variables required to generate data for analyses involving time-related factors

Variable	Comments
YOB	Decimalized date of birth
YIN	Decimalized date of hire
YOUT	Decimalized date of termination
YRIN	Decimalized starting date of follow-up
YROUT	Decimalized end date of follow-up
DEAD	1 = dead, 0 = alive or unknown status
ICD	3-digit ICD code for cause of death
CUM40—CUM75	Cumulative exposure, one variable for each year the overall cohort has been followed (from 1940 to 1975 in this instance)

Table 8–3. Records for a hypothetical worker for whom follow-up started on January 1, 1954 (at age 26.1 years), and finished on January 1, 1964

Variable	1954	1955	1956	1957	1958	1959	1960	1961	1962	1963
Age at risk	26.6	27.6	28.6	29.6	30.6	31.6	32.6	33.6	34.6	35.6
Calendar year	54.5	55.5	56.5	57.5	58.5	59.5	60.5	61.5	62.5	63.5
Year of follow-up	0.5	1.5	2.5	3.5	4.5	5.5	6.5	7.5	8.5	9.5
Cumulative exposure	0.1	0.2	0.6	1.2	1.3	2.6	2.6	2.6	2.6	2.6

during this first year of follow-up. The total follow-up time was ten years.

Person-time data are created for each individual by considering each year of follow-up in turn and generating a separate record with values for the following variables: calendar year, in seven five-year groupings (1940–44, 1945–49, . . . , 1970–75); age at risk, in 14 five-year groupings (20–24, 25–29, . . . , ≥85); length of follow-up, in five-year groupings (0–4, 5–9, 10–14, 15–19, ≥20); and cumulative exposure, in five groupings. The exposure data may be lagged by a specified duration, such that a worker's person-time of observation for a given age, year, and follow-up time are classified according to the cumulative exposure category achieved a certain number of years previously. The lag period has been set to zero unless otherwise indicated.

The program used here (Pearce and Checkoway, 1987) rounds off the number of years of follow-up so that ten records are created for a person who has been followed for 9.6 years but only nine are created for a person followed for 9.4 years. Data for each worker were classified in this manner, and the person-time contributions were accumulated accordingly. Table 8–4 lists the deaths and person-years in each exposure category, using various lag periods.

The Poisson likelihood can be calculated using an iteratively reweighted least squares algorithm (Frome, 1983). GLIM (Baker and Nelder, 1978) was used for the example presented here. Some commonly used programs for Cox's partial likelihood estimation procedure cannot handle time-related factors. A limited time-related analysis can be performed using the BMDP program 2L (BMDP, 1979), but a full-time related analysis required a FORTRAN subroutine to augment the BMDP procedure (Hopkins and Hornung, 1985). Harrell's (1983b) PHGLM procedure was used

Table 8–4. Person-years at risk and deaths in each cumulative exposure category for various lag periods

Cumulative exposure (1,000 fibers/cc × days)	0-yr lag		5-yr lag		15-yr lag	
	Person-years	Deaths	Person-years	Deaths	Person-years	Deaths
<1	13,146	5	16,253	5	23,126	7
1–9	12,823	10	10,915	10	6,554	13
10–39	4,976	7	4,148	10	2,262	9
40–99	1,270	11	925	9	362	6
≥100	139	2	113	1	0	0

for conditional logistic regression, and his (1983a) LOGIST procedure was used for unconditional logistic regression analysis.

6.3. Importance of Time-Related Analysis

Before defining the model, we first illustrate the importance of time-related analyses. The proportional hazards model was used for this purpose because programs for both time-related (Hopkins and Hornung, 1985) and fixed (Harrell, 1983b) analyses are available. Table 8–5 contrasts the findings. In the fixed (i.e., non-time-related) analysis workers were classified according to their *final* cumulative exposures and years at risk, rather than according to the values at the appropriate ages involved in each risk set comparison. The two analytic methods produced markedly different results. This occurs partly because the fixed analysis involves comparing the cumulative exposure of each case with the final cumulative exposure of persons at risk at the age the case occurred. Thus, the exposure of each case is estimated correctly, but that of the corresponding risk set is inflated, since it includes exposure obtained during subsequent periods. This problem was also discussed in Chapter 5, where we indicated that incorrect person-years attribution in a fixed analysis can result in a dampened exposure–response curve (Enterline, 1976).

6.4. Model Definition

The first decision in model construction is the definition of the main exposure variable(s). In Section 5.2 of this chapter we argued that it is preferable to use a categorical classification, since this best

Table 8–5. Relative risk estimates obtained using the Cox model with time-related and fixed analyses, adjusted for calendar year, with age as the time variable

Cumulative exposure (1,000 fibers/cc × days)	Time-related		Fixed	
	R	95% confidence interval	R	95% confidence interval
<1[a]	1.00	—	1.00	—
1–9	1.83	0.63, 5.36	1.69	0.57, 4.98
10–39	1.86	0.58, 5.94	1.08	0.31, 3.71
40–99	6.82	2.34, 19.85	3.24	1.10, 9.52
≥100	8.10	1.52, 43.21	4.58	0.85, 24.70

[a]Reference category.

Table 8–6. Relative risk estimates obtained using Poisson regression with continuous and categorical exposure classifications, adjusted for age and calendar year

Cumulative exposure (1,000 fibers/cc × days)	Mean level of cumulative exposure	Continuous		Categorical	
		R	95% confidence interval	R	95% confidence interval
<1[a]	0.5	1.00	—	1.00	—
1–9	3.4	1.04	1.02, 1.06	1.87	0.64, 5.48
10–39	21.2	1.32	1.15, 1.51	1.96	0.61, 6.25
40–99	60.0	2.20	1.48, 3.27	6.79	2.33, 19.77
≥100	173.0	9.83	3.12, 30.98	8.81	1.64, 47.25

[a]Reference category.

enables the estimation of the observed exposure–response curve. We illustrate this with separate analyses using continuous and categorical classifications of cumulative asbestos exposure. It was initially intended to do these analyses with the Cox model so that each worker's exact cumulative exposure data could be used. However, it was found that the continuous analysis was unduly affected by two influential data points, representing two noncases with cumulative asbestos exposures of approximately 250,000 fibers/cc × days. To circumvent this problem we categorized the exposure data from the outset. The continuous analysis was then based on the mean scores for the person-time data in each category. (This yielded a coefficient for one unit of cumulative exposure of 0.0133, compared with a coefficient of 0.0091 obtained using the Cox model with individual exposure data.) The analyses were performed with Poisson regression, adjusting for age and calendar year. Table 8–6 and Figure 8–2 contrast the findings of the categorical and continuous analyses.

The continuous approach produced apparently better precision, as indicated by narrower confidence intervals. However, the validity of the confidence intervals generated by the continuous model is suspect, since they do not include the observed effect estimates for several exposure categories. For example, the cumulative exposure category of 40,000 to 99,000 fibers/cc × days yields a relative risk of 6.79 (Table 8–6) in the observed categorical data, but the continuous model yields a predicted relative risk (based on the mean exposure level for the category of 60,000 fibers/cc × days and compared to the lowest exposure level that had a mean of 500 fibers/cc × days) of 2.20 with a 95-percent confidence interval of 1.48, 3.27.

For very low or very high exposures, the continuous approach gives effect estimates markedly different from the observed data.

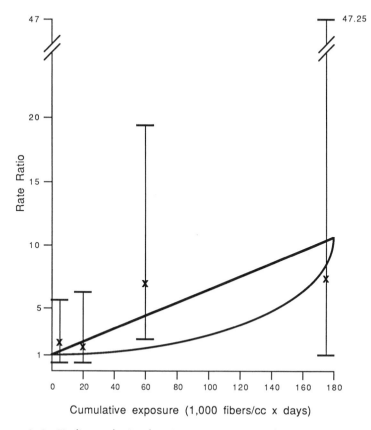

Figure 8-2. Findings obtained using continuous and categorical cumulative exposure classifications (x = observed rate ratio).

For example, a cumulative exposure of 1,000 fibers/cc × days yields a predicted relative risk of 1.0133 under the exponential model, obtained by exponentiating the coefficient (0.01325) associated with one unit (1,000 fibers/cc × days) of cumulative exposure. The corresponding estimate under the linear model is 1.054 (see Figure 8–2), obtained by fitting an inverse variance weighted linear regression to the categorical effect estimates. (A similar estimate was obtained by fitting an additive Poisson regression model using GLIM.) This small difference becomes magnified when extrapolating the study findings to large, nonoccupational populations with low exposures. On the other hand, the exponential and linear models, respectively, predict relative risks of 748.7 (= exp[0.01325 × 500]), and 27.0 (= 1 + 0.054 × 500) for a cumulative exposure of 500,000 fibers/cc × days.

Table 8–7. Effect estimates obtained with Poisson regression using various lag intervals, adjusted for age and calendar year

Cumulative exposure (1,000 fibers/cc × days)	0-yr lag		5-yr lag		15-yr lag	
	R	95% confidence interval	R	95% confidence interval	R	95% confidence interval
<1[a]	1.00	—	1.00	—	1.00	—
1–9	1.87	0.64, 5.48	1.97	0.67, 5.78	2.89	1.08, 7.72
10–39	1.96	0.61, 6.25	2.85	0.96, 8.40	3.40	1.19, 9.70
40–99	6.79	2.33, 19.77	7.31	2.42, 22.08	11.19	3.54, 35.40
≥100	8.81	1.64, 47.25	5.03	0.68, 37.38	—	—

[a]Reference category.

If the exposure–response relationship is linear, as it often appears to be for asbestos exposure and lung cancer (Liddell and Hanley, 1985), then the exponential model using continuous data produces a distorted exposure–response curve. This problem is avoided in a categorical analysis because the model is permitted to fit the data pattern actually observed, and, if desired, a linear exposure–response relationship can be estimated subsequently. Hence, the main exposure variable was defined categorically in all subsequent analyses.

Another decision in the definition of the main effect variable is the choice of an appropriate lag period for exposure. Occupationally-related lung cancer mortality usually does not occur until at least 10–15 years after first exposure to asbestos (Selikoff et al., 1979). Therefore, it might be expected that the rate ratios for asbestos exposure would be greater if "irrelevant" exposures during more recent years were ignored. Table 8–7 shows the findings for lag periods of 0, 5, and 15 years. Except for the highest exposure category, which involves very small numbers, the relative risk for each exposure category increases with lag time. Thus, there would be some justification for using a 15-year lag period throughout the analysis. However, the zero-year lag provides the largest numbers of person-years and deaths in the higher cumulative exposure categories, and for purposes of illustration, a zero-year lag has been used here.

Confounders were also defined categorically. These were age at risk, calendar year, and length of follow-up. Table 8–8 summarizes the confounder assessment. Model 2 is the full model involving cumulative exposure, age, year and follow-up duration. Models 3–5 show the effects of deleting any one of the latter three factors

Table 8-8. Assessment of confounding in Poisson regression analysis

Model	Rate ratio for each exposure category (1,000 fibers/cc × days)				
	<1[a]	1–9	10–39	40–99	≥100
1. Cumulative exposure	1.00	2.05	3.70	22.77	37.83
2. Cumulative exposure, age, year, follow-up	1.00	1.75	1.62	5.21	6.36
3. Cumulative exposure, age, year	1.00	1.77	1.96	6.79	8.81
4. Cumulative exposure, age, follow-up	1.00	1.93	2.17	7.17	9.57
5. Cumulative exposure, year, follow-up	1.00	1.98	2.75	11.34	21.36

[a]Reference category.

from the full model. The effect estimates change markedly if age is deleted from the model, suggesting that age is a strong confounder. The changes in risk estimates are smaller if calendar year or follow-up duration were deleted from the full model, but these changes are still large enough to suggest that the full model is preferable. However, follow-up duration had the smallest effect on the exposure risk estimates, and thus is the prime candidate for deletion.

There was no a priori reason to investigate the joint effects of asbestos exposure with any of the other factors included in the model; therefore, no interaction terms were defined. However, we did examine the asbestos exposure effect in the context of the Armitage–Doll multistage model of carcinogenesis (Armitage and Doll, 1961); these findings are presented in Chapter 10.

6.5. Comparison of Modeling Methods

These initial analyses suggested that the final model should contain the following factors: cumulative exposure, age, year, and length of follow-up. Unfortunately, it was found that the proportional hazards model failed to converge when all four factors were modeled. Consequently, the comparative analysis was restricted to cumulative exposure, age, and year.

Poisson regression and the proportional hazards model yield very similar findings (Table 8–9), the only discrepancy being for the highest exposure category that contains very small numbers. The minor discrepancies for the other exposure levels arise from the different degree of control of confounding by age, since there are 14 age strata with Poisson regression, whereas the proportional hazards model effectively required creating 35 age strata (one for each lung cancer death). Logistic regression analysis yielded effect estimates

Table 8–9. Effect estimates for various methods of analysis of cohort data, adjusted for age and calendar year

Cumulative exposure (1,000 fibers/cc × days)	Poisson regression		Proportional hazards model		Unconditional logistic regression	
	R	95% confidence interval	R	95% confidence interval	R	95% confidence interval
<1[a]	1.00	—	1.00	—	1.00	—
1–9	1.87	0.64, 5.48	1.83	0.63, 5.36	2.03	0.67, 6.14
10–39	1.96	0.61, 6.25	1.86	0.58, 5.94	2.40	0.71, 8.05
40–99	6.79	2.33, 19.77	6.82	2.34, 19.85	7.85	2.42, 25.44
≥100	8.81	1.64, 47.25	8.10	1.52, 43.21	12.50	1.51, 103.83

[a]Reference category.

that were larger and less precise. This commonly occurs in logistic regression analyses of cohort studies when the follow-up period is relatively long (Green and Symons, 1983; Abbott, 1985).

The case–control findings using conditional and unconditional logistic regression (Table 8–10) differ from the cohort study findings because of sampling error, but once again, similar results were obtained with the different analytic methods (except for the highest exposure category). The findings in Table 8–10, obtained using maximum likelihood estimation (conditional and unconditional), differ to some extent from those obtained with the adjusted Mantel–Haenszel estimates (Table 6–14). These minor differences are presumably due to differences in weightings given to the stratum-specific odds ratios by these estimation procedures.

Table 8–10. Effect estimates for various methods of analysis of case–control data, adjusted for age and calendar year

Cumulative exposure (1,000 fibers/cc × days)	Conditional logistic regression		Unconditional logistic regression	
	R	95% confidence interval	R	95% confidence interval
<1[a]	1.00	—	1.00	—
1–9	2.24	0.70, 7.23	2.36	0.72, 7.72
10–39	2.19	0.59, 8.08	2.12	0.58, 7.79
40–99	6.86	1.74, 27.04	6.86	1.84, 25.61
≥100	5.55	0.62, 49.39	6.88	0.80, 60.68

[a]Reference category.

6.6. Discussion

This example has illustrated the interrelationships between Poisson regression, the proportional hazards model, and logistic regression on the same data set. Poisson regression and the proportional hazards model yielded very similar findings, whereas logistic regression tended to yield effect estimates that were too large. Case–control sampling from the risk sets used in proportional hazards analysis has been recommended as an inexpensive alternative analytic method (Liddell et al., 1977). However, in the preceding example computational simplicity was gained at the expense of some loss of precision.

The proportional hazards model is rarely used in occupational cohort studies because of its computational complexity. Computer time itself is no longer of major importance with the advent of high-speed microcomputers, but the practical complexities of running the proportional hazards model with time-related factors are still of concern. However, theoretical analyses have shown the inherent link between Poisson regression and the proportional hazards model, and this has been illustrated in the analyses presented here. Poisson regression was found to have computational advantages with costs of approximately $10 (U.S.) for an initial run (the generation of the person-time data) and just a few dollars for each GLIM analysis. These analyses were only marginally more expensive than the case–control analyses. In contrast, the proportional hazards analyses were more expensive, costing approximately $50 per model when time-related factors were analyzed appropriately. Furthermore, Poisson regression follows directly from elementary person-time analyses; time-related factors can be handled relatively easily, and incidence rate estimates can be generated directly. Hence, these considerations suggest that Poisson regression may be an efficient method for time-related analyses of occupational cohort data when mathematical modeling is required.

7. SUMMARY OF ADVANTAGES AND DISADVANTAGES OF MODELING

The major advantage of mathematical modeling is that it can handle a larger number of confounders and effect modifiers than conventional stratified analysis (e.g., SMRs or SRRs). Even with categorical variables, mathematical models smooth the data and permit adjustment for a larger number of factors than in a stratified analysis. In particular, it is possible to adjust for the various time-related confounders that are common in occupational studies. Furthermore, modeling permits straightforward calculation of effect estimates for each factor in the model.

The advantages of mathematical modeling are also sources of potential disadvantages. Inappropriate use of continuous variables may lead to incomplete control of confounding and may distort the exposure–disease relationship. Furthermore, mathematical modeling may obscure relationships within the data (e.g., the influence of just one or two strata with small cell sizes). Thus, mathematical modeling can be a very powerful tool, but it should always be preceded by the simpler stratified analyses presented in Chapters 5–7.

Glossary

Cox model   A specific form of the proportional hazards model in which the underlying time-dependent incidence rate is treated as an unknown nuisance parameter.

goodness of fit   A statistic that reflects the extent to which the model correctly predicts the observed data.

hazard rate   Incidence rate.

influential data point   A data point whose inclusion or exclusion changes the effect estimate "considerably."

likelihood statistic   Minus twice the log of the maximized likelihood.

logistic regression   A mathematical model in which the log odds is modeled as a linear combination of a set of risk factors.

maximum likelihood estimate   A method for calculating parameters that maximizes the probability of obtaining the data actually observed.

multicollinearity   Instability in an effect estimate(s) resulting from a strong correlation between one or more risk factors.

Poisson regression   A mathematical model in which the log of the incidence rate is modeled as a linear combination of a set of risk factors.

proportional hazards model   A mathematical model in which specified risk factors are assumed to affect the incidence rate in a multiplicative manner.

risk set   The set of all persons included in follow-up and free of the disease of interest at a particular "time."

time-related factor   A risk factor or effect modifier that varies as a person ages.

Notation

b_i	The coefficient associated with risk factor i in the exponential model
$Cov(X_1, X_2)$	The covariance of X_1 and X_2
Exp	Number of expected events
N_{0i}	Number of person-years in the non-exposed group of stratum i

Obs	Number of observed events
P_0	The proportion of non-exposed persons who are cases
P_1	The proportion of exposed persons who are cases
R	Relative risk
R_{00}	The baseline relative risk (1.0) in the absence of exposure
R_{10}	The relative risk for factor 1 in the absence of factor 2
R_{01}	The relative risk for factor 2 in the absence of factor 1
R_{11}	The relative risk for exposure to both factors 1 and 2, relative to exposure to neither factor
t	The "time" variable (usually age) used to define risk sets in the proportional hazards model
$Var(b_i)$	The variance of the coefficient $((b_i)$ for a variable (X)
X_i	A risk factor in a mathematical model
Y	The rate or odds of disease
Y_E	The rate or odds of disease in the exposed group
$Y_{\overline{E}}$	The rate or odds of disease in the non-exposed group
Y_0	The rate or odds of disease in persons with zero values for all variables in the model
λ	The incidence rate in a group; or the mixture parameter in a generalized relative risk model
$\lambda(t)$	The incidence rate at age t
λ_{0i}	The incidence rate in the non-exposed group in stratum i
λ_{1i}	The incidence rate in the exposed group in stratum i

References

Abbott RD (1985): Logistic regression in survival analysis. *Am J Epidemiol* 121:465–471.

Anderson EB (1970): Asymptotic properties of conditional maximum likelihood estimators. *J R Stat Soc (B)* 32:283–301

Armitage P., and Doll R (1961): Stochastic models for carcinogenesis. In: Neyman J (ed). *Proceedings of the Fourth Berkeley Symposium on Mathematical Statistics and Probability,* Vol. 4. Berkeley: University of California Press, pp 19–38.

Baker RJ, and Nelder JA (1978): *Generalized Linear Interaction Modeling (GLIM).* Release 3, Oxford, England: Numerical Algorithms Group.

Belsey DA., Kuh E., and Welsch RE (1980): *Regression Diagnostics.* New York: John Wiley & Sons.

Berry G (1983): The analysis of mortality by the subject years method. *Biometrics* 39:173–184.

Biomedical Computer Programs P-Series (1979): BMDP-79. Berkeley: University of California Press.

Breslow N E (1986): *Logistic Regression and Related Methods for the Analysis of Chronic Disease Risk in Longitudinal Studies.* Technical Report No. 76. Seattle, WA: Department of Biostatistics.

Breslow NE, and Day NE (1980): *Statistical Methods in Cancer Research. Volume I: The Analysis of Case-Control Studies.* Lyon, France: International Agency for Research on Cancer.

Breslow NE, and Day NE (1987): *Statistical Methods in Cancer Research. Volume II:*

The Analysis of Cohort Studies. Lyon, France: International Agency for Research on Cancer.

Breslow NE, and Storer BE (1985): General relative risk functions for case-control studies. *Am J Epidemiol* 122:149–162.

Breslow NE, Lubin JH, Marek P, et al. (1983): Multiplicative models and cohort analysis. *J Am Stat Assoc* 78:1–12.

Cornfield J (1962): Joint dependence of risk of coronary heart disease on serum cholesterol and systolic blood pressure: a discriminant function analysis. *Fed Proc 21:58–61.*

Cox DR (1972): Regression models and life tables. *J R Stat Soc (B)* 34:187–220.

Cox DR (1975): Partial likelihood. *Biometrika* 62:269–276.

Dement JM, Harris RL, Symons MJ, and Shy CM (1983): Exposures and mortality among chrysotile asbestos workers. Part II: Mortality. *Am J Ind Med* 4:421–433.

Enterline PE (1976): Pitfalls in epidemiologic research: an examination of the asbestos literature. *J Occup Med* 18:150–156.

Frome EL (1983): The analysis of rates using Poisson regression models. *Biometrics* 39:665–674.

Frome EL, and Checkoway H (1985): Use of Poisson regression models in estimating incidence rates and ratios. *Am J Epidemiol* 121:309–323.

Green MS, and Symons MJ (1983): A comparison of the logistic risk function and the proportional hazards model in prospective epidemiologic studies. *J Chronic Dis* 26:715–724.

Greenland S (1979): Limitations of the logistic analysis of epidemiologic data. *Am J Epidemiol* 110:693–698.

Greenland S, and Robins JM (1985): Estimation of a common effect parameter from sparse follow-up data. *Biometrics* 41:55–68.

Guerrero VM, and Johnson RA(1982): Use of the Box–Cox transformation with binary response models. *Biometrika* 69:309–314.

Harrell F (1983a): The LOGIST procedure. In: *SAS Supplemental Library User's Guide.* Cary, NC: SAS Institute, Inc.

Harrell F (1983b): The PHGLM procedure. In: *SAS Supplemental Library User's Guide.* Cary, NC: SAS Institute, Inc.

Hopkins A, and Hornung R (1985): *New 2L Features with Illustrative Examples.* Technical Report No. 80. Los Angeles, CA: BMDP Statistical Software.

Kalbfleisch JD, and Prentice RL (1980): *The Statistical Analysis of Failure Time Data.* New York: John Wiley & Sons.

Lemeshow S, and Hosmer DW (1982): A review of goodness of fit tests for use in the development of logistic regression models. *Am J Epidemiol* 115:91–106.

Liddell FDK, and Hanley JA (1985): Relations between asbestos exposure and lung cancer SMRs in occupational cohort studies. *Br J Ind Med* 42:389–396.

Liddell FDK, McDonald JC, and Thomas DC (1977): Methods of cohort analysis: appraisal by application to asbestos mining. *J R Stat Soc (A)* 140:469–491.

McKinlay SM (1977): Pair matching—a reappraisal of a popular technique. *Biometrics* 33:725–735.

Mantel N. (1966): Evaluation of survival data and two new rank order statistics arising in its consideration. *Cancer Chemother Rep* 50:163–170.

Mantel N, and Haenszel W (1959): Statistical aspects of the analysis of data from retrospective studies of disease. *J Natl Cancer Inst* 22:719–748.

Miettinen OS (1972): Standardization of risk ratios. *Am J Epidemiol* 96:383–388.

Miettinen OS (1982): Causal and preventive interdependence. Elementary principles. *Scand J Work Environ Health* 8:159–168.

Moolgavkar SH, and Venzon DJ (1987): General relative risk regression models for epidemiologic studies. *Am J Epidemiol* 126:949–961.

Pearce NE, and Checkoway H (1987): A simple computer program for generating person–time data in cohort studies involving time-related factors. *Am J Epidemiol* 125:1085–1091.

Pearce NE, Checkoway H, and Shy CM (1986): Time-related factors as potential confounders and effect modifiers in studies based on an occupational cohort. *Scand J Work Environ Health* 12:97–107.

Prebigon D (1981): Logistic regression diagnostics. *Ann Stat* 9:705–724.

Prentice RL, and Breslow NE (1978): Retrospective studies and failure time models. *Biometrika* 65:153–158.

Robins JM, and Greenland S (1986): The role of model selection in causal inference from nonexperimental data. *Am J Epidemiol* 123:392–402.

Rosenbaum PR, and Rubin DB (1984): Difficulties with regression analyses of age-adjusted rates. *Biometrics* 40:437–443.

Rothman KJ (1986): *Modern Epidemiology.* Boston, MA: Little, Brown. & Co.

Scotto J, Kopf AW, and Urbach F (1974): Non-melonoma skin cancer among Caucasians in four areas of the United States. *Cancer* 34:1333–1338.

Selikoff IJ, Hammond EC, and Seidman H (1979): Mortality experience of insulation workers in the US and Canada, 1943–1976. *Ann NY Acad Sci* 330:91–116.

Storer BE, and Crowley J (1985): A diagnostic for Cox regression and general conditional likelihoods. *J Am Stat Assoc* 80:139–147.

Thomas DC (1981): General relative risk models for survival time and matched case-control analysis. *Biometrics* 37:673–686.

Thomas DC (1983): Statistical methods for analyzing effects of temporal patterns of exposure on cancer risks. *Scand J Work Environ Health* 9:353–366.

Thomas DC, and Greenland S (1983): The relative efficiencies of matched and independent sample designs for case-control studies. *J Chron Dis* 36:685–697.

Wallenstein S, and Bodian C. (1987): Inferences on odds ratios, relative risks, and risk differences based on standard regression programs. *Am J Epidemiol* 126:346–355.

Whittemore AS (1985): Analyzing cohort mortality data. *Am Stat* 39:437–441.

9 Dose and Exposure Modeling

1. OVERVIEW

Estimation of dose–response relationships between occupational exposures and human health effects is central to understanding disease induction mechanisms. Ultimately, dose–response relationships are used to predict effects in populations other than those studied, and therefore form the bases of occupational and nonoccupational exposure guidelines.

In Chapter 2 we introduced some of the important concepts involved in dose–response estimation and offered conceptual definitions of such parameters as exposure concentration, burden, and dose. In this chapter we discuss these and related concepts more formally. We then present mathematical expressions for calculating the exposure and dose parameters required for modeling. The modeling procedures are illustrated first with examples of radionuclides that emit alpha radiation. In the second example we use data from the asbestos textile workers cohort study.

2. FUNDAMENTAL DEFINITIONS OF EXPOSURE AND DOSE PARAMETERS

The unifying notion of exposure and dose modeling that leads to dose–response function estimation is that biological effects arise from damage induced in specific targets, where the targets may be particular organs, cells, or subcellular sites. Our ability to specify precisely the ultimate target sites is limited by the state of knowledge of disease pathogenesis. Thus, in some situations we may feel confident that the biological targets are certain gene loci on DNA, as might be the case for cancer induction, but in other situations we may have to be content with identifying less specific targets, such as bronchial epithelium or the central nervous system.

During some small time interval the damage caused by an environmental substance can be assumed to be related directly to the amount of the substance present at the target during the same interval. The observable effect of the damage, such as cell death, malignant transformation, or metabolic disturbance, often is not apparent until some later time. Predicting the probability or severity of an effect requires estimation of the concentration of the substance at the target as a function of time. For some substances, the concentration at the target at any time is proportional to the concentration in the environment. As the speed with which a material is removed from the body increases, the ratio of dose to exposure intensity approaches a constant throughout the period of exposure. However, this proportionality does not always hold true. Thus, we would like to know what the concentrations at the target have been at various times, rather than simply relying on environmental concentration data.

2.1. Exposure Variables

We can recall from Chapter 2 that *exposure* refers to the presence of substances in the environment external to the body. By contrast, doses and organ burdens are measures of the amount of the substance within the body. It is convenient to define exposures according to two dimensions: intensity and duration. *Intensity* represents the magnitude of the amount of a substance that potentially can enter the body and be delivered to the biological target(s). (It should be noted here that one substance can have multiple targets and modes of activity.) The environmental concentration that can be measured with sampling devices provides an observable estimate of the intensity. More generally, intensity is the *rate* at which a substance is brought into contact with the body. The terms *exposure intensity* and *exposure rate* therefore are synonymous. The second exposure variable is *duration,* which is the length of time during which a given intensity is maintained.

The *cumulative exposure* (E) accumulated during the time interval for which a constant intensity (I) occurred is simply the product of the intensity and duration (T), which can be expressed as

$$E = IT \qquad (9.1)$$

Expression (9.1) refers only to one particular time interval, during which the intensity is assumed to be constant. More generally, when I varies over time, cumulative exposure between times t_1 and t_2 is

$$E = \int_{t_1}^{t_2} I(t) \, dt \tag{9.2}$$

where the duration of exposure is the interval (t_1, t_2). If all of the important environmental and biological factors other than intensity are assumed to be constant during the duration of exposure and if the concentration in the environment remains directly proportional to the concentration at the target, then either E or I will be a reliable predictor of dose.

2.2. Dose Variables

Exposure variables may give imprecise and misleading estimates of concentrations and cumulative amounts of substances reaching body targets. This limitation arises because environmental concentrations are not the only determinants of the quantity of a substance that reaches a biological target. Other factors such as particle size and chemical forms of a substance are physical characteristics that can influence bodily concentrations. Some of the biological factors that determine target concentrations include characteristics of retention, excretion, and metabolism. Thus, the temporal pattern of dose may be different from the temporal pattern of exposure. Also, exposure intensities may not reflect amounts reaching biological targets when protective devices, such as filtering masks, are used.

The concept of *dose* arises, then, because of the limitations of exposure variables in quantifying the amount of a substance that actually is delivered to a biological target and that remains there in an active state. Dose (D) is defined as the amount of a substance that reaches the biological target during some specified time interval. This amount will be related to the concentration of the substance at (or near) the target and to the time interval considered. The rate of delivery is referred to as the dose rate, or *dose intensity* (I_D). The dose delivered to a target during some time interval (t_1, t_2) is given by

$$D = \int_{t_1}^{t_2} I_D(t) \, dt \tag{9.3}$$

where I_D is given the subscript D to distinguish dose intensity from exposure intensity. In general $I_D(t)$ is considered to be proportional to the concentration of the substance at the target. It should be borne in mind that doses are not directly measurable, but instead are estimated by mathematical models that include exposure variables as well as biological factors.

Dose intensity is related closely to the concept of *burden,* where we can consider burdens for the entire body, for individual organs, or for specifically identified biological targets. For simplicity, we shall consider only organ burdens. The organ burden, $B(t)$, at time t is defined as the concentration of the substance in the organ. We can thus note that organ burden can vary over time. For many substances, including most chemicals and all radionuclides, the dose rate is directly proportional to the burden, and the dose is proportional to the integral of the burden over some time interval. This relationship can be expressed as follows:

$$D = K \int_{t_1}^{t_2} B(t) \, dt \qquad (9.4)$$

where K is the proportionality constant relating $I_D(t)$ [from expression (9.3)] and $B(t)$. In other words, K is the rate at which the substance "strikes" the target per unit burden. For radionuclides, K is referred to as the "S-Factor." K is less easily specified for most chemicals, dusts, and fibers and is typically left as an unknown constant. The latter situation is not of concern in that all one needs is some measure of the rate at which damage is produced, and this measure only needs to be proportional to the actual (and generally unknown) rate of damage.

Relationships between exposure and dose variables are perhaps best understood for ionizing radiations; consequently, we illustrate some of these concepts in that context. For ionizing radiations, dose takes on a specialized meaning that is easily related to the more general definition given earlier. It is reasonably well established in radiobiology that the extent of biological damage in an organ, cell, or subcellular site is related directly to the amount of radiation energy absorbed per unit mass of biological material (i.e., the energy density). Thus, the rate of damage is directly proportional to the dose rate. As a result, radiation dose is defined as the energy deposited in biological materials (usually cells) divided by the mass of the material. The dose rate is the rate at which this energy is delivered. The unit of radiation dose is referred to as the rad (ICRP, 1977), which is defined rather arbitrarily as being equal to a density of 100 ergs per gram of biological material (where ergs is a unit of energy). In recent years the rad has been replaced by the gray as a unit of dose, where 1 gray is equal to 100 rads.

The value of K in expression (9.4) thus has units of rads per unit time per unit of organ burden. Thus, the product of K and the organ burden equals the dose rate or dose intensity. No similar specialized meanings for dose are available for chemicals or other physical agents, although it is conceivable that common systems of dose units will be adopted as the mechanisms of action for such materials become more clear. Again, this presents no problem, provided that the rate of damage is proportional to the organ burden.

The organ burden at any time is a function of both the history of past intakes and the biological retention of these intakes. *Retention,* which includes metabolism, absorption, uptake, and clearance by various organs and tissues, can be modeled collectively as *retention functions.* Retention functions, denoted generally as $R(t)$, specify the fraction of a substance present in an organ after a time interval t following entry into the organ. Related to the retention function is the *uptake rate,* which is the amount of a substance entering an organ per unit exposure per unit of time. The organ burden thus is a function of both the uptake rate and the retention function.

The kinds of models that specify retention functions are known generally as *biokinetic (pharmacokinetic) models,* or more specifically for toxic substances, *toxicokinetic models.* These models describe the relationships between exposures in environmental media and the resulting concentrations in target organs and tissues. Biokinetic or toxicokinetic models can be distinguished from pharmacodynamic models, where the latter relate tissue concentrations to biological responses (Smith, 1987). Biokinetic models treat the body as a series of compartments, between which substances are exchanged. These compartments might, for instance, consist of organs, classes of cells, or even complex physiologic entities (e.g., the immune system).

3. BIOMATHEMATICAL MODELS OF ORGAN BURDEN AND DOSE

Biomathematical models permit prediction of doses to targets for a given exposure. We can begin by depicting the models that are used to estimate doses from exposure data. Figure 9–1 shows a schematic representation of some bodily compartments through which materials enter the body, the bloodstream, and other organs that transport or take up materials. This diagram is simplified so as to represent compartments by specific organs.

In general, we can let $I(t)$ be the exposure intensity in an environmental medium that is encountered by a worker at time t, where the exposure intensity is given in units of concentration such as parts per million of air. The substance then enters the skin, gastrointes-

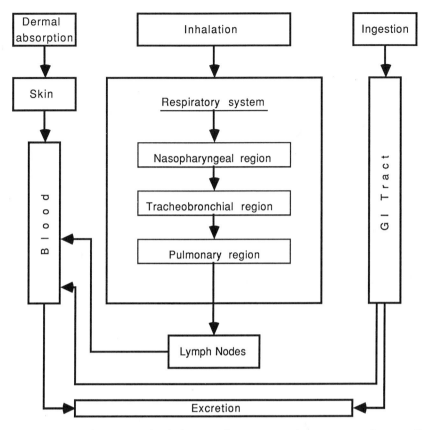

Figure 9-1. Schematic of inhalation, clearance, and excretion of internally deposited substances.

tinal tract, or lungs. For substances entering through the skin, the rate of deposition onto the skin usually can be characterized by a deposition coefficient, λ_D, expressed in units of mass per unit environmental concentration. The rate of movement from the environment onto the skin at some time t is equal to $\lambda_D I(t)$. For movement into the gastrointestinal tract from ingested materials, the rate of entry is given as $V_I I(t)$, where V_I is the rate at which material is ingested and $I(t)$ is the concentration of the substance in ingested material.

The respiratory system offers a somewhat more complicated case because substances in air that ultimately impart physiologic doses enter, are deposited, and can be removed from the lung. Furthermore, the respiratory system can be divided into three distinct subregions, which are characterized by separate retention functions and amounts of deposited material. These subregions are the naso-pharyngeal (NP), the tracheobronchial (TB), and the pulmonary (P) regions (ICRP, 1966). Inhaled particles or other materials (except gases) are deposited in the respiratory system subregions with different deposition fractions. The deposition fractions, in turn, are determined by the physical properties of the inhaled material. We can denote these fractions as f_{NP}, f_{TB}, and f_P for the nasopharyngeal, tracheobronchial, and pulmonary subregions, respectively. The corresponding rates of deposition into the three subregions for a substance in air are $ff_{NP}V_B I(t)$, $ff_{TB}V_B I(t)$, and $ff_P V_B I(t)$. In these three quantities the leading term f is the fraction of the substance inhaled after managing to circumvent protective devices (e.g., masks), V_B is the volumetric breathing rate in liters per minute (averaged over the period of exposure), and $I(t)$ is the environmental concentration of the substance, as before.

Once the material has entered the skin, gastrointestinal tract, or respiratory system, it will be retained in each compartment with a characteristic retention function $R(t)$. As mentioned earlier, these retention functions give estimates of the fractions of atoms or molecules of the substance remaining in the organ after time t following intake. If we let $B_S(t)$, $B_{GI}(t)$, $B_{NP}(t)$, $B_{TB}(t)$, and $B_P(t)$ represent the organ burdens at time t in the skin, gastrointestinal tract, and the three lung subregions, respectively, then these terms can be expressed mathematically as follows:

$$B_S(t) = \int_0^t \lambda_D I(T) R_S(t - T) \, dT \tag{9.5}$$

$$B_{GI}(t) = \int_0^t V_I I(T) R_{GI}(t - T) \, dT \tag{9.6}$$

$$B_{NP}(t) = \int_0^t ff_{NP} V_B I(T) R_{NP}(t - T) \, dT \tag{9.7}$$

$$B_{TB}(t) = \int_0^t ff_{TB} V_B I(T) R_{TB}(t - T) \, dT \tag{9.8}$$

$$B_P(t) = \int_0^t ff_P V_B I(T) R_P(t - T) \, dT \tag{9.9}$$

In expressions (9.5) through (9.9) the retention functions have been indexed to indicate that they are specific to each organ or respiratory system subregion, and it is assumed that exposure starts at time equal to 0. Values for f_{NP}, f_{TB}, and f_P for various persons' ages and for different sizes of solid particles can be found in papers by Crawford-Brown (1982) and Crawford-Brown and Eckerman (1983). The retention functions for the gastrointestinal tract and the respiratory system subregions for particles (primarily radioactive) of different sizes and solubilities in body fluids are given in publications by the International Commission on Radiological Protection (1966; 1972).

For the five organ systems mentioned earlier, the dose of some substance delivered between times t_1 and t_2 is proportional to the integral of the corresponding organ burden for the same time interval. Thus, using K as the proportionality constant, the doses for these five organs and lung subregions can be expressed in general forms as

$$D_S = K_S \int_{t_1}^{t_2} B_S(t)\, dt$$

$$= K_S \int_{t_1}^{t_2} \int_0^t \lambda_D I(T) R_S(t-T)\, dT\, dt$$

(9.10)

$$D_{GI} = K_{GI} \int_{t_1}^{t_2} B_{GI}(t)\, dt$$

$$= K_{GI} \int_{t_1}^{t_2} \int_0^t V_I I(T) R_{GI}(t-T)\, dT\, dt$$

(9.11)

$$D_{NP} = K_{NP} \int_{t_1}^{t_2} B_{NP}(t)\, dt$$

$$= K_{NP} \int_{t_1}^{t_2} \int_0^t ff_{NP} V_B I(T) R_{NP}(t-T)\, dT\, dt$$

(9.12)

$$D_{TB} = K_{TB} \int_{t_1}^{t_2} B_{TB}(t)\, dt$$

$$= K_{TB} \int_{t_1}^{t_2} \int_0^t ff_{TB} V_B I(T) R_{TB}(t-T)\, dT\, dt$$

(9.13)

$$D = K_P \int_{t_1}^{t_2} B_P(t)\, dt$$

$$= K_P \int_{t_1}^{t_2} \int_0^t ff_P V_B I(T) R_p(t-T)\, dT\, dt$$

(9.14)

The dose rate, and hence dose, at any time can then be assumed to be directly proportional to the calculated organ burden. This approach has been described for estimation of organ doses of alpha radiation from inhaled radionuclides (Checkoway and Crawford-Brown, 1987).

Equations describing organ burdens and doses in systemic organs (i.e., organs not in direct contact with the environment) are more complicated than those given earlier for the skin, gastrointestinal tract, and lungs. This complexity arises because some substances continuously transfer materials back and forth between systemic organs via the blood and the lymphatics. Biokinetic models that allow for cycling of material between systemic organs are known as *mammilary models*. These models are mathematically more complex than the models described earlier and are thus not generally useful in occupational epidemiology studies. The necessary equations for mammilary models described by Bernard (1977) and Skrable et al. (1980) could be developed for broader application.

Invocation of only a few assumptions reduces the complicated mammilary models to a set of models referred to as *catenary models* (Leggett, 1984). A catenary model describes the cascading movement of substances from one organ to the next, where the direction of movement is assumed to be only in one direction, terminating in excretion of the substance from the body. Catenary models simplify even further if it is assumed that the substance enters and is cleared from each systemic organ on a time scale that is rapid compared with the smallest time unit considered in the study. Since many occupational epidemiology studies do not consider time intervals smaller than single years, this second simplifying assumption will apply whenever the substance is removed from an organ with a half-life of a few months or less. If this assumption holds true, then the systemic organ burden at any point in time is directly proportional to the burden in the portal of entry (e.g., skin, gastrointestinal tract, or respiratory system) at that time.

It should be noted that the time lag between intake at the portal of entry and transport to a systemic organ is assumed to be negligible, relative to the duration of exposure. When the interval between intake and transport is delayed, as occurs when the substance is sequestered in adipose tissue or bone, a separate term for the lag time will be required in the model. Fortunately, most substances that are not sequestered satisfy this assumption. If, in addition, the substances are cleared rapidly from the skin, gastrointestinal tract, and lungs, then the systemic organ burdens are directly proportional to the exposure intensity. It should be appreciated that the numerical value of the proportionality between exposure intensity and organ burden still depends on the presence of exposure barriers and the physical properties of the environment that control intake and deposition into organs that act as portals of entry.

Many substances encountered occupationally move rapidly from the skin and gastrointestinal tract, and all but very insoluble substances (e.g., lead) are cleared rapidly from the lungs. Thus, in typical situations the rates at which substances enter the bloodstream are proportional to the rates of movement into the skin, gastrointestinal tract, or lungs. A certain fraction of a substance that enters the bloodstream will then be distributed to the systemic organs, with each organ receiving a characteristic uptake fraction. The rate at which material moves into a systemic organ can therefore be expressed as the product of the rate of discharge from the portal of entry organ into the blood (and lymphatics) and the uptake fraction. When the substance also is removed rapidly from the skin, gastrointestinal tract, or lungs, the rate of movement into the bloodstream from the portal organs will be proportional to the rates of intake by these organs. As a result of this relationship, substances that pass quickly through the skin, gastrointestinal tract, or lungs display a systemic organ burden at time t given by the following expression:

$$B_k(t) = \int_0^t Gf_B f_k I(T) R_k(t - T)\, dT \qquad (9.15)$$

where G is the proportionality constant relating exposure intensity and the rate of deposition into either the skin, gastrointestinal, tract or lungs; f_B is the fraction of the substance moving into the bloodstream, given that it has deposited in the portal of entry organ; f_k is the fraction of the substance that is deposited into the kth systemic organ, given that it has entered the bloodstream; and $R_k(t)$ is the retention function for the substance in the kth systemic organ. Values for f_B, f_k, and $R_k(t)$ for most radionuclides and many nonradioactive elements can be found in the report by the ICRP (1979). Models useful for specifying G for the lung for dusts and other physical substances are described by Cuddihy et al. (1979), Gerrity et al. (1983), and Smith (1985). Pharmacokinetic models are also available for solvents and other volatile chemicals (Fiserova-Bergerova et al., 1974; Perbellini et al., 1986), although these models tend to be complicated because they incorporate considerations of transport to and metabolism (e.g., biotransformation) in multiple body compartments.

Expression (9.15) can be applied regardless of how long the substance in question remains in a systemic organ, provided that the transport from the portal of entry organ is rapid. Retention times in the pulmonary subregions of the lungs can be quite long (at times, with half-lives extending to decades) for very insoluble substances, such as amphibole asbestos fibers. A slightly more complicated catenary model is required for very insoluble substances because the rate of movement into the bloodstream no longer is proportional to exposure intensity. Instead, the rate of entry into the bloodstream is proportional to the burden in the portal of entry organ. To illustrate, let f_B be the fractional rate at which the substance leaves the portal of entry and enters the bloodstream. Thus, the burden in the kth systemic organ at time t can be expressed as

$$B_k(t) = \int_0^t f_B f_k B_e(T) R_k(t - T)\, dT \qquad (9.16)$$

where $B_e(T)$ is the burden for the portal of entry organ and the constants are as defined earlier. $B_e(T)$ usually can be obtained from expression (9.9) because equation (9.16) really is needed only for substances that enter the pulmonary subregion of the respiratory tract.

This completes our general discussion of organ burdens. Next, we can turn our attention to dose estimation using organ burden models.

Doses can be estimated from any of the preceding organ burden models in conjunction with the relationship between burden and dose given in expression (9.4). Thus, organ burdens are computed first and then integrated to arrive at doses. To this point we have merely mentioned how retention functions are incorporated into organ burden models, without offering an explicit form for retention. Retention functions usually are assumed to be exponential or series of exponential functions (the exponential form facilitates integration). A typical exponential retention function is as follows:

$$R(t) = A_1 \exp[-\lambda_1 t] + A_2 \exp[-\lambda_2 t] + \cdots + A_m \exp[-\lambda_m t] \quad (9.17)$$

where λ_m is the fractional rate at which the substance leaves the mth compartment of an organ and A_m is the fraction of the substance reaching the organ in the mth compartment. Other, more complicated retention functions are not discussed here because their use in occupational epidemiology is restricted by their complexity.

Summary of Organ Burden and Dose Modeling

We have described four situations of organ burden and dose modeling. In the interest of simplifying the discussion, we have considered body organs as the biological targets, although the presentation of modeling approaches also applies to more specific targets, such as subpopulations of cells or intracellular sites. Another sim-

plifying assumption is that the exposure or dose index to be estimated is an average for a given year of exposure. Summaries of the
four modeling cases follow.

1. The first case is when all of the material moves out of all organs with
   a halftime that is short in comparison to one year (e.g., a few months
   or less). Under this condition, the organ burden and, hence, the dose
   are directly proportional to the average exposure intensity for the
   year. This proportionality is a function of the physical and chemical
   properties of the substance, the route of entry into the body, and the
   uptake and metabolism of the target organ.
2. The second case arises when the material moves quickly out of the
   portal of entry organs (e.g., skin, gastrointestinal tract, or lungs) but
   is retained significantly in a systemic organ(s) for times longer than
   one year. As in the first case, the burdens for the portal of entry
   organs are proportional to exposure intensity. However, this proportionality does not hold for systemic target organs; consequently,
   equation (9.15) must be used.
3. The third situation is when the material moves slowly out of the portal of entry organs but is rapidly cleared from systemic organs. This
   case generally pertains to entry through the pulmonary subregion of
   the lung. Here systemic organ burdens are directly proportional to
   burdens in the portal of entry organs. The relationships are specified
   adequately by equations (9.5) through (9.9). The necessary proportionality constant also depends on the physical characteristics of the
   substance.
4. Finally, there is the case in which substances are retained for long
   periods of time in both the portal of entry and systemic organs.
   When this situation arises, burdens and doses must be computed
   using equation (9.16) in conjunction with expressions (9.5) through
   (9.9). This situation is uncommon but may be encountered in occupations involving inhalation of highly insoluble materials that are
   deposited in the pulmonary subregion of the lungs and are trans-
   ported to the bone. Examples are inhaled plutonium or lead.

One complicating feature that arises in estimating doses for many
chemicals is metabolic activation (or deactivation). By metabolic
activation we mean chemical alterations of the substance in the body
to a different chemical species. Conversions of polycyclic aromatic
hydrocarbons from precarcinogens to ultimate carcinogens, by
means of hydroxylation and epoxidation, is one such example (Harris et al., 1985). Many substances not only cascade through the various body organs, but also undergo chemical transformations as
they move. We can therefore consider the *biologically effective dose* as
the integral of the target (organ) burden for the transformed sub-

stance. If the substance is transformed rapidly upon entering the body, then the biologically effective organ burden is directly proportional to the organ burden calculated from the equations given earlier. When this assumption is not valid, burden and dose estimation becomes substantially more difficult. As a practical guideline, we suggest that variable rates of chemical activation can be ignored in most epidemiologic analyses.

4. EXAMPLES OF DOSE MODELING

Thus far, we have been describing exposure and dose modeling in abstract terms. Some examples should help to illustrate modeling principles and techniques.

4.1. Example 1: Inhaled Soluble Uranium Compounds

The first example comes from ionizing radiation epidemiology and concerns exposures to dusts of uranium compounds. Although this example is hypothetical, the exposure levels are similar in magnitude to those encountered in uranium processing facilities.

First, we can assume that workers at some facility are exposed to airborne uranium dust. The form is uranium hexafluoride, which is very soluble in body fluids and leaves the lungs rapidly with a retention half-life on the order of 0.5 day. The uranium enters the bloodstream after clearance from the lung and is deposited in bone with a 22.3-percent efficiency (i.e., f_K is 0.223 for uranium in bone) (ICRP, 1979). The remainder is excreted promptly via the kidneys. Once in the bone, the uranium remains with a retention function (ICRP, 1979) equal to

$$R(t) = 0.897 \exp\left[\frac{-0.693t}{20}\right] + 0.103 \exp\left[\frac{-0.693t}{5000}\right]$$

where $R(t)$ is the fraction of the substance remaining in the bone t days after entry into the bone, 0.897 and 0.103 represent the fractions of uranium deposited, respectively, in two separate compartments of the bone, 20 and 5,000 are half-lives (in days) for uranium in these compartments, and 0.693 is the natural logarithm of 2. The retention function is the same for all forms of uranium because they are metabolized to a common form, hexavalent uranium, in the bloodstream prior to bone deposition.

Assume that a worker is exposed only to the very soluble uranium

(^{238}U) fluoride at an air concentration of 10^{-4} μCi/.n^3, during the years 1940 and 1941. [The microcuric (μCi) is a unit of radioactivity that is proportional to the number of atoms of uranium.] During each of these years the worker is exposed for 2,000 hours, based on employment for 40 hours per week for 50 weeks. The average breathing rate of air V_B is assumed to be a constant, 10 m^3/day, which is typical for light activity (ICRP, 1975). Assume that the worker wears a respirator that stops 75 percent of the uranium dust. Our objective is to compute the organ burden for, and dose to, the lungs for each year starting with 1940.

For soluble (and insoluble) uranium, deposition in the pulmonary subregion of the respiratory tract is far greater than in either the nasopharyngeal or tracheobronchial subregions. A typical deposition fraction for uranium dust particles in the pulmonary subregion is 0.30 (ICRP, 1966). The value for f in equation (9.9) is 0.25, representing the 25 percent of airborne dust reaching the lungs, $I(t)$ is 10^{-4} μCi/m^3 during both years of exposure, and V_B is 10 m^3/day. The retention function for soluble uranium in the pulmonary subregion of the lung is

$$R_P(t) = \exp[-0.693t/0.5]$$

where t is in days. Inserting the known values into equation (9.9) gives a pulmonary burden function of

$$B_P(t) = \int_0^t (0.25)(0.3)(10)(10^{-4})\exp[-0.693T/0.5]\, dT$$

or

$$B_P(t) = \frac{(0.25)(0.3)(10)(10^{-4})(1 - \exp[-0.693t/0.5])}{(0.693/0.5)}$$

$$= (5.4 \times 10^{-5})(1 - \exp[-1.39t])$$

where $B(t)$ is in units of μCi.

The dose delivered during the first year of exposure, 1940, can be calculated using equation (9.4), with K equal to 0.24 rad/day/ μCi (Dunning et al., 1980). Performing this integration yields

$$D_{1940} = \int_0^{365} (0.24)(5.4 \times 10^{-5})(1 - \exp[-1.39t])\, dt$$

$$= (0.24)(5.4 \times 10^{-5})\left[365 - \frac{(1 - \exp[-1.39(365)])}{1.39} \right]$$

$$= 4.7 \times 10^{-3}\ \text{rads}$$

The dose delivered during 1941 will also be 4.7×10^{-3} rads.

Exposure to soluble uranium stops at the end of 1941, and the material is removed from the lungs very rapidly. As a result, soluble uranium inhaled in 1940 and 1941 contributes a negligible dose during the years after 1941. To see this, consider that the average lung burden throughout 1940 is roughly the same as the burden at the end of the year. Hence

$$B_{1940} = (0.25)(0.3)(10)(10^{-4}) \int_0^{365} \exp[-0.693t/0.5] \, dt$$

$$= 5.4 \times 10^{-5} \, \mu Ci$$

For 1941 the estimated lung burden is

$$B_{1941} = (0.25)(0.3)(10)(10^4) \int_0^{365} \exp[-0.693/0.5] \, dt$$

$$= 0 + 5.4 \times 10^{-5} = 5.4 \times 10^{-5} \, \mu Ci,$$

which applies at the end of 1941 (or the beginning of 1942).

Thus, the burden approximation for soluble uranium in the lung is nearly identical for both years of exposure. Also, the dose in each year is proportional to exposure intensity. For years after 1941, the contribution from material inhaled in 1940 and 1941 is negligible, also because of the short half-life of soluble uranium in the lungs, as indicated by the very rapidly decreasing exponential terms in the two lung burden equations.

The dose in 1942 will be

$$D_{1942} = \int_0^{365} (0.24)(5.4 \times 10^{-5}) \exp[-1.39t] \, dt$$

$$= \frac{0.24(5.4 \times 10^{-5})}{1.39} (1 - \exp[-1.39(365)])$$

$$\simeq 0 \text{ rad}$$

It may be noted, therefore, that exposure intensity is directly proportional to dose for these three years.

For the lung, exposure acts as an almost perfect surrogate for dose. Consider now the case of organ burden and dose to bone. In general, expression (9.16) for burden in a systemic organ can be applied. However, expression (9.15) can also be used because soluble uranium moves quickly through the lungs. In expression (9.15), G is equal to $ff_P V_B$, which is equal to $(0.25)(0.3)(10) = 0.75$. Equation (9.15) then yields

$$B_k(t) = \int_0^t (0.75) f_B f_k I(T) R_k(t - T) \, dT$$

which, after insertion of the expression for $R_k(t)$ for bone, and set-ting $f_k = 0.223$ and $f_B = 1.0$, yields

$$B_k(t) = \int_0^t (0.75)(1.0)(10^{-4})(0.223)\{(0.897)\exp[-0.693T/20]$$

$$+ (0.103)\exp[-0.693T/5000]\}\, dT$$

or

$$B_k(t) = (7.5 \times 10^{-5})\{(0.2(20)/0.693)(1 - \exp[-0.693t/20])$$

$$+ (0.023(5000)/0.693)(1 - \exp[-0.693t/5000])\}$$

This last expression holds for any time up to the end of 1941 because exposure intensity was constant during the period before that year. Assuming an S-factor of 6.4×10^{-6} rads/day/μCi for uranium in bone (Dunning et al., 1980) and assuming that the uranium is located in cancellous bone, the bone dose for 1940 is

$$D_{1940} = 6.4 \times 10^{-6} \int_0^{365} B_k(t)\, dt$$

$$= 6.4 \times 10^{-6} \int_0^{365} \{(4.3 \times 10^{-4})(1 - \exp[-0.693t/20])$$

$$+ (0.0124)(1 - \exp[-0.693t/5000])\}\, dt$$

$$= (0.258)(6.4 \times 10^{-6}) = 1.7 \times 10^{-6}\ \text{rads}$$

The dose in 1941 is

$$D_{1941} = 6.4 \times 10^{-6} \int_{365}^{730} B_k(t)\, dt$$

$$= (0.487)(6.4 \times 10^{-6}) = 3.1 \times 10^{-6}\ \text{rads}$$

Note that, unlike the lung where material is removed rapidly, the dose to the bone in each year is no longer proportional to the exposure intensity in that year. This is seen most dramatically for years after 1941, when exposure had since stopped. Consider the year 1942, for example. The bone burden at the end of 1941 is $1.63 \times 10^{-3}\ \mu$Ci, which is divided between the two bone compartments, with $4.3 \times 10^{-4}\ \mu$Ci in the 20-day compartment and $1.2 \times 10^{-3}\ \mu$Ci in the 5,000-day compartment.

Hence, the bone dose for 1942 is

$$D_{1942} = (6.4 \times 10^{-6})(4.3 \times 10^{-4}) \int_0^{365} \exp[-0.693t/20]\, dt$$

$$+ (6.4 \times 10^{-6})(1.2 \times 10^{-3}) \int_0^{365} \exp[-0.693t/5000]\, dt$$

$$= 2.8 \times 10^{-6}\ \text{rads}$$

In other words, the bone dose in 1942 is approximately the same as that in 1941, despite the fact that exposure ceased in 1941. This results from the long retention of even soluble uranium compounds in bone. Dose delivery to the bone would persist for some years after exposure ended. By contrast, the lung doses in 1942 and subsequent years would be virtually nil because of rapid clearance from that organ.

4.2. Example 2: Inhaled Asbestos Fibers

The second example involves an analysis of the data from the historical cohort study of mortality among asbestos textile plant workers (Dement et al., 1983). The objective here is to develop an index of exposure that, in part, reflects the subsequent temporal pattern of dose. Exposure modeling for asbestos presents a more typical situation than dose modeling for radionuclides (from the preceding example) because estimation of the kinetics parameters for asbestos is much more difficult than that for uranium compounds. As a result, exposure modeling, rather than burden and dose modeling, is more practical for studies of asbestos-exposed workers. Thus, despite the large body of experimental evidence demonstrating the fibrogenic and carcinogenic potential of the various types of asbestos fibers in the lungs (and possibly some systemic organs in the case of carcinogenesis), quantitative dose estimation remains an uncertain proposition.

In general terms, exposure modeling consists of applying various weighting schemes to exposure intensity data. Weighting is designed to relate exposure in a given year to an effect (damage) produced subsequently. The simplest approach is to compute a cumulative exposure (E) index, which is merely the summed products of environmental concentrations and the durations of time spent at those concentrations. Cumulative exposure as of some point in time t is given by expression (9.2).

Cumulative exposure is the most commonly used index in studies of chronic diseases, and in fact, it was the index used by Dement et al. (1983) in their original analysis. However, there are some shortcomings to cumulative exposure measures, as we pointed out in Chapter 5. To review briefly, cumulative exposure often provides little information about the temporal course of the rate of exposure delivery, one result of which is that effects of peak exposures can go unnoticed (Copes et al., 1985). Furthermore, the simple cumulative exposure measure will not take into account retention in target organs or tissues, and thus may be a poor surrogate for dose for slowly cleared or metabolized substances. These problems can be mitigated partially by weighting exposures to reflect the ultimate dose that is delivered.

A general form for a weighted cumulative exposure (E_j) at the end of year j (Y_j) from exposures received in the preceding i years ($i = 1,2, \ldots, j$) is given by

$$E_j = \sum_i^j I_i w_i \tag{9.18}$$

where I_i are the yearly exposure concentrations and the w_i are the assigned weights. (Note that we are using yearly time intervals, although smaller units may be required in studies of acute effects.) Ideally, we would choose weights that account best for effect induction time and retention of the substance in the target organ or tissues. Hence, exposures that theoretically are most etiologically important should be weighted most heavily. One approach is to let w_i equal the fraction of the substance inhaled or ingested in year i, which is still present in year j ($j \geq 1$). In this instance, E_j will be proportional to the dose rate in year j.

We can recognize that the latency analysis described in Chapter 5, where exposures are lagged by an assumed latency interval, is a form of exposure weighting. In the simplest, most common case of exposure lagging, the w_i for exposures during the estimated latency period are set to 0, whereas weights of 1.0 would be assigned for exposures in all other years. Considerations of substance retention are thus ignored in this approach. Another approach involves setting weights equal to 1.0 for the assumed etiologically relevant "time window" and assigning weights of 0 to all other years. This second approach to latency analysis requires the assumption that the most recent and the most distant exposures are unrelated to disease induction (Rothman, 1981).

Conventional latency analysis does not address retention of the substance explicitly. However, an exposure weighting method described by Jahr (1974) was devised for this purpose. According to this approach, each exposure is weighted in direct proportion to the time since occurrence. Thus, the w_i in expression (9.18) become

$$w_i = Y_j - Y_i + 0.5 \tag{9.19}$$

where Y_i is the year of exposure, Y_j is the year when damage is being measured ($Y_j > Y_i$), and 0.5 allows for delivery of exposure throughout year Y_i, rather than all at once at the beginning of the year.

Table 9-1. Hypothetical example of Jahr model of exposure weighting for a worker exposed for three years and followed for ten years

Year	Exposure intensity (I_i)	E_i^a (1950)	E_i (1951)	E_i (1952)	$E_j = \Sigma E_i$
1950	10	5	—	—	5
1951	5	15	2.5	—	17.5
1952	2	25	7.5	1	33.5
1953	0	35	12.5	3	50.5
1954	0	45	17.5	5	67.5
1955	0	55	22.5	7	84.5
1956	0	65	27.5	9	101.5
1957	0	75	32.5	11	118.5
1958	0	85	37.5	13	135.5
1959	0	95	42.5	15	152.5

^{a}Jahr model with no clearance: $E_i = I_i(Y_j - Y_i + 0.5)$.

Jahr's method theoretically is most useful for examining dose–response relationships when the substance under study is tenaciously retained in the body (e.g., amphibole asbestos fibers).

The Jahr model of exposure weighting is illustrated in Table 9–1. In this hypothetical example, a worker is exposed for three years to environmental concentrations of 10, 5, and 2 units of some substance, and follow-up extends for a ten-year period from first exposure. Thus, in 1950 the worker receives a total of 5 units of cumulative exposure, and it is assumed that there is a constant contribution of 10 units from this year's exposure in all successive years. In other words, the burden resulting from the first year's exposure is 5 at the end of that year and stays constant at 10 in all subsequent years. It should be noted that this formulation of the Jahr approach assumes no clearance of the substance (i.e., retention time approaches the end of the worker's lifetime). The contributions from exposures occurring in 1950, 1951, and 1952 can be computed using expression (9.18), as shown in the rightmost column of Table 9–1.

Expression (9.18) can be refined to allow for clearance of the substance, while still maintaining the Jahr scheme of weighting exposures in proportion to time since occurrence. The equation is given as

$$E_j = \sum_i^j I_i\{1/k - 1/k^2(1 - \exp[-k])(\exp[-k(Y_j - Y_i)])\} \quad (9.20)$$

where $k = \ln 2/T_{1/2}$, with $T_{1/2}$ being the half-life in the target organ. The main uncertainty of using a clearance model for many substances is that there are insufficient data to estimate values for half-lives in the body as a whole or in particular target organs. This difficulty has been noted by other investigators who have applied approaches similar to Jahr's method (Berry et al., 1979; Finkelstein, 1985). Also, the clearance model depicted in expression (9.20) assumes a constant rate of clearance, irrespective of the exposure rate and the organ burden. More complex models that allow for variable rates of clearance could be constructed, but estimation of rate constants would be subject to great uncertainty. The problem of half-life estimation becomes even more difficult for systemic organs, particularly when the kinetics require a model with transport to and from more than one organ (i.e., multicompartment models).

Weighting exposures in the manner suggested by Jahr makes an implicit assumption about the induction and latency periods for a delayed effect of exposure. Thus, according to Jahr's scheme, observed health effects are assumed to be most strongly related to the earliest exposures during a worker's employment, and it is assumed that the effect of these exposures becomes evident later in life. We should point out that the weights need not be constrained to be linear or necessarily in direct proportion to the time since exposure occurred. Geometrical weights can be assigned, or one might, for example, assign weights so that the most recent exposures are weighted more heavily than those in the past if there is reason to believe that recent exposures are more etiologically important (Axelson, 1985). Another alternative would be to weight exposures by the square of time since occurrence, if there were reason to assume that the earliest exposures were substantially more important than those received in later years. Complex weighting schemes involving higher-order polynomials are seldom justified in most practical applications, however.

Some approaches to exposure weighting are illustrated with data from the asbestos textile plant workers cohort study (Dement et al., 1983). Trends of lung cancer mortality were assessed in relation to the following exposure indices: (1) simple cumulative exposure; (2) cumulative exposure with a ten-year lag; (3) cumulative exposures attained during the time period 10–25 years previously [i.e., truncation of exposures more than 25 years before the year of evaluation (year j), as well as a ten-year lag]; (4) the simplest case of the Jahr model, with weights assigned in direct proportion to time since occurrence and no clearance; and (5) the Jahr model, but with an assumed ten-year half-life of asbestos in the lungs. The results are summarized in Table 9–2.

For these analyses the cohort was divided into seven exposure

Table 9–2. Exposure–response relationships for asbestos exposure and lung cancer mortality using various exposure weighting models

Stratum[a]	(1) Cumulative exposure, 0-yr lag	(2) Cumulative exposure, 10-yr lag	(3) Cumulative exposure time window, 10–25 yr	(4) Jahr model, no clearance	(5) Jahr model, $T_{1/2} =$ 10 yr
1[b]	1.00	1.00	1.00	1.00	1.00
2	2.08	2.31	2.64	1.53	1.92
3	1.46	2.41	1.97	2.26	1.96
4	3.35	5.24	3.33	6.34	4.32
5	4.28	4.03	5.94	3.46	3.76
6	5.70	6.92	9.84	5.72	6.68
7	11.17	15.27	16.96	13.33	13.57
$\chi^2_{df=6}$	17.9	19.5	23.0	20.0	19.0

[a]Each stratum contains five deaths.
[b]Reference category.

strata, where each stratum contains five lung cancer deaths. Thus, the stratum boundaries were specified by the exposure levels attained by the cases. This approach to exposure stratification was used instead of a more customary procedure, such as setting exposure boundaries on the basis of quartiles of the cohort's exposure distribution, to assure maximum stability in the comparison of rates between strata. Relative risk estimates (rate ratios) were computed by means of Poisson rate regression (Frome, 1983), and the magnitude of the exposure–response association was evaluated with a chi-square statistic with 6 degrees of freedom (one less than the number of exposure categories). The relative risks were adjusted for age, calendar year, and duration of follow-up, each in five-year intervals.

There are marked gradients of lung cancer mortality with increasing exposure level for all weighting schemes, which is consistent with the originally reported findings (Dement et al., 1983). It can also be noted that the chi-square results for an overall effect are all similar in magnitude. Model 3, the 10–25-year cumulative exposure window, yields the highest relative risks for the last two exposure strata, although the trend is slightly dampened by a relatively high rate ratio in the second stratum (2.64). We also performed an analysis similar to model 5, assuming a 30-year rather than a ten-year retention half-life (data not shown); the results differ only slightly.

In this example it appears that each of these exposure weighting schemes is consistent with a linear trend of relative risk. Had there been substantial differences in the patterns of the relative risks, there might be some clear choice of the best model, at least on statistical grounds. In any event, the choice of a best model should be made with regard not only to the data being analyzed, but also to findings from previous epidemiologic and experimental research. It should be appreciated that we have been using exposure rather than dose modeling in this example; consequently, the conclusions drawn from such an analysis need to be tempered with caveats about the suitability of exposure variables as surrogates for dose parameters.

5. SUMMARY

Dose–response models for occupational exposures and disease risks can provide insights into mechanisms of disease induction and are necessary for predicting adverse health effects in populations with varying exposure levels. In Chapter 2 we defined exposure and dose variables in conceptual terms, stressing that exposure refers to the presence of a substance in the environment external to the body, whereas organ or body burdens and doses refer to the amount of a substance within the body. In this chapter we have taken a more mathematical approach to defining these terms in order to lay the groundwork for deriving dose–response models.

Ultimately, we would like to know the concentrations of substances at specific biological targets that are sufficient to induce disease. Identifying specific biological targets and measuring concentrations that change over time at these targets impose practical constraints in most instances. Instead, we are forced to use mathematical models that depict first the relationships between environmental exposure intensities and organ (or tissue) burdens, and second the relationships between burdens and doses. Modeling requires estimation of intake rates, retention in the portal-of-entry organ(s), and transport to and retention in remote (systemic) organs. An understanding of the metabolic fates of substances in the body will assist in determining biologically effective doses. However, for most substances either the "active" metabolites are not known or the predictors of individuals' metabolic responses are unknown. Consequently, modeling usually ends with somewhat uncertain dose estimation.

Ionizing radiation is a valuable paradigm for dose modeling because there is a vast body of experimental and epidemiologic data from which models have been developed depicting deposition and retention in various body organs. Our first example concerning uranium compounds illustrates some methods for estimating organ burdens and doses from exposure data.

This first example also illustrates some of the uncertainties that arise in dose modeling. For example, an air concentration of uranium dust (or alpha radiation activity) is measured with some error, perhaps because of defects in instrumentation. Next, we need to be concerned about whether the measurements made in various areas of a facility adequately represent workers' actual exposure intensities. Poorly located sampling devices can result in exaggerated or underestimated intensities. If we are confident that environmental concentrations can be linked validly to individual workers, then we must make a series of assumptions regarding the effectiveness of protective devices, breathing rates, and deposition patterns in portal-of-entry organs (e.g., all routes other than inhalation are irrelevant). Next, intake rates are estimated and are used in conjunction with knowledge of the physical and chemical properties of the substances considered (e.g., solubility in body fluids) to estimate retention functions in the lungs. These retention functions are used to model organ burdens and ultimately doses, which represent time-integrated burdens. The modeling can be extended further to include estimation of doses to systemic organs, such as the bones, that have their own characteristic retention functions.

Thus, modeling provides average expected doses, and the validity of the estimates depends on the validity of a number of assumptions. Misclassification of workers into dose categories occurs when some of these assumptions are violated or when the study population is small and expected average doses are likely to be inaccurate. An alternative to modeling doses from exposure data is to obtain direct biological measurements from which organ burdens can be estimated for individual workers. This alternative, although desirable, involves greatly added costs to a study and has its own shortcomings relating to uncertainty of the metabolic modeling that must be performed to relate biological measurements to organ burdens.

Exposure modeling is required when biokinetic models are not well specified or are fraught with extreme computational complexities. In this situation, the time-dependent delivery of exposures is modeled to provide dose surrogates.

The most common approach is to compute simple cumulative exposure as the dose surrogate, where cumulative exposure is the time-integrated exposure intensity. As we discussed in Chapter 5, simple cumulative exposure is a valuable surrogate for dose when the probability or severity of the disease of interest is directly proportional to the amount reaching biological targets. However, cumulative exposure often does not reveal important temporal patterns in the rates of exposure delivery. Exposure weighting is one strategy for enhancing the informativeness of a cumulative exposure index. For example, weights can be assigned to account for disease latency, as is done when cumulative exposures are lagged or restricted to particular time windows. Also, weighting schemes are available to estimate retention half-times of substances in various organs and tissues. We illustrated various weighting schemes with data on lung cancer mortality from the asbestos textile plant cohort study. In this example, similarly strong gradients of lung cancer risk were seen for all exposure weighting schemes, as would be expected given the strength of the association between asbestos exposure and lung cancer. Consequently, we could not decide unequivocally which of the exposure models best describes the underlying biological process. In the absence of compelling prior reasons to use a particular model, the simple cumulative exposure and lagged exposure models appear to be preferable on the grounds of conceptual and computational simplicity.

It is arguable whether dose modeling or exposure modeling is to be preferred. The two approaches address related but somewhat different issues. Dose modeling is clearly preferable when the metabolism of substances is well understood, whereas exposure modeling can serve as a substitute for dose modeling when biokinetic and metabolic models are less certain. There are situations where exposure modeling is not a good substitute for dose modeling. This was seen in the example of estimating bone doses from soluble uranium, where the proportionality between exposure and dose is nonlinear. In addition, dose modeling will be important when conclusions drawn from studies of workers experiencing one route of exposure are to be extrapolated to persons exposed by different routes. Exposure modeling, however, is important in its own right because protection standards for most substances are more easily based on exposure levels that can be measured in the environment than on doses that are estimated indirectly from mathematical models. Increasingly, there is interest in developing and refining dose models for a wide range of substances, including radiations, dusts, and chemicals.

Glossary

biologically effective dose   Dose of the active metabolite of a chemical or physical agent.

biokinetic models   Models that describe the relationships between exposures and target concentrations.

burden   The amount of a substance in the body or in some particular target (e.g., organ) at time t.

catenary models   Models describing the movement of substances between body organs, where movement is assumed to be unidirectional.

cumulative exposure   The integral of exposure intensity over time.

dose   The amount of a substance that is delivered to a target during some specified time interval.

dose intensity   The rate of delivery of a substance to the target.

dose rate   A synonym for dose intensity.

exposure rate   The rate at which a substance is brought into contact with the body, estimated by the environmental concentration.

half-life   The time required for half of the substance to be removed from the target organ or tissues.

intensity   The concentration of a substance in the environment that potentially can enter the body and be delivered to biological targets.

pharmacodynamic models   Models relating target concentrations of substances to biological responses.

portal-of-entry organs   Organs through which substances enter the body.

retention function   A model that specifies the amount of a substance remaining in an organ or tissue as a function of time since uptake.

systemic organs   Organs not in direct contact with the environment (i.e., remote from portal-of-entry organs).

uptake fraction   The fractional amount of a substance that enters an organ, given prior entrance into the bloodstream.

Notation

A_m The fraction of a substance reaching the mth part of an organ.

$B(t)$ The organ burden at time t.

$B_e(t)$ The burden at the portal-of-entry organ at time t (e.g., $B_P(t)$ is the burden in the pulmonary region of the lung).

$B_k(t)$ The burden in the kth systemic organ at time t.

D Dose to a target organ or tissue.

E Cumulative exposure during the interval (t_1,t_2).

E_j Cumulative exposure at the end of year j from exposures delivered during the preceding $i(i < j)$ years.

f The fraction of the substance that enters the body from the environment.

f_B The fraction of the substance moving from the portal-of-entry organ to the bloodstream.

f_k The fraction of the substance deposited in the kth organ (e.g., f_P is the fraction deposited in the pulmonary region of the lung).

G A proportionality constant relating exposure intensity and deposition into a portal-of-entry organ.

I_D Dose intensity or dose rate.

I_i Exposure intensity for year i.

$I(t)$ Exposure intensity at time t.

k $\ln2/T_{1/2}$, where $T_{1/2}$ is the half-life of the substance in the target organ.

K A proportionality constant relating dose intensity and organ burden.

$R_k(t)$ The retention function of a substance in the kth organ (e.g., R_P is the retention function for the pulmonary region of the lung).

t Time.

T Duration of exposure.

V_B Volumetric breathing rate in liters per minute.

V_I Rate at which a substance is ingested.

w_i Weight assigned to exposure delivered in year i.

Y_i Year i, during which exposure occurred.

Y_j The year in which damage is being measured.

References

Axelson O (1985): Dealing with exposure variable in occupational health epidemiology. *Scand J Soc Med* 13:147–152.

Bernard SR (1977): Dosimetric data and a metabolic model for lead. *Health Phys* 32:44–46.

Berry G, Gibson JC, Holmes S, et al. (1979): Asbestosis: a study of dose-response relationships in an asbestos textile factory. *Br J Ind Med* 36:98–112.

Checkoway H, and Crawford-Brown DJ (1987): Metabolic modeling of organ-specific doses to carcinogens, as illustrated with alpha-radiation emitting radionuclides. *J Chron Dis* 40(Suppl 2):191S–200S.

Copes R, Thomas D, and Becklake MR (1985): Temporal patterns of exposure and nonmalignant pulmonary abnormality in Quebec chrysotile workers. *Arch Environ Health* 40:80–87.

Crawford-Brown DJ (1982): Identifying critical human subpopulations by age groups: radioactivity and the lung. *Phys Med Biol* 27:539–552.

Crawford-Brown DJ, and Eckerman KF (1983): Modifications of the ICRP Task Group Lung Model to reflect age dependence. *Radiat Prot Dosim* 2:209–220.

Cuddihy RG, McClellan RO, and Griffith WC (1979): Variability in target organ deposition among individuals exposed to toxic substances. *Toxicol Appl Pharmacol* 49:179–184.

Dement JM, Harris RL, Symons MJ, and Shy CM (1983): Exposures and mortality among chrysotile asbestos workers. Part II: Mortality. *Am J Ind Med* 4:421–433.

Dunning DE, Pleasant JC, and Killough GG (1980): S-factor: a computer code for calculating dose equivalent to a target organ per microcurie-day residence of a radionuclide in a source organ. ORNL/NUREG/TM-85/S1. Oak Ridge, TN: Oak Ridge National Laboratory.

Finkelstein MM (1985): A study of dose-response relationships for asbestos associated disease. *Br J Ind Med* 42:319–325.

Fiserova-Bergerova V, Blach J, and Singhal K (1974): Simulation and prediction of uptake, distribution and exhalation of organic solvents. *Br J Ind Med* 31:45–52.

Frome EL (1983): The analysis of rates using Poisson regression models. *Biometrics* 39:665–674.

Gerrity TR, Garrard CS, and Yeates DB (1983): A mathematical model of particle retention in the air-spaces of human lungs. *Br J Ind Med* 40:121–130.

Harris CC, Vahakangas K, Newman MJ, et al. (1985): Detection of benzo[a]pyrene diol epoxide-DNA adducts in peripheral blood lymphocytes and antibodies to the adducts in serum from coke oven workers. *Proc Natl Acad Sci* (USA) 82:6672–6676.

International Commission on Radiological Protection, ICRP Task Group on Lung Dynamics (1966): Deposition and retention models for internal dosimetry of the human respiratory tract. *Health Phys* 12:173–207.

International Commission on Radiological Protection (1972): *ICRP Publication 19: The Metabolism of Compounds of Plutonium and Other Actinides.* Oxford: Pergamon Press.

International Commission on Radiological Protection (1975): *ICRP Publication 23: Reference Man.* Oxford: Pergamon Press.

International Commission on Radiological Protection (1977): *ICRP Publication 26: Recommendations of the International Commission on Radiological Protection.* Oxford: Pergamon Press.

International Commission on Radiological Protection (1979): *ICRP Publication 30: Limits for Intakes of Radionuclides by Workers.* Oxford: Pergamon Press.

Jahr J (1974): Dose-response basis for setting a quartz threshold limit value: a new simple formula for calculating the "lifetime dose" of quartz. *Arch Environ Health* 29:338–340.

Leggett RW (1984): On estimating dose rates to organs as a function of age following internal exposure. ORNL/TM-8265. Oak Ridge, TN: Oak Ridge National Laboratory.

Perbellini L, Mozzo P, Brugnone F, and Zedde A (1986): Physiologicomathematical model for studying human exposure to organic solvents: kinetics of blood/tissue *n*-hexane concentrations and 2,5-hexanedione in urine. *Br J Ind Med* 43:760–768.

Rothman KJ (1981): Induction and latent periods. *Am J Epidemiol* 114:253–259.

Skrable KW, Chabot GE, French CS, et al. (1980): Blood–organ transfer kinetics. *Health Phys* 39:193–210.

Smith TJ (1985): Development and application of a model for estimating alveolar and interstitial dust levels. *Ann Occup Hyg* 29:495–516.

Smith TJ (1987): Exposure assessment for occupational epidemiology. *Am J Ind Med* 12:249–268.

10 Special Applications of Occupational Epidemiology Data

1. OVERVIEW

In the preceding chapters, the emphasis has been on ascertaining whether a particular occupational exposure poses an increased risk of disease. Complex mathematical models are not usually necessary for this type of analysis, since the focus is more on detecting the presence of an excess risk than extrapolating to other exposure levels or populations. However, if an excess risk is found and assumed to be causally related, then more complex analyses may be warranted. As in other areas of epidemiology, these further studies involve two main activities: scientific inference and public health decision making. The use of occupational data in scientific inference is intended to increase etiologic understanding by determining which of the currently available biological models are consistent with the observed data, or perhaps to formulate a new model. Such etiologic considerations can also have important public health implications. For example, if a carcinogen appears to act at an early stage of the disease process, then this suggests the possibility of preventing disease in previously exposed workers if an agent can be found that prevents the later stage events from occurring. A further use of occupational epidemiology data in public health decision making is in the field of risk assessment, which may involve extrapolating the available findings to other populations or other exposure levels.

The use of occupational data in both etiologic research and risk assessment usually involves some form of biological model. It is important to emphasize at the outset that epidemiologic or experimental data alone cannot completely confirm or refute a biological model. Epidemiologic data often are quite limited and subject to large statistical fluctuations, whereas experimental data only pertain to restricted environmental conditions. Most biological models are derived deductively using theoretical considerations in conjunction with findings from previous epidemiologic and experimental studies. The task is then to assess a particular theory, or group of theories, in light of the observed epidemiologic data. Unfortunately, for many diseases (e.g., cancer) current biological understanding of disease mechanisms is very crude. Few detailed biological models are available, and the existing models all enjoy some degree of support. Many applications of occupational epidemiologic data involve cancer research; hence, models of carcinogenesis are used here for illustration.

Most biological models of cancer assume that exposure to more than one factor is necessary for disease induction. This assumption is appealing, since it is known that complete carcinogens are rare (i.e., very few agents can cause cancer in all exposed subjects, even at very high doses). This finding could be explained as arising from the need for a single probabilistic "hit," but it does appear that more than one factor is needed to produce most cancers. Rothman (1976) has generalized this viewpoint with the concept of *causal constellations*. These are combinations of "causes" that together are sufficient for disease to occur. Each causal constellation is composed of a number of component causes, each of which cannot cause disease by itself but is effective in combination with the other component causes. A disease may have many different causal constellations, and a particular factor may be a component of more than one constellation.

Specific theories can be derived by introducing restrictions into this general framework. In particular, if it is assumed that the disease process involves a certain number of distinct events, then the various causal constellations may be viewed as different ways of producing the same events. For example, one necessary event in a carcinogenic process might be the activation of a specific proto-oncogene (Franks and Teich, 1986), and this might be achieved either by a virus infection or by exposure to a chemical. Thus, the virus and chemical would be components of separate causal constellations. On the other hand, if each exposure activated a separate proto-oncogene, each of which was necessary for carcinogenesis, then they would be common components of at least one causal constellation. Biological models, particularly those with a mathematical formulation, usually are oriented toward elucidating necessary events rather than specific causal constellations. For example, a theory might assume that cancer occurs through a fixed number of sequential events, and a particular factor might be assessed in terms of whether it can cause one or more of the events.

The intention of this chapter is to illustrate the use of occupational epidemiologic data in models of this type. No attempt is made to be comprehensive. Instead, some fundamental issues are illustrated with several examples. We start with a discussion of the multistage model of carcinogenesis proposed by Armitage and Doll (1961). We discuss this model in some detail because this form of multistage model is assumed most commonly in occupational epidemiology. Also, the discussion of this relatively simple model lays the groundwork for the more complex models that follow (and that contain the Armitage–Doll model as a special case). Our intention is not to review evidence supporting or against the validity of the Armitage–Doll model, but rather to illustrate currently available methods for examining such models with occupational epidemiologic data. In particular, these methods will be illustrated by applying the Armitage–Doll model in further analyses of data from the cohort study of asbestos textile workers (Dement et al., 1983).

The second half of the chapter discusses the mathematical development and use of various models of carcinogenesis in extrapolating the findings of occupational epidemiology studies to other populations. This area is commonly referred to as *risk assessment.* Clearly defined models of carcinogenesis are usually required for this task, since the populations "at risk" may have quite different exposure patterns from those examined in previous studies. For example, the general population may experience a low level of exposure throughout life, rather than the relatively high exposure levels during the working years of life that characterize occupational populations. In addition, it is necessary for risk assessments to show that a model follows logically from a set of assumptions about the nature of the disease process.

A brief introduction is followed by an outline of the mathematics of risk assessment. Several models of carcinogenesis are presented, and their applications to the calculation of lifetime risk and probability of causation are outlined. The application of these methods is then illustrated with published risk assessments for exposures to ionizing radiation and benzene. Finally, we discuss some of the qualitative and quantitative features required of occupational epidemiology data if they are to be suitable for risk assessment.

2. THE ARMITAGE–DOLL MULTISTAGE MODEL OF CARCINOGENESIS

2.1. Introduction

One of the most commonly used models for predicting cancer incidence in a population exposed to a carcinogen is the Armitage–Doll model. This model assumes that, for cancer ultimately to occur, at least one cell must pass through k distinct, heritable changes in a particular sequence. The simplest model assumes that the background rate for a particular transition j is constant, although in more sophisticated models the background rate may vary with factors such as age, the condition of the neighboring cells, or the time since that cell experienced a previous change(s). The underlying theory thus assumes that cellular change j occurs with a background rate R_j that is independent of age. It can be shown (Whittemore and Keller, 1978) that at age t the background cancer incidence rate (among non-exposed) $B(t)$ satisfies the following condition in the absence of confounding:

$$B(t) \simeq R_1 R_2 \cdots R_k (t - w)^{k-1}/(k - 1)! \qquad (10.1)$$

or

$$B(t) \simeq (t - w)^{k-1} \qquad (10.2)$$

where w is the time for a fully transformed cell to develop into a clinically detectable cancer (i.e., latency). This approximation may be inaccurate if the transition rates are much larger than 10^{-4} per cell per year (Moolgavkar, 1978), but a larger transition rate should not alter the general patterns of effect modification and induction time to be discussed here.

Usually it is further assumed that the cellular change j occurs in excess with a carcinogen-induced $R'_j I_D(t)$ that is proportional to the dose rate $I_D(t)$ at age t. Note that the model is based on the dose rate to the relevant target cells. The actual dose rate is indeterminable but can be estimated either by bioassay methods (e.g., urinalysis) or from modeling exposure monitoring data.

The transition rate in the exposed population of cells is

$$R_j^*(t) = R_j + R'_j I_D(t) = (R_j)(1 + a_j I_D(t)) \qquad (10.3)$$

where a_j is the increase in transition rate j (relative to R_j) per unit dose rate. The model can be simplified by assuming that the latency interval (w) is zero and that the dose rate at a particular age is either zero or a constant (I_D). Note that R_j and a_j are both assumed to be constant and not dependent on age. Thus, if an exposure occurs throughout life, the incidence rate at age t takes the form:

$$B(t) + E(t) \simeq (1 + a_1 I_D)(1 + a_2 I_D) \cdots (1 + a_k I_D) R_1 R_2 \cdots R_k t^{k-1} \qquad (10.4)$$

where $E(t)$ is the excess incidence rate due to exposure. Hence, the incidence rate at a particular age (t) is of the form:

$$B(t) + E(t) \simeq (b_0 + b_1 I_D + b_2 I_D^2 + \cdots + b_k I_D^k) t^{k-1} \qquad (10.5)$$

In general, if a carcinogen only affects n of the k stages ($n < k$), then equation (10.5) is of order n, rather than k (i.e., $b_0, b_1, \ldots, b_n$ are all nonzero, whereas $b_{n+1}, b_{n+2}, \ldots, b_k$ are all zero). Thus, if a carcinogen only affects one stage, then the incidence rate in the exposed population is a linear function of the dose rate. (This is implicit in the preceding assumption that each cellular change occurs with an excess rate that is proportional to the dose rate.) In general, it can be shown (Guess and Crump, 1976) that the lifetime risk $P(I_D)$ in an individual continuously exposed at a constant dose rate (I_D) is expressed as

$$P(I_D) \simeq 1 - \exp[-(q_0 + q_1 I_D + q_2 I_D^2 + \cdots q_k I_D^k)] \qquad (10.6)$$

Once again, the polynomial only contains terms of the order of I_D^n or less if a carcinogen affects exactly n stages ($n < k$).

Equation (10.6) is widely used in risk assessment (Anderson et al., 1983), which is discussed in the second part of this chapter. Next we introduce the further simplifying assumption that only one of the cellular changes (j) is affected by the exposure of interest and examine various methods for assessing the temporal relationship between exposure and subsequent disease risk. However, it should be noted that some carcinogens (most notably, cigarette smoke) appear to affect both an early and a later stage (Doll and Peto, 1978). Other agents, such as arsenic (Brown and Chu, 1983) and nickel (Kaldor et al., 1986), may also affect more than one stage.

2.2. Lifetime Exposure

One special case is when exposure occurs throughout life. In this situation it can be shown (Whittemore, 1977) that the excess incidence rate $E(t)$ at age t is proportional to t^{k-1} for all $j < k$. (It should be remembered that we are assuming that exposure affects only one stage and that the transition rate coefficient a_j is constant with age and is a linear function of the dose rate.) Since the background rate $B(t)$ is also proportional to t^{k-1}, it follows that the excess rate is proportional to the background rate at all ages, and the rate ratio is constant throughout life.

2.3. Exposure Commencing Subsequent to Birth

Occupational exposures generally begin at some age subsequent to birth. (Exceptions are exposures to genetic material causing heritable changes or in utero exposure.) To derive the age-specific incidence rate for an exposed individual we assume that the occupa-

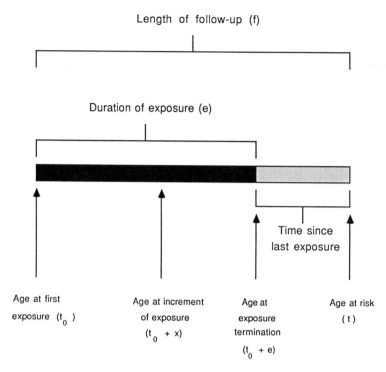

Figure 10–1. Exposure history of a hypothetical worker.

tional (additional) exposure begins at age t_0, remains at a constant level I_D for a time period e until age $t_0 + e$, and increases the cellular event rates from R_j to $R_j + R'_j I_D$. The individual is then observed for a further period. At age t the individual has been followed for a period $f(= t - t_0)$. This exposure pattern is represented in Figure 10–1.

Exposure duration (e) is important in at least two respects. At a constant dose rate (I_D), exposure duration is a surrogate measure of the total dose. A longer duration also implies an increased likelihood that exposure will occur at some time subsequent to the completion of the $j - 1$ necessary prior transitions. In this latter situation duration of exposure is acting as a surrogate for age at exposure. For simplicity, duration of exposure initially is regarded as fixed; the situation of continuing exposure is discussed later.

2.4. Fixed Duration of Exposure

When the stage affected is the last, then the excess rate is zero immediately following cessation of exposure (assuming a zero latency period). When the stage affected is not the last, and a cell receives an increment of exposure at age $t_0 + x$ (see Figure 10–1), the likelihood that this will cause the cell to become fully transformed at age t depends on four factors: (1) the likelihood that the cell has undergone the $j - 1$ prior transitions by age $t_0 + x$ (proportional to $(t_0 + x)^{j-1}$) (2) the likelihood that the exposure will cause transition j to occur (proportional to I_D), (3) the likelihood that the $k - 1 - j$ subsequent transitions will occur by age t (proportional to $(t - (t_0 + x)^{k-1-j})$), and (4) the likelihood that the final transition will occur at age t (a constant). The excess cancer incidence (derived from Whittemore, 1977) is thus of the form

$$E(t) \sim I_D \int_0^e (f - x)^{k-1-j}(t_0 + x)^{j-1} \, dx \qquad (10.7)$$

The implications of this formulation will be illustrated for the situations $j = 1$ and $j = k - 1$.

When $j = 1$,

$$E(t) \sim I_D \int_0^e (f - x)^{k-2} \, dx$$
$$= I_D[f^{k-1} - (f - e)^{k-1}] \qquad (10.8)$$

Hence, the excess rate increases markedly with length of follow-up (f) and is independent of age at first exposure (t_0). The excess rate ratio (i.e., the ratio of the excess incidence rate to the background incidence rate) is

$$\frac{E(t)}{B(t)} \sim \frac{I_D[f^{k-1} - (f - e)^{k-1}]}{(t_0 + f)^{k-1}} \qquad (10.9)$$

The excess rate ratio decreases with increasing age at first exposure (t_0). It can be shown (Pearce et al., 1986) that $E(t)/B(t)$ increases with increasing length of follow-up (f) for a relatively long period of time before eventually beginning to decrease.

When $j = k - 1$,

$$E(t) \sim I_D \int_0^e (t_0 + x)^{k-2} \, dx$$
$$= I_D[(t_0 + e)^{k-1} - t_0^{k-1}] \qquad (10.10)$$

The excess rate ($E(t)$) increases with increasing age at first exposure (t_0) and is independent of length of follow-up (f) for fixed duration of exposure (e). The excess rate ratio is

$$\frac{E(t)}{B(t)} \sim \frac{I_D[(t_0 + e)_n^{k-1} - t_0^{k-1}]}{(t_0 + f)^{k-1}} \qquad (10.11)$$

The excess rate ratio decreases with increasing length of follow-up (f). The relationship with age at first exposure (t_0) depends on the relative lengths of follow-up and exposure. When the length of follow-up is very much greater than the exposure duration, the excess rate ratio increases with increasing age at first exposure, for fixed length of follow-up. However, when exposure is still continuing or has just been terminated (i.e., $f = e$), the excess rate ratio will decrease with increasing age at first exposure (Pearce et al., 1986).

2.5. Continuing Exposure

For exposures that continue until the end of follow-up, the length of follow-up (f) is equal to the duration of exposure (e). Thus, the latter term should be substituted for length of follow-up (f) in the preceding formulas. This situation can occur when studying workers who are still employed or workers who are exposed to a substance with a long biological half-life. It can then be shown that, for fixed duration of exposure, the general patterns for age at first exposure are the same as the preceding. As would be expected, when duration of exposure is permitted to vary, the excess rate and excess rate ratio increase with duration of exposure. When a carcinogen acts at an early stage, or exposure commences early in life, $E(t) \sim e^{k-1}$. This pattern was observed by Doll and Peto (1978), who found the incidence of lung cancer in cigarette smokers to be proportional to the fourth or fifth power of duration of smoking, for a fixed level of daily cigarette consumption.

2.6. Implications

Figures 10–2 and 10–3 illustrate the preceding findings for a hypothetical five-stage carcinogenic process. Figure 10–2 illustrates the relationship of the rate difference and excess rate ratio to age at first exposure, given a fixed duration of employment (five years) and a fixed length of follow-up (20 years). Figure 10–3 illustrates the relationship of the same two effect measures to length of follow-up, given a fixed duration of employment (five years) and a fixed age at first exposure (15 years). The patterns for carcinogens affecting intermediate stages (not shown) are intermediate to those for first-stage and penultimate-stage carcinogens.

Figure 10–2 demonstrates that age at first exposure is an important potential effect modifier. In particular, if a carcinogen acts at any stage other than the first, then the rate difference will increase with increasing age at first exposure, since the necessary prior tran-

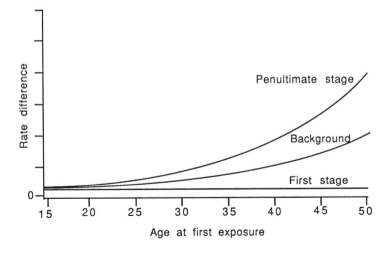

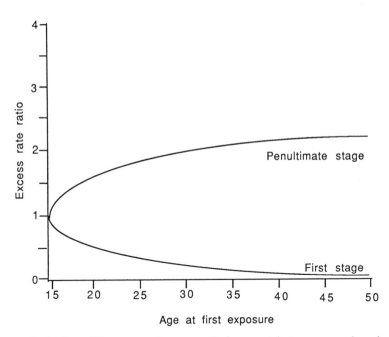

Figure 10-2. Rate difference and excess ratio by age at first exposure, for a fixed duration of exposure (five years) and length of follow-up (20 years), for a hypothetical five-stage carcinogenic process.

sitions will be more likely to have occurred. This pattern has been observed in studies of solid tumors in heavily irradiated organs (Darby et al., 1985) and in a study of bladder cancer in dyestuff workers (Case et al., 1954), although in the latter instance the increase was relatively moderate.

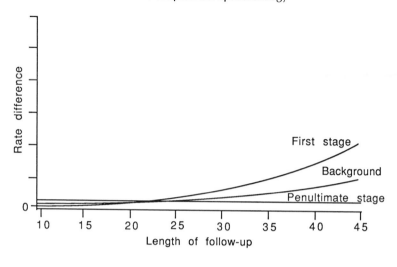

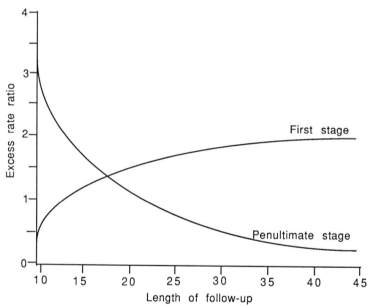

Figure 10–3. Rate difference and excess rate ratio by length of follow-up, for a fixed duration of exposure (five years) and age at first exposure (15 years), for a hypothetical five-stage carcinogenic process.

Figure 10–3 demonstrates that length of follow-up is also an important potential effect modifier. The effect of exposure to an early-stage carcinogen is small until sufficient time has elapsed for the later-stage transitions to occur. For example, if the atomic bomb survivor studies had been terminated after about 15 years, the leukemia excess would have been detected but not the increased risks for solid tumors (Boice and Land, 1982). On the other hand, the rate difference associated with a carcinogen affecting the penultimate stage remains approximately constant after exposure stops. This pattern has been observed in studies of cigarette smoking (Peto, 1977). Thus, cigarette smoking appears to be both an early- and a late-stage carcinogen (Doll and Peto, 1978).

Although the factors of age at risk and duration of exposure do not enter directly into the simple formulation of the Armitage–Doll model, they may be effect modifiers if some of the simplifying assumptions are relaxed. For example, the background transition rate for a late-stage transition might be a function of age at risk rather than constant. In particular, if a carcinogen acts at an early or intermediate stage and one of the later-stage transitions generally occurs at a specific age, then exposed persons will only develop disease when they become old enough for some target cells to have undergone the relevant transitions, irrespective of the age at which they were first exposed. Peto et al. (1975) have presented evidence suggesting that cancer does not appear to be a natural consequence of aging. However, other studies have suggested that transition rates corresponding to a given exposure are higher in young persons and may also depend on age-related endogenous factors, such as hormone levels for certain cancers (Whittemore, 1977). Such a phenomenon has been suggested for breast cancer, where radiation appears to have an early-stage effect but operates in conjunction with a strong hormonally mediated promoting action (Moolgavkar et al., 1980). In other words, radiation appears to initiate cellular changes that increase the likelihood that other, age-related events later in life result in breast cancer, with excess incidence rates proportional to the age-specific background incidence rates (Land and Tokunaga, 1980).

Duration of exposure will be an effect modifier if the effect of a given cumulative exposure depends on the delivery rate [i.e., if $R_j^*(t)$ is not a linear function of $I_D(t)$]. For example, a given nonlethal radiation dose may be less effective (due perhaps to different cellular repair probabilities) if an equivalent dose is delivered in smaller fractions over a lengthy period than if it is delivered over a relatively short period. On the other hand, if the overall dose is very large, then it will be less effective if it is delivered over a relatively short period, as cell killing may occur (Beebe, 1982).

The findings for duration of exposure in the simpler model are also of importance, as duration is predicted to be more important (in terms of excess cancer incidence) than exposure intensity for a carcinogen that affects only one or two stages (Doll and Peto, 1978). This suggests that the characterization of dose as some function (usually assumed to be linear) of the simple product of intensity and duration may not be optimal (Breslow and Day, 1980).

3. APPLICATION TO STUDY OF ASBESTOS TEXTILE PLANT WORKERS

The implications of the Armitage–Doll model for asbestos-induced lung cancer will be explored, using the cohort study of lung cancer in 1,261 white male workers from an asbestos textile manufacturing plant (Dement et al., 1983), described in Chapter 5. Three approaches will be illustrated here: (1) induction time analyses, (2) analysis of the relationship of the excess risk to age at first employment and length of follow-up, and (3) direct fitting of the Armitage–Doll model.

3.1. Induction Time Analyses

One approach to considering induction time has been described by Rothman (1981). This method involves taking the expected contribution of exposure to be constant over some "window" of time and zero outside of it. Thus, this approach only considers exposures during some specified time interval, while ignoring other exposures. This can be regarded as an extension of the exposure lagging approach (see Chapter 5) in that not only are recent exposures considered to be etiologically irrelevant, but so are exposures that occurred in the distant past. For example, we might consider exposures 10–25 years prior to a particular person-year at risk as potentially most relevant etiologically; as a result, exposures before and after this time window would be assigned values of zero. Thus, Rothman's method does not attempt to evaluate total cumulative exposure, but only the cumulative exposure delivered during the etiologically relevant period. Table 10–1 shows the rate ratio estimates for lung cancer mortality for a cumulative exposure of ≥5,000 fibers/cc × days versus <5,000 fibers/cc × days, obtained using various exposure time windows. Using a window of 15–19 years, a particular person-year (or death) would be classified as "exposed" if the individual accumulated ≥5,000 fibers/cc × days during the period 15–19 years previously. Note that the exposure windows are

Table 10–1. Rate ratios for lung cancer for ≥5,000 versus <5,000 fibers/cc × days for various exposure "windows"

Exposure "window"	Exposed		Non-exposed		Rate[a] ratio	95% Confidence interval	Adjusted[b] rate ratio	95% Confidence interval
	Deaths	Person-years	Deaths	Person-years				
0–4	13	4,341	22	28,013	1.5	0.5,3.9	0.8	0.3,2.3
5–9	16	4,123	19	28,231	2.8	1.3,6.0	1.3	0.5,3.6
10–14	19	3,375	16	28,979	3.9	1.9,7.9	1.3	0.5,3.9
15–19	17	2,609	18	29,745	4.9	2.5,9.7	1.4	0.4,4.8
20–24	14	1,871	21	30,483	5.7	2.9,11.3	4.6	1.3,16.3
25–29	10	1,186	25	31,168	3.9	2.0,7.5	0.7	0.2,2.5
≥30	5	725	30	31,629	3.4	1.7,6.3	1.2	0.4,3.5

[a] Adjusted for age and calendar year.
[b] Adjusted for age, calendar year, and exposures occurring in other exposure windows.

not mutually exclusive but are treated as separate, independent exposures [i.e., a particular person-year (or death) is assessed seven times, once for each exposure window]. Thus, each line of Table 10–1 contains all the person-years and lung cancer deaths in the cohort.

Table 10–1 gives two sets of rate ratio estimates. In the first, the effect of exposure in a particular time window was assessed without considering exposures in other time periods. The rate ratios are particularly elevated for exposures occurring 10–29 years previously but are still elevated above the null value when considering more recent exposures or those occurring more than 30 years previously. This pattern is consistent with other published reports of relative risks for asbestos workers that declined but that are still elevated more than 30 years after commencement of exposure (Walker, 1984). However, this pattern can be misleading in that the effect of exposure in a particular time window may be confounded by the effects of exposures in other windows. Hence, the rate ratio estimates for each window were also calculated with adjustment made for the effects of exposures in other windows. The resulting estimates are imprecise, because of the strong correlation between exposures in the various windows. Nevertheless, Table 10–1 suggests that the increase in the rate ratio is primarily due to exposures occurring 15–24 years previously, whereas there is little effect from exposures occurring 0–14 or ≥25 years previously. Intuitively this suggests that asbestos may act at an intermediate stage, but many alternative explanations are available. For example, the same pattern might be observed if asbestos acted at an initial stage, but death of the cancerous cells could occur because of immune surveillance or from direct cell killing by the asbestos fibers, or if asbestos affected a late stage with the long lag resulting from prolonged retention.

3.2. Relationship of Risk with Age at First Employment and Length of Follow-up

Induction time analyses can assist in determining whether a carcinogen appears to operate at an early or late stage in the etiologic process. However, if attention is being focused on a particular model, such as that proposed by Armitage and Doll, then it is desirable to explore the exposure–disease relationship in more depth and to determine which forms of the model are most consistent with the relationship of incidence to age at first employment and time

Table 10-2. Person-years and observed and expected numbers of lung cancer deaths among asbestos textile workers

Variable	Person-years at risk	Observed	Expected	SMR
Age at first employment				
<20	13,554	6	1.83	3.28
20–24	8,817	6	2.14	2.80
25–29	3,995	5	1.67	2.99
30–34	2,841	9	1.81	4.97
≥35	3,147	9	3.38	2.66
Time since first employment				
<15	21,933	6	2.57	2.34
15–19	4,393	6	1.98	3.06
20–24	3,369	5	2.62	1.91
25–29	2,090	14	2.61	5.36
≥30	569	4	1.06	3.77
Cumulative exposure[a]				
<1	13,146	5	3.73	1.34
1–9	12,823	10	3.69	2.71
10–39	4,976	7	2.18	3.21
40–99	1,270	11	1.10	10.00
≥100	139	2	0.13	15.39

[a] 1,000 fibers/cc × days.

since first employment (Brown and Chu, 1983; Kaldor et al., 1986). The assessment should involve both relative and excess rate estimates to explore fully the relationships predicted in Figures 10–2 and 10–3.

Since age at risk and calendar year are potential confounders, the usual procedure is to calculate observed and expected deaths, with adjustments made for these two factors. Thus, in our analysis of the asbestos textile plant workers' cohort data, the numbers of person-years at risk and observed lung cancer deaths were calculated according to three factors: age at first employment in five five-year age-groups, time since first employment in five five-year groupings, and cumulative exposure in five groupings (Table 10–2). For each of the 125 combinations of these factors, the expected numbers of lung cancer deaths were calculated using rates for U.S. white males, jointly stratified by age and calendar year, in five-year categories of each.

Table 10–2 summarizes the observed and expected deaths for each of the three study factors separately. However, the most appropriate analysis involves calculating the effect estimates for each factor, adjusted for the other two (as well as for age and calendar year). This analysis was accomplished using Poisson regression (see Chapter 8) implemented with GLIM (Baker and Nelder, 1978). Two models were fitted. The first is the rate ratio model described in Chapter 8:

$$\text{SMR} = \frac{\text{Obs}}{\text{Exp}} = \exp(b_1 X_1 + b_2 X_2 + \cdots + b_j X_j) \qquad (10.12)$$

The second is the rate difference (excess rate) model suggested by Kaldor et al. (1986):

$$\text{EMR} = \frac{\text{Obs} - \text{Exp}}{\text{PYRS}} = \exp(b_1 X_1 + b_2 X_2 + \cdots + b_j X_j) \qquad (10.13)$$

where EMR is the excess mortality ratio, Obs is the observed number of deaths, Exp is the expected number on the basis of national rates, PYRS is the person-years at risk, and $X_1, X_2, \ldots, X_j$ represent various categories of age at first employment, time since first employment, and cumulative exposure. If cumulative exposure data had not been available, then separate terms for exposure duration (in years) or exposure intensity (e.g., "high," "medium," and "low") could have been substituted.

The findings from both models are displayed in Table 10–3. The association of lung cancer mortality with cumulative asbestos exposure is strong and consistent with that shown in Chapter 8. The

Table 10–3. Estimated adjusted rate ratios (SMRs) and excess rate ratios (EMRs) for lung cancer among asbestos textile workers

Variable	Rate ratio (SMR)	Relative excess rate (EMR)
Age at first employment		
<20	1.0[a]	1.0[a]
20–24	0.9	1.6
25–29	0.8	0.8
30–34	1.5	7.4
≥35	1.1	11.7
Time since first employment		
<15	1.0[a]	1.0[a]
15–19	1.1	2.5
20–24	0.7	5.6
25–29	1.7	26.9
≥30	0.6	15.4
Cumulative exposure		
<1	1.0[a]	1.0[a]
1–9	2.0	10.3
10–39	2.4	13.0
40–99	7.6	48.6
≥100	18.0	163.5

[a] Reference category.

excess rate appeared to increase with increasing age at first exposure. If the Armitage–Doll model is applicable, then this finding
suggests that asbestos does not act solely at the first stage because
the excess rate should be constant across age at first exposure categories if that were the case, assuming that the rates for the additional transitions are not affected by age (see Figure 10–2). Similarly, the excess rate appeared to increase with increasing time since
first employment, suggesting that asbestos does not act solely at the
penultimate stage (see Figure 10–3). Alternatively, asbestos might
affect an intermediate stage, rather than both an early and a late
stage.

3.3. Direct Fitting of the Armitage–Doll Model

The preceding methods for assessing the relationship of risk with
factors such as age at first employment and time since first employment are widely used. However, most results from analyses of this
type are inconclusive in that they typically only indicate that a particular agent does not act solely at the first or penultimate stages of
the carcinogenic process. Identifying specific intermediate stages
cannot be accomplished. Furthermore, such analyses do not allow
for changes in exposure intensity over time.

These problems can be mitigated to some extent when quantitative exposure data are available to assess the relationship of each
increment of exposure to later increases in risk. The assessment is
carried out for each possible stage of the model in order to ascertain
which stages of action are consistent with the observed data. Thus,
for a particular person-year at risk occurring at age $t_0 + x$, the expo-
sure obtained in each preceding year is weighted by $(f - x)^{k-1-j}(t_0 + x)^{j-1}$ [see equation (10.7)], and the contributions from each preceding year are summed. This procedure is analogous to that used
for calculating cumulative exposure, except that the exposure for
each year is weighted by its expected contribution to excess incidence on the basis of the Armitage–Doll model. This weighted sum
is calculated a number of times, each time assuming that the carcinogen acts at a different stage. Thus, the calculations are performed
for each possible value of j [e.g., from $j = 1$ to $j = 6$ (assuming a
six-stage process)]. These weighted exposure estimates are then
applied to the observed data.

Table 10–4 shows rate ratio estimates (standardized for age and
calendar year) obtained using both a categorical exposure classification and those obtained with a continuous exposure classification.

Table 10-4. Age-standardized rate ratios and chi-squares obtained by assuming that asbestos acts at various stages of a six-stage carcinogenic process

Stage at which asbestos acts	Categorical								Continuous	
	Exposure category							Chi-square (6 df)	R[b]	Chi-square (1 df)
	1[a]	2	3	4	5	6	7			
1	1.0	1.8	8.2	3.5	8.0	11.4	9.1	19.4	1.27	2.5
2	1.0	2.2	7.3	6.1	5.8	13.1	12.7	19.8	1.37	3.7
3	1.0	1.6	9.4	9.8	4.9	8.7	15.2	24.9	1.39	5.4
4	1.0	1.6	9.3	6.3	5.7	13.5	12.1	24.0	1.44	6.6
5	1.0	2.0	4.8	5.3	7.1	14.7	13.6	20.1	1.50	8.8
6	1.0	1.1	2.2	3.7	7.0	5.3	6.4	16.1	1.23	8.2

[a] Reference category.

[b] Based on estimate for mean exposure level.

The categorical analysis involved grouping the values for each exposure variable into seven categories, from lowest to highest, with each containing five deaths. Equal allocation of deaths was used to yield the greatest statistical precision. The continuous exposure classification was achieved by assigning scores to each of the exposure categories, based on the mean exposure score for the person-time data in the category. It should be noted that the rate ratio estimates for the continuous analysis are based on the mean exposure levels for the person-time data. These are considerably lower than the mean exposure levels for the lung cancer cases, and the rate ratio estimates for the categorical analysis (which grouped the exposure data so as to ensure an adequate number of cases in each category) are thus considerably higher.

The findings in Table 10-4 should be regarded with reservation because of the relatively small number (35) of lung cancer deaths. However, the chi-square values for the categorical analyses suggest that the best fit to the data is obtained by assuming that asbestos acts at stages 3, 4, or 5, whereas the continuous analyses suggest that asbestos acts at stages 4 or 5. The continuous analysis is theoretically more valid, since it is assessing the strength of the linear trend suggested by the Armitage–Doll model. However, it should be remembered that we used exposure rather than dose data and that the relationship between an exposure and the resulting organ dose may not be linear (Hoel et al., 1983). Hence, the observed exposure–response relationship may be nonlinear, even though the actual (unmeasurable) dose–response relationship is linear. The categorical analysis may therefore be more appropriate. In fact, all the different exposure classifications fitted the data well, and this small data set does not contain enough deaths to differentiate between the various models. However, if it is assumed that the Armitage–Doll model is valid, then the data are generally consistent with Thomas' (1983) finding that asbestos appears to act at the fourth stage of a six-stage process of lung carcinogenesis.

3.4. Some Additional Comments on the Armitage–Doll Model

The preceding discussion has illustrated the application of the Armitage–Doll model to occupational data and has demonstrated two problems of such analyses. First, most occupational studies do not generate enough cases of site-specific cancers to distinguish between the various forms of the model. (This is also true for modeling other diseases in many instances.) Second, the model has an empirical derivation but lacks a biological foundation. It is of particular concern that the model does not allow for multiplication and death of cells in any preneoplastic stage. Armitage and Doll (1957) have also proposed a two-stage model in which cells that have undergone the first transition grow exponentially, but this model still cannot account for the age-specific incidence patterns for embryonal cancers or leukemia (Peto, 1977). Additionally, no more than two separate stages have been demonstrated experimentally (Moolgavkar and Knudson, 1981), in apparent contradiction with the suggestion of a five- or six-stage process obtained using the standard Armitage–Doll (1961) model. Furthermore, there is reason to doubt the assumption that the transition rates do not depend on age, at least for some cancers.

Despite concerns regarding the interpretation of the Armitage–Doll model, analyses of the type presented above can at least suggest whether a carcinogen appears to act at an early, intermediate, or late stage. Furthermore, the general statistical methods illustrated here will retain their usefulness as further models are developed.

4. INTRODUCTION TO RISK ASSESSMENT

In the second part of this chapter, we discuss the use of occupational data in risk assessment using multistage models. The task of a risk assessment is to estimate the effects that might occur following an exposure. This might be achieved using theories, extrapolations, direct experience, judgments, or some combination of these. Thus, the focus is not limited to the predictions of a particular model, but includes assessments of predictions from several competing models and their relative degrees of support.

In some countries, such as the United States, the result of a risk assessment is typified by criteria documents prepared in support of regulatory standards. Such documents describe (1) existing exposures to the substance of interest, (2) routes by which a population is exposed, (3) how the substance behaves in the body, (4) the mechanism by which the substance produces health effects, (5) the kinds of health effects likely to occur as a result of exposures at the levels of interest, (6) the expected incidence of such effects in the population, and (7) methods for controlling exposures. An epidemiologist is most likely to be involved in developing an understanding of features 5 and 6, although epidemiologic information might also be sought for any of the other features.

Risk assessment often requires extrapolation of epidemiologic findings to other age groups, to different levels or routes of exposure, and to the end of the normal human lifespan. Ideally, inferences of risk should be supported by a clearly detailed line of reasoning, proceeding from empirical observations through development and testing of theory and associated mathematical models (Crawford-Brown and Pearce, 1989). It must then be shown how other inferences might arise if a different choice of data, theory, or model had been made. Finally, a degree of support should be assigned to each step in the line of reasoning leading to each inference. The degree of support may be quantitative, but usually arises from qualitative judgments.

5. THE MATHEMATICS OF RISK ASSESSMENT

Often risk assessments are performed in anticipation of regulatory action, which can be based on either of two forms of inference. If the regulatory action is designed to limit a risk below a prescribed level, the regulatory approach is considered to be *probability-based*. It is necessary then to develop the mathematical functions required for calculating lifetime risk resulting from various patterns of exposure. This approach will be illustrated with a detailed example of risks associated with radon exposures. At other times, the relevant information may not be of sufficient quality to warrant a detailed calculation of the probability of an effect at exposure levels below those encountered occupationally. In that case, epidemiologic data may be used only to determine the lowest exposure level (or dose) that has been associated with a consistent elevation in incidence in an occupationally exposed population. Such an approach is said to rely on the concept of a *no observed effects level* (NOEL). An example of this approach concerning occupational exposures to benzene will be presented briefly near the end of this chapter. In the meantime, we will focus on probability-based risk assessments and look first at some of the requisite mathematical functions.

The risk assessment process can be divided conceptually into two distinct steps (Anderson et al., 1983). The first questions addressed are, "Is there evidence that exposure to substance X produces effect Y?" and, "What is the strength of this evidence?" The second step asks, "If such evidence is firm, then what is the lifetime risk (i.e., the cumulative incidence up to the end of the "normal" lifespan) imposed by exposure to substance X at level D throughout life?" In this section we explore how the lifetime risk is estimated in a risk assessment. We focus on the form that the necessary mathematical models might take in such an assessment. There are three questions of principal interest:

1. What is the form of the dose–response curve for the substance?
2. What is the shape of the temporal function describing the appearance of the effect after exposure?
3. What is the influence of age at exposure on questions 1 and 2?

5.1. Dose–Response Models

In an earlier section of this chapter, we discussed the application of the Armitage–Doll model to epidemiologic studies. The Armitage–Doll model is a special case of a more general category of models known as *hit-target models* that specify that an organ or cell contains some finite number of targets that must be hit in a prescribed sequence. The present section develops the general mathematical relations underlying the hit-target models and shows how the Armitage–Doll model, linear model, and several other related mathematical models are derived from a common conceptual framework. This development should aid in demonstrating the assumptions (or approximations) underlying such models and suggests the form more general models would take if the approximations are deemed inadequate. Other models, based on quite different assumptions from those involved in hit-target models are available but are not discussed here.

Most risk assessments assume a linear dose–response model for acute exposures. In addition, it is assumed that the dose delivered during the course of each year (i.e., the integral of the dose rate over the year) is the independent variable for predicting the lifetime risk imposed by exposures in that year. A final important assumption is that risks imposed by each year of exposure are additive and independent. These assumptions are used because they simplify the necessary mathematics and because they appear to be valid for many carcinogenic substances.

The linear dose–response function is a special case of a more general multistage model. We will derive the equations for a system in which cells are believed to exist in one of three states, although any number of states may be assumed. This general approach produces the Armitage–Doll model as a special case. It is then possible to describe the condition of an organ or tissue by specifying the fraction of cells in each of the three states. The resulting model is referred to generally as a *state-vector model*. The first state is assumed to consist of cells that have received no damage from the substance. The second state consists of cells that have had one of two necessary targets damaged, but not the other. Such cells are considered to have received subeffectual damage. The third state consists of those cells in which each of the two targets has been damaged. Only cells in the third state will manifest the effect; thus, the response of the organ is assumed to be related functionally to the number of cells in the third state.

Let D be the dose delivered to the organ in a given year. In general, D is proportional to the integral of the organ burden throughout the year. There are assumed to be rate constants, k_{12}, k_{23}, and k_{13}, that describe the fraction of cells per unit dose transferring from one state to the next. In other words, k_{ij} is the fraction of cells moving from state i to state j per unit dose, interpreted here as the probability per unit dose that a chemical molecule, a fiber, or a radiation unit strikes the target associated with the transition. At times, a single molecule, fiber, or unit of radiation might strike several targets simultaneously, resulting in a transition by more than one state. This case probably is more relevant to radiation than chemicals or other physical substances, so k_{13} should be zero for most substances. In addition, there might be a repair process that moves cells from a higher to a lower state (e.g., from state 2 to state 1), but this consideration can be ignored to simplify matters in this discussion. The general model then looks like the following:

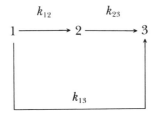

Before reviewing the equations specifying this model, it will be useful to examine various sets of biophysical assumptions that can be made. Each set is part of the class of hit-target models, in which the transitions are assumed to occur as a result of distinct hits to some cellular target, with the rate of hits assumed to be proportional to the concentration (or density in the case of radiation) of a substance (or its active metabolite) at the target. Organ or cell concentrations can serve as surrogates of subcellular target concentrations. Thus, there are two ways to view the resulting model. Both approaches assume that the model applies to individual cells; therefore, the probability of producing an effect in an organ is given approximately by the product of the probability of producing an effect in a cell times the number of cells.

In the first approach, transitions must occur in a specific temporal sequence such that state 2 corresponds to cells sustaining a hit to a very specific target. The rate constant k_{12} then applies to this particular transition, and the rate constant k_{23} applies to hitting the next target in the sequence, given that the first has been hit. For example, such a model might apply if a molecule can cause the transition from the second to third state only if a prior hit has changed the shape of the target into a suitable form.

A second approach is to view the transitions as independent events that can occur in any sequence. In this case, state 2 corresponds to cells that have had any one transition, and state 3 corresponds to cells that have had both necessary transitions. (Note that this model can easily be extended to n states.) Therefore, the transition rate constant k_{12} in the model is the sum of the rate constants for all transitions, whereas the transition rate constant k_{23} is equal to this sum minus the rate constant associated with whichever transition occurred to place the cell in the second state. It is easier mathematically, however, to divide such a three-state model into two separate two-state models, with state 1 being common to each model. In that case, k_{12} is the transition rate for a particular transition, and the number or fraction of cells in state 2 is found for each separate transition. The probability of both transitions occurring then is equal to the product of the individual probabilities associated with movement to the second state for each transition.

Consider first the case where the transitions must occur in a specific sequence (the assumption of the Armitage–Doll model). We can now write differential equations describing the rate of change of cells in each state as a function of the dose (D) as it accumulates during a year. Assume that the first approach is adopted and that the transitions must occur sequentially. These equations are

$$\frac{dN_1(D)}{dD} = -k_{12}N_1(D) - k_{13}N_1(D) \tag{10.14}$$

$$\frac{dN_2(D)}{dD} = k_{12}N_1(D) - k_{23}N_2(D) \tag{10.15}$$

$$\frac{dN_3(D)}{dD} = k_{13}N_1(D) + k_{23}N_2(D) \tag{10.16}$$

Equations (10.14) to (10.16) may be solved serially using the Bernoulli formula (Kells, 1960) to yield

$$N_1(D) = N_1(0) \exp[-(k_{12} + k_{13})D] \tag{10.17}$$

$$N_2(D) = \frac{k_{12}N_1(0) \{\exp[-(k_{12} + k_{13})D] - \exp[-k_{23}D]\}}{(k_{23} - k_{12} - k_{13})}$$

$$+ N_2(0)(\exp[-k_{23}D]) \tag{10.18}$$

$$N_3(D) = N_1(0) + N_2(0) + N_3(0) - N_1(0) \exp[-(k_{12} + k_{13})D]$$

$$- N_2(0) \exp[-k_{23}D] - \frac{k_{12}N_1(0) \{\exp[-(k_{12} + k_{13})D] - \exp[-k_{23}D]\}}{(k_{23} - k_{12} - k_{13})}$$

$$\tag{10.19}$$

In these equations, $N_i(0)$ is the number of cells in the ith state at the beginning of exposure in the year, and $N_1(0)$ generally is a function of age as the various organs grow. The solution for any state greater than three can be obtained through the repeated use of the Bernoulli solution. When $N_1(0)$ remains constant, equation (10.19) may be shown to reduce to equation (10.1) of the Armitage–Doll model. This result has also been reported by Whittemore and Keller (1978) and Moolgavkar (1978).

When all the transitions are assumed to be independent, so that they need not occur in any sequence, the preceding model is particularly simple. Only states 1 and 2 exist, and if we focus on a particular transition, the fraction of cells with that transition will be given by

$$f_i = 1 - \exp[-k_i D] \tag{10.20}$$

where i refers to the ith kind of transition and k_i corresponds to the rate constant associated with that transition. If there are two necessary transitions, the fraction (f) of cells with the potential for yielding the effect of interest is

$$f = f_1 f_2 = (1 - \exp[-k_1 D])(1 - \exp[-k_2 D]) \tag{10.21}$$

This expression is easily generalized for n transitions. At low values of D, it reduces to equation (10.6), which is specified by the Armitage–Doll model. In fact, equation (10.21) is identical to the Armitage–Doll model if the latter is generalized to apply to any dose regardless of magnitude.

Because of the complexity of the preceding equations, and the scarcity of data usually available from occupational epidemiology studies, essentially all risk assessments use a one-hit model that gives rise to a linear dose–response curve at low doses. Under a one-hit model, there are only two states (1 and 2), as discussed earlier, and the equations are

$$N_1(D) = N_1(0) \exp[-k_{12} D] \tag{10.22}$$

$$N_2(D) = N_1(0)(1 - \exp[-k_{12} D]) + N_2(0) \tag{10.23}$$

The response then is proportional to $N_2(D)$, which for small values of $k_{12} D$ yields

$$N_2(D) \simeq (k_{12} D) N_1(0) + N_2(0) \tag{10.24}$$

which is the familiar linear model.

5.2. Lifetime Risk

Two forms of risk coefficients have been used frequently in epidemiologic risk assessments. The first is the *relative risk coefficient,* which specifies the fractional increase above the natural rate of an effect produced by a given dose $((RR - 1)/D)$. The relative risk coefficient can be a function of age at exposure. If $R(D)$ is the function relating the relative risk coefficient and the dose, and if $I_n(t)$ is the natural incidence rate at a time t, after delivery of the dose, then the excess incidence rate I_e at time t is

$$I_e(D,t) = R(D) I_n(t) \tag{10.25}$$

In most risk assessments, $R(D)$ is assumed to be constant at all times after dose delivery, with only a few modifications. It is also important that $R(D)$ be calculated from epidemiologic data using values of assumed latency and risk plateau (see the following discussion).

A second approach is to estimate the *absolute risk coefficient,* which assumes no explicit causal link between the excess incidence rate and the natural incidence rate. Instead, this second approach assumes a fixed excess incidence rate that remains constant in time after delivery of the dose, at least until the end of some finite period of disease expression. Let this absolute risk coefficient be given as $G(D)$, with units of excess incidence rate. The excess incidence rate at time t after delivery of the dose (D) then is simply

$$I_e(D,t) = G(D) \qquad (10.26)$$

Two modifications are necessary in equations (10.25) and (10.26). Most effects are characterized by a latency (empirical induction) period l and a plateau period p. The plateau period is the time during which the excess incidence rate is assumed to hold and, for solid tumors, usually is assumed to be infinite. For leukemia and bone sarcomas, p may be in the range of 10–20 years. If a dose is delivered at t equal to zero, then the excess incidence rate rises to the level given by equations (10.25) or (10.26) abruptly at t equal to l, remains at these levels until t equal to $l + p$, and then immediately drops back to zero.

These considerations can be combined to determine the lifetime risk imposed by an environment or action that delivers an annual dose $D(A)$ as a function of age A. In other words, the dose may be different at each age due to differences in exposure timing, metabolism, and so on. For the relative risk approach, the excess incidence rate at any age X will be

$$I(X) = \int_{X-p}^{X-l} R_A(D(A))I_n(X)\, dA \qquad (10.27)$$

where $R_A(D(A))$ indicates the relative risk coefficient at age A (subscript) and for an annual dose at age A $(D(A))$. The lower bound of the integral arises because a dose delivered at an age separated from X by more than the plateau period cannot contribute to the excess incidence rate at age X. The value of $X - p$ cannot be less than zero. The upper bound arises because a dose delivered at an age separated from X by less than the latency period cannot contribute to the excess incidence rate at age X. This approach is similar to the use of exposure "windows" for induction time assessment, demonstrated in Section 3.1 of this chapter. It should be stressed that the estimate of $R_A(D)$ should be obtained by analyzing the epidemiologic data with the same assumptions about l and p as will be used in the risk assessment. The analogous equation for an absolute risk model is

$$I_e(X) = \int_{X-p}^{X-l} G(D(A))\, dA \tag{10.28}$$

The lifetime risk then may be calculated by integrating $I_e(X)$ from age 0 to the end of life, given here as age E. (The value of E usually is chosen as 70 or 75 years.) The lifetime risk L may then be shown to be

$$L = \int_{X=0}^{E} I_e(X)\, dX = \int_{X=0}^{E} \int_{A=X-p}^{X-l} R_A(D(A))I_n(X)\, dA\, dX \tag{10.29}$$

for the relative risk approach, and

$$L = \int_{X=0}^{E} I_e(X)\, dX = \int_{X=0}^{E} \int_{A=X-p}^{X-l} G_A(D(A))\, dA\, dX \tag{10.30}$$

for the absolute risk approach.

Alternatively, competing risks can be incorporated, and the model adapted to measure true lifetime risk (rather than risk to age E), by using

$$L = \int_{X=0}^{\infty} I_e(X)S(X)\, dX \tag{10.31}$$

where $S(X)$ is the probability of surviving to age X, derived either from the current general population lifetable or from modeled death rates. Here we discuss only the simpler approach of calculating the lifetime risk using equations (10.29) or (10.30). Several functions must be determined. First, it is necessary to calculate $D(A)$, the dose delivered during each year of life, through the use of equations described in Chapter 9. The dose–response function at age A, $R_A(D)$, is best determined through epidemiologic studies involving short-term exposures at various ages. In practice, however, a linear dose–response function usually is assumed a priori, and maximum likelihood estimates of the parameters are determined from the categorical data. Determining the age dependence of $R(D)$ requires either: (1) that doses in the study population in each age group extend only over time periods that are short compared to the time scale of significant changes in $R(D)$ or (2) that $R(D)$ be determined from data obtained on chronic exposures by deconvolution of equations (10.29) or (10.30) to yield $R_A(D)$ from the value of L in different exposure groups. Some simpler approaches will be examined in the example of radiation exposures in Section 6.4, which will also illustrate the use of the mathematical relations presented here.

5.3. Probability of Causation

The findings of a risk assessment may be brought to bear on a loosely related question that typically arises in court cases (Shavell, 1980): "Given the fact that exposure X and effect Y occurred in an individual, what is the probability that X caused Y?" Such a question asks for a calculation of *probability of causation*. The simplest case of probability of causation is when the effect only occurs after a particular form of exposure and never is produced otherwise. In that case, the appearance of X and Y in the history of an individual implies with certainty (or as close to certainty as can be obtained) that X caused Y. The only remaining issue is whether a particular source produced the exposure X. It should be appreciated that apparent disease causation by one and only one exposure may simply reflect incomplete understanding of etiology. Moreover, some diseases fit this description because of etiologic diagnoses (e.g., silicosis).

More generally, we are concerned with studying the etiology of diseases with multiple causative factors, some of which may operate in combination. Two different sets of assumptions might then be adopted for computing the probability of causation. The first is where the sources of risk are mutually exclusive, often referred to as the assumption of "disjoint" causes. In other words, there may be n sources of exposure that could yield the effect, but it is believed that only one source resulted in the effect that appeared in an individual. This is conceptually analogous to assuming a single hit model for the effect, with the effect occurring whenever the first stage is produced. A second approach assumes that the effect occurs only after several stages and that each of the sources can act at some subset of these stages, with the various subsets perhaps being different. The more simple problem of disjoint causes is considered first.

Let $P(Y \mid X)$ be the *excess* probability of developing a disease at a specific age as a result of an exposure X at another specific age or during some past period of time. For disjoint causes, the probability that X caused Y (P_c) is

$$P_c = P(Y \mid X)/P(Y \mid X + U) \tag{10.32}$$

where $P(Y \mid X + U)$ is the probability of developing the effect at the age of interest, given an exposure X and all other causes (U) of that effect (i.e., the cumulative incidence up to the age of interest in persons exposed to X). For example, if the effect is cancer, $P(Y \mid X + U)$ is the probability of an individual developing cancer at a particular age as a result of an exposure X or any other source. The probability $P(Y \mid X + U)$ may be subdivided into the individual probabilities (assuming all the probabilities are small):

$$P(Y \mid X + U) = P(Y \mid X) + \Sigma P(Y \mid S_i) + P(Y \mid N) \qquad (10.33)$$

where $P(Y \mid N)$ is the probability of developing cancer at the age of interest from background sources (the "natural" incidence), and $P(Y \mid S_i)$ is the excess incidence from exposures to other substances S_i that might appear in the history of an individual. For example, let the effect be lung cancer. If X is exposure to uranium and the individual also smoked and was exposed to asbestos, then $P(Y \mid N)$ would be the probability of a nonsmoker who had not experienced exposures X or S developing lung cancer, $P(Y \mid S_1)$ would be the incremental risk associated with exposure to cigarettes of magnitude S_1, and $P(Y \mid S_2)$ would be added risk contributed by exposure to asbestos at magnitude S_2. This approach clearly assumes disjoint causes since $P(Y \mid S_1)$ is not a function of the exposures S_2 or X, and vice versa. This approach becomes conceptually flawed when the various probabilities approach unity because the excess incidence ceases to be an appropriate measure of the fraction of individuals who develop disease from exposure X. In that case, the probability of causation can be underestimated.

The situation is considerably more complex when at least two exposures are not disjoint (i.e., when they are a part of at least one common causal constellation). We will only examine the situation where there is one main exposure (X) and one other exposure (S). First consider the situation where exposure S is absent. Then from equations (10.32) and (10.33),

$$P_c = \frac{P(Y \mid X,\overline{S})}{P(Y \mid X,\overline{S}) + P(Y \mid N)} \qquad (10.34)$$

where $P(Y \mid X,\overline{S})$ is the incremental probability (over background) that an individual will develop the effect at the age of interest due to exposure X, in the absence of S. If we then define R_X as the incidence rate ratio (relative risk) at the age of interest associated with exposure to X in the absence of S, then R_X satisfies the relation

$$R_X = \frac{P(Y \mid X,\overline{S}) + P(Y \mid N)}{P(Y \mid N)} \qquad (10.35)$$

Inserting this into equation (10.34) yields

$$P_c = \frac{R_X - 1}{R_X} \tag{10.36}$$

Again, this relation is only valid when the individual probabilities are small.

The relevant equations are more complex when S is present, and we will only consider the case when X and S have a multiplicative joint effect (i.e., when $R_{XS} = R_X R_s$). Here R_{XS} is the rate ratio due to X and S in combination, relative to the background incidence; R_X is the rate ratio, relative to the background incidence, in persons exposed to X but not S; and R_s is the rate ratio, relative to the background incidence, in persons exposed to S but not X. This could occur under the Armitage–Doll model (e.g., if X and S act at different stages of the same multistage process). In this situation it can be shown that the formula for P_c [equation (10.32)] reduces to equation (10.36). In other words, when the rate ratio for X and S combined (relative to background) is simply the product of their independent rate ratios, then the probability that disease Y was caused by exposure X only depends on the independent effect of X and does not depend on whether the individual in question was exposed to S.

When probability of causation calculations are developed, an epidemiologic study must be designed to give the values for the individual conditional probabilities found in equation (10.32). There are several problems that an epidemiologist might encounter in specifying the necessary probabilities. The first problem is the reliability and completeness of data. Specifying each of the probabilities in equation (10.32) requires that the level of exposure to each substance be given for the individual of interest. This can prove difficult, particularly for an individual with a complicated work history.

Another problem concerns the dose–response model to be used in specifying $P(Y \mid X)$ or $P(Y \mid S_i)$. The choice of model can result in a variation of as much as 10^4–10^5 when probabilities at low levels of exposure are extrapolated from high levels. It has been typical in the past to adopt the single-hit model [equation (10.20)], as the basis for calculating the probabilities in equation (10.32), by simply ignoring other models or at least arguing that the single hit is the best available model.

A third problem concerns how the background probability $P(Y \mid N)$ should be assigned. The background incidence rates in subgroups of reference populations can differ, depending upon factors such as diet, socioeconomic status, or quality of health care. For any individual, the national incidence rate at any age might be used as a baseline. However, there are potentially numerous modifiers to background rates, and it never is clear how far one should carry the adjustments for the modifiers on an individual basis (especially when the uncertainties in these adjustments can be large). Furthermore, individuals who differ from the average value of $P(Y \mid N)$ may also differ in their susceptibility to incremental exposures. National averages provide values for $P(Y \mid N)$, and corrections can be made only for important risk factors such as smoking. The task is simplified if a relative risk model is adopted, since equation (10.32) reduces to equation (10.36).

The classification of disease also can produce uncertainties. For example, in some instances a diagnosis of leukemia should be recategorized as one of the subtypes of leukemia. This process, in turn, can affect the probability of causation calculation, since the effect on $P(Y \mid X)$ can be quite different from the effect on $P(Y \mid N)$ or $P(Y \mid S_i)$. It is important to ensure that the level of specificity for an effect is constant across each of the probabilities appearing in equation (10.32).

6. EXAMPLES OF OCCUPATIONAL EPIDEMIOLOGY IN RISK ASSESSMENT

This section illustrates some relatively straightforward methods that have been used in past risk assessments. The example chosen is from a risk assessment concerning the induction of lung cancer following exposure to environmental levels of radon (^{222}Rn), a radioactive gas present in most buildings throughout the world. In a risk assessment performed by the United States Environmental Protection Agency (1986), a full range of mathematical models and sets of epidemiologic data were examined for their influence on risk estimates. The final risk estimate then was given as a probability distribution over all possible inferences of risk identified in the risk assessment (Crawford-Brown and Cothern, 1987). To simplify matters, only one model for each of two central issues will be examined in the following examples. These issues are (1) specification of the dose–response function and (2) lifetime risk extrapolation.

6.1. The Dose–Response Curve

For the risk assessment of ^{222}Rn, it was determined that the occupational epidemiology data concerning uranium miners (e.g.,

Archer et al., 1976; Kunz et al., 1979) were not sufficiently precise to determine the shape of the dose–response curve at low doses (or cumulative exposures). From a combination of theoretical radio-biological arguments and experimental data (as well as purely legal concerns), it was decided that a linear model was the most reasonable option. The epidemiologic data thus determined the parameters of the model, but the model itself was generated and supported by a compilation of data from several fields of study.

A summary of the available dose–response data for the uranium miners can be fit by a function of the form

$$P(D) = 1 - e^{-kD} \qquad (10.37)$$

Note that individuals in this study were simply placed into dose categories based on total doses received over the course of employment. Thus, the function $P(D)$ is given as the average excess incidence rate in a group characterized by a dose D during the period represented by follow-up. The units for $P(D)$ are excess lung cancers per year per 10^6 persons per unit dose (actually cumulative exposure was used as a dose surrogate). This is assumed to be equal to the probability of an individual dying in a given year per unit dose. The best fit to the composite data (using a least-squares procedure) was determined to be given by a value of k equal to 10 cases per 10^6 person-years per working level month. [The working level month (WLM) is a unit of cumulative exposure.]

A summary of the data for the U.S. uranium miners can be found in Table 10–5, with follow-up extending until 1974. All lung cancer deaths and person-years occurring within ten years of the start of

Table 10-5. A summary of epidemiologic data for U.S. uranium miners

Cumulative exposure (WLM)	Person-years	Lung cancers		Absolute risk, cases per 10^6PY per WLM[a]	Relative risk, % increased risk per WLM
		Observed	Expected		
60	5,183	3	3.96	—	—
180	3,308	7	2.24	8.0	1.2
300	2,891	9	2.24	7.8	1.0
480	4,171	19	3.33	7.8	1.0
720	3,294	9	2.62	2.7	0.3
1,320	6,591	40	5.38	4.0	0.5
2,760	5,690	49	4.56	2.8	0.4
7,000	1,068	23	0.91	3.0	0.3

Source: Derived from BEIR (1980).

[a] Working level month.

mining were excluded because of considerations of latency. (A preferable approach would have been to lag all exposures by ten years.) To illustrate, consider only the group characterized by a mean exposure of 180 WLM. The absolute risk coefficient derived for this group is

$$k = \frac{Obs - Exp}{PY \times WLM} = \frac{7 - 2.24}{(3,308) \times (180)} = 8 \times 10^{-6} \text{ per PY per WLM}$$

For the uranium miner data, the data at exposures greater than 300 WLM were not used, since the dose–response curve begins to "turn over" due to cell killing and competing causes of death.

6.2. Temporal Extrapolation

Most of the uranium miners had not yet reached the end of life when the study ended. As a result, it was necessary to determine the extent to which increasing the length of follow-up would influence the coefficient k in equation (10.37). The simplest assumption, and one that commonly is used in estimating lifetime risk, is that the absolute risk coefficient remains constant in time during any plateau period. Hence, the factor of 10 cases per 10^6 person-years per WLM was assumed to continue to be constant at times after the end of follow-up for the population of miners.

Such an assumption may be unwarranted for several reasons. First, the period of follow-up in an epidemiologic study may not be characterized by a constant excess incidence rate within any dose group. This could occur if, for example, doses were accumulated over a long period of time and, hence, yielded a continuously increasing incidence rate during the period of follow-up. The average excess incidence rate during follow-up then would not be representative of the excess incidence rate that will occur after follow-up; the excess incidence rate may begin to rise as the natural rate increases. This problem may be avoided by calculating a relative risk coefficient instead of an absolute risk coefficient (see Table 10–5). The excess relative risk then is assumed to apply until the end of life. Some support for the validity of the relative risk approach can be gained by noting that the excess incidence rate in the mining population increased from 10 cases per 10^6 PY per WLM for the age group 35–39 at diagnosis to 50 cases PY per WLM for those older than age 65 at diagnosis (BEIR, 1980). This pattern is similar to the increase in the natural rate of lung cancer. A third consideration is that competing risks may change dramatically after the end of follow-up for a population. If competing risks are important, equation (10.37) can be replaced by

$$P(D) = (1 - e^{-kD})(1 - P(0))\qquad(10.38)$$

where $P(0)$ is the probability of death (from all causes) in a non-exposed population. Equation (10.38) then is used both to calculate the value of k from the study population during the period of follow-up and to calculate $P(D)$ in all years after the period of follow-up. Since the natural death rate generally increases with age, it is possible that $P(D)$ will decrease for a population after the end of a period of incomplete follow-up.

6.3. Lifetime Risk

It now is possible to combine the dose–response function and the temporal pattern of risk into a single example. Suppose that we want to estimate the lifetime risk of dying from lung cancer as a result of radiation exposure for a ten-year-old child who is exposed to 1 WLM of ^{222}Rn during the course of a year. For this example we will use the relative risk model and assume that the natural rate of lung cancer is insignificant until age 20 but is given by the following averages within the prescribed age groups: 5×10^{-5} per year for ages 21–40 years, 5×10^{-4} per year for ages 41–60, and 1.2×10^{-3} per year for ages 61–70. The use of such broad age groups is designed only to make this example simpler.

From the data in Table 10–5, it will be assumed that the adult relative risk coefficient indicates a 1-percent excess incidence per WLM for adult exposures. An induction period of ten years will be assumed, after which the relative risk rises instantaneously to a plateau value and stays constant until age 70 (the end of time for the risk assessment). The relative risk coefficient for a ten-year-old child then will be 2.5 percent/WLM (Crawford-Brown, 1983a). Since the assumed cumulative exposure is 1 WLM, the child in this example will experience a 2.5-percent increase in lung cancer incidence at all ages greater than 20 years (ten years of age at exposure plus a latency period of ten years). The excess incidence rate for this child from age 21 to age 40 will then be

$$R_1 = (0.025)(5 \times 10^{-5}) = 1.25 \times 10^{-6}$$

The probability of death during this 20-year period will be

$$P_1 = R_1 T_1 = (1.25 \times 10^{-6})(20) = 2.5 \times 10^{-5}$$

For ages 41–60 years, the exposed child will experience an excess incidence rate of

$$R_2 = (0.025)(5 \times 10^{-4}) = 1.25 \times 10^{-5}$$

or a probability of death equal to

$$P_2 = R_2 T_2 = (1.25 \times 10^{-5})(20) = 2.5 \times 10^{-4}$$

Finally, from ages 61–70 years the excess incidence rate will be

$$R_3 = (0.025)(1.2 \times 10^{-3}) = 3 \times 10^{-5}$$

or a probability of death equal to

$$P_3 = R_3 T_3 = (3 \times 10^{-5})(10) = 3 \times 10^{-4}$$

The total lifetime probability of death from the exposure at age ten then is

$$P = P_1 + P_2 + P_3 = 5.75 \times 10^{-4}$$

In the actual risk assessment for ^{222}Rn (U.S. EPA, 1986), this approach was used to calculate the lifetime risk imposed by each year of exposure. The risks from each year then were summed to predict the lifetime risk from exposure at a level of 1 WLM per year throughout the lifetime.

6.4. Probability of Causation

We now will consider a probability of causation calculation. Assume that a white male of age 45 years dies from leukemia. His work history indicates that he was exposed at age 35 to benzene at a concentration of 10 ppm for a period of one year. The baseline incidence rate for this form of leukemia at age 45 is taken to be 69 per 10^6 persons per year. What is the probability that his leukemia resulted from the exposure to benzene? To answer this question it is necessary to collect (or extrapolate) data on a group of persons with the preceding characteristics and then to assume that the individual under study has been chosen at random from this group.

Several risk assessments have been performed for occupational benzene exposure and leukemia (Austin et al., 1988), and they have yielded somewhat conflicting results. For purposes of illustration, we consider only the risk assessment done by White et al. (1982), who attempted to develop a probability-based standard for benzene exposure. To perform this task, the authors collected data on exposure to benzene in air for rubber industry workers (Infante et al.,

1977) and chemical manufacturing workers (Ott et al., 1978). These data were used to obtain rough estimates of the average benzene levels in air during distinct time periods. A single-hit model for leukemia production by benzene then was assumed, and an excess risk coefficient of about 0.0002 cases per ppm-yr was obtained. (ppm-yr is the measure of cumulative exposure.) This excess risk is the lifetime risk. Assuming a plateau period of about 20 years in the study population, the excess incidence rate would be 1×10^{-5} per year per ppm-yr. Multiplying this by the preceding risk coefficient, the probability of death from leukemia at age 45 due to benzene exposure is

$$P(D) = (1 \times 10^{-5})(10) = 10^{-4}$$

Since the natural incidence rate at age 45 is 69×10^{-4}, the probability of causation would be

$$P_c = \frac{P(D)}{P(D) + P(0)} = \frac{10^{-4}}{10^{-4} + (0.69 \times 10^{-4})} = 0.59$$

or a 59-percent probability of causation.

If, however, the exposure had occurred at age 55 and the death at age 65 (when the natural incidence rate is about 2.4×10^{-4}/year), the probability of causation would have been

$$P_c = \frac{10^{-4}}{10^{-4} + (2.4 \times 10^{-4})} = 0.29$$

or 29 percent. For the death at age 45, a court might consider benzene to be the cause of death, or at least "more likely than not" to be the cause. For the death at age 65, a different decision would be reached.

6.5. The No-Observed-Effects Level

We now briefly consider regulatory standards based on an empirical demonstration of an effect. This approach (no-observed-effects level) is typified by the 1987 U.S. EPA standard for benzene, in which it simply was argued that no effect had been observed below 100 ppm. Next, a safety factor of 10 was applied to produce a standard of 10 ppm. The safety factor used depended upon whether the epidemiologic interferences are considered "strong" or "weak." Strong studies are taken as an indication that a safety factor of 10 is warranted, whereas weak studies often require a safety factor of 100. What a regulatory agency considers strong or weak is judgmental and is dictated by the manner in which the risk assessor assigns weight to various forms of evidence.

Some general guidelines for evaluating relative strength of epidemiologic studies for risk assessment are as follows:

1. There are numerous consistent epidemiologic studies of effects related to exposure to the substance under a variety of conditions.
2. The epidemiologic results do not appear to change dramatically under different competing assumptions of how to analyze the data or assign exposure categories, and the uncertainties introduced by analytic assumptions are understood.
3. The inferences do not rely heavily on a simple accumulation of case histories, but rather involve formal epidemiologic studies.
4. The onset (decline) of a disorder can be shown to coincide with the use (removal) of a substance by a study population.
5. The exposures or doses have been assigned accurately to all groups displaying an elevated level of the health effect, and the potential errors in assignment are understood in magnitude and direction.
6. Separate risk coefficients are available for a wide range of ages at the start of exposure.
7. An internal comparison group has been included in a cohort study.
8. The estimates of exposure or dose allow grouping of workers into relatively narrow categories.
9. The temporal course of appearance of the effect (particularly the features of latency and plateau periods) has been determined and found to be in keeping with prior expectations based on available information, such as clinical and experimental studies or a knowledge of the etiology of the disease.
10. There is little reason to suspect that factors not included in a particular epidemiologic study (such as socioeconomic status) would compromise the applicability of results to other populations.

7. DISCUSSION

This chapter has illustrated some uses of occupational epidemiologic data in scientific inference and public health decision making. We have not attempted to be comprehensive in our review of available methods, but rather have focused on the central issues. The emphasis in this chapter is on understanding the etiologic process that produces the effect, both for scientific inference and valid extrapolations of the findings to other populations. Such applications of epidemiologic data necessarily involve the use of particular theories of disease processes. The importance of theory is that it involves the formalization of experience, permitting more abstract, and therefore more general, principles to be developed.

It is important to emphasize that applications of the type presented in this chapter are often not the primary goal of an occupational epidemiology study. The goal of many studies is to measure the excess disease incidence in persons employed in a particular industry, or exposed to a particular substance. The resulting methodologic considerations may be quite different from those of a study intended to be used in risk assessment. For example, the age range of the study subjects may be restricted for reasons of validity or statistical efficiency, whereas a study oriented toward risk assessment would usually require the broadest possible age range among study subjects.

The assumptions and reasoning underlying any models and theories should be stated formally. For example, if an epidemiologic observation at one facility, or among a particular group of workers, is used as a predictor of expected results elsewhere, then extrapolation is more justified when the same underlying processes are believed to be occurring in each instance. Thus, most applications of occupational epidemiologic data will require not just the epidemiologic results, but also a description of (1) the assumptions used in generating the results, (2) other assumptions that might have been employed, and (3) the degree of support that can be offered for any given assumption, relative to competitors. It is thus particularly valuable to conduct the analysis under several sets of assumptions (e.g., the relative risk and absolute risk models).

An epidemiologic study may find application in the assessment of the effects of a route of exposure other than that found in the study population. For example, a regulatory agency may require a standard for benzene in drinking water, but may be forced to rely on the epidemiologic data from studies of benzene in the air of workplaces. It becomes necessary, therefore, to extrapolate risk coefficients from one route of exposure to another. This extrapolation is facilitated when dose data, rather than exposure data, are available. Epidemiologic studies are thus most widely applicable when they yield risk coefficients that are as general as possible. This usually requires that the measure of potential for causing damage is the dose to specific biological targets, rather than the concentration in an environmental medium (i.e., exposure intensity).

In the past, the lack of appropriate dose data has restricted the applications of occupational epidemiologic data. Furthermore, even when appropriate data were available, the lack of suitable statistical methods has limited their usefulness. However, as occupational epidemiology matures as a scientific discipline, better methods are being developed both for gathering appropriate dose data and for using such data in investigating broader scientific and public health issues.

Glossary

absolute risk coefficient   Excess incidence rate above background per unit dose or exposure.
background incidence   Incidence that would occur in the absence of exposure.
excess incidence   Incidence due to exposure.
hit-target model   An approach to biophysical modeling that assumes that an effect is produced when a certain number of biologically distinct targets are "struck" by a substance or its metabolite.
lifetime risk   The cumulative probability of an individual dying, as a result of an exposure, prior to the end of a normal lifespan.
multistage model   A biological model that assumes that disease occurs as a result of a fixed number of distinct sequential steps, which may or may not be reversible.
plateau period   The length of time during which a risk is found following an acute exposure.
relative risk coefficient   Percent increase above background incidence rate per unit dose or exposure.
state vector model   A model that conceives of a cell as existing in one of several states that are reached by successive transitions.
transition rate   The rate at which a particular stage of a multistage process occurs.

Notation

a_i	Age-dependent risk coefficient
$B(t)$	Background incidence rate
C	Cumulative exposure
D	Dose
D_i	Dose delivered during ith year of life
e	Duration of exposure $(= t_1 - t_0)$
$E(t)$	Excess incidence rate
f	Length of follow-up $(= t - t_0)$
f_i	Fraction of cells with transition i
$F(t)$	Relative fractional incidence rate any time t after delivery of dose
I_D	Dose rate
$I_D(t)$	Dose rate at age t
$I_n(t)$	Natural incidence rate at time t after delivery of dose
$I_e(D,t)$	Excess incidence rate at time t after delivery of dose (D)
k	Number of stages in a multistage process
k_{ij}	Fraction of cells moving from state i to state j per unit dose

l	Empirical induction time (latency period)
L	Lifetime risk
N	Normal lifespan
N_0	Number of cells in the organ or tissue prior to the onset of dose
N_c	Number of cells that have produced the effect
$N_i(0)$	Number of cells in the ith state at the beginning of exposure in a particular state
$N_i(D)$	Number of cells in the ith state as a function of dose (D)
$P(0)$	Background disease risk
$P(D)$	Excess disease risk
$P_i(D)$	Probability that the target receives i hits at dose D
P_c	Probability that exposure X caused disease Y
P_e	Probability that the target receives n or more hits and produces the effect
$P(Y \mid N)$	Background probability of developing disease Y due to "normal" background exposure by the age of interest
$P(Y \mid X)$	Incremental probability of developing disease Y by the age of interest due to exposure X
R	Relative risk
$R(D)$	Relative risk coefficient
R_j	Background transition rate of cellular change j
R'_j	Change in stage j transition rate induced by one unit of dose
R_X	Rate ratio (compared to background) of disease in persons independently exposed to X
t	Age at risk ($= t_0 + f$)
t_0	Age at first exposure
t_1	Age at termination of exposure
w	Latency period

References

Anderson EL, and the Carcinogen Assessment Group of the U.S. Environmental Protection Agency (1983): Quantitative approaches in use to assess cancer risk. *Risk Anal* 3:277–295.

Archer VE, Gillam JD, and Wagoner JK (1976): Respiratory disease mortality among uranium miners. *Ann NY Acad Sci* 271:280–293.

Armitage P, and Doll R (1957): A two-stage theory of carcinogenesis in relation to the age distribution of human cancer. *Br J Cancer* 11:161–169.

Armitage P, and Doll R (1961): Stochastic models for carcinogenesis. In: Neyman J (ed). *Proceedings of the Fourth Berkeley Symposium on Mathematical Statistics and Probability*, Vol. 4. Berkeley: University of California Press, pp. 19–38.

Austin A, Delzell E, and Cole P (1988): Benzene and leukemia: a review of the literature and a risk assessment. *Am J Epidemiol* 127:419–439.

Baker RJ, and Nelder JA (1978): *Generalized Linear Interactive Modeling (GLIM)* Release 3. Oxford: Numerical Algorithms Group.

Beebe GW (1982): Ionizing radiation and health. *Am Sci* 70:35–44.

Beebe GW, Kato H, and Land CE (1978): Studies of the mortality of A-bomb survivors. *Radiat Res* 75:138–201.

BEIR, Committee on the Biological Effects of Ionizing Radiation (BEIR III) (1980): *The effects on populations of exposure to low levels of ionizing radiation.* Washington, D.C.: National Academy of Sciences.

Boice JD, and Land CE (1982): Ionizing radiation. In: Schottenfeld D, Fraumeni JF (eds). *Cancer Epidemiology and Prevention.* Philadelphia: WB Saunders.

Breslow NE, and Day NE (1980): *Statistical Methods in Cancer Research. Volume I: The Analysis of Case-Control Studies.* Lyon, France: International Agency for Research on Cancer.

Brown CC, and Chu KC (1983): A new method for the analysis of cohort studies: implications of the multistage theory of carcinogenesis applied to occupational arsenic exposure. *Environ Health Perspect* 50:293–308.

Case RAM, Hosker ME, McDonald DB, et al. (1954): Tumors of the urinary bladder in workmen engaged in the manufacture and use of certain dyestuff intermediates in the British chemical industry. *Br J Ind Med* 11:75–104.

Crawford-Brown DJ (1983a): The impact of radiobiological considerations on epidemiological inferences of age-dependent radiosensitivity. In: *Epidemiology Applied to Health Physics.* CONF-830101. National Technical Information Service, pp. 504–517.

Crawford-Brown DJ (1983b): On a theory of age dependence in the induction of lung carcinomas following inhalation of a radioactive atmosphere. In: *Current Concepts in Lung Dosimetry.* CONF-820492. Washington, DC: U.S. Department of Energy, pp. 178–187.

Crawford-Brown DJ, and Cothern CR (1987): A discussion of the Bayesian analysis or scientific judgment for the uncertainties involved in the estimated risk due to the occurrence of Radon-222 in U.S. public drinking water supplies. *Health Phys* 53:11–21.

Crawford-Brown, DJ, and Pearce NE (1989): Sufficient proof in the scientific justification of environmental actions. *Environ Ethics* (in press).

Darby SC, Nakashima E, and Kato H (1985): A parallel analysis of cancer mortality among atomic bomb survivors and patients with ankylosing spondylitis given X-ray therapy. *J Natl Cancer Inst* 75:1–21.

Dement JM, Harris RL, Symons MJ, and Shy CM (1983): Exposures and mortality among chrysotile asbestos workers: Part II: Mortality. *Am J Ind Med* 4:421–433.

Doll R, and Peto R (1978): Cigarette smoking and bronchial carcinoma: dose and time relationships among regular smokers and lifelong non-smokers. *J Epidemiol Community Health* 32:303–313.

Franks LM, and Teich NM (eds) (1986): *Introduction to the Cellular and Molecular Biology of Cancer.* Oxford: Oxford University Press.

Guess HA, and Crump KS (1976): Low-dose extrapolation of data from animal carcinogenesis experiments: analysis of a new statistical technique. *Math Biosci* 32:15–36.

Hoel DG, Kaplan NL, and Anderson MW (1983): Implication of non-linear kinetics on risk estimation in carcinogenesis. *Science* 219:1032–1037.

Infante PF, Rinsky RA, Wagoner JK, et al. (1977): Leukaemia in benzene workers. *Lancet* ii:76–78.

Kaldor J, Peto J, Easton D, et al. (1986): Models for respiratory cancer in nickel refinery workers. *J Natl Cancer Inst* 77:841–848.

Kells LM (1960): *Elementary Differential Equations.* New York: McGraw-Hill.

Kunz E, Sevc J, Placek V, et al. (1979): Lung cancer in man in relation to different time distribution of radiation exposure. *Health Phys* 36:699–706.

Land CE, and Tokunaga M (1984): Induction period. In: Boice JD, Fraumeni JF (eds). *Radiation Carcinogenesis: Epidemiology and Biological Significance.* New York: Raven Press.

Moolgavkar S (1978): The multistage theory of carcinogenesis and the age distribution of cancer in man. *J Natl Cancer Inst* 61:49–52.

Moolgavkar SH, and Knudson AG (1981): Mutation and cancer: a model for human carcinogenesis. *J Natl Cancer Inst* 66:1037–1052.

Moolgavkar SH, Day NE, and Stevens RG (1980): Two-stage model for carcinogenesis: epidemiology of breast cancer in females. *J Natl Cancer Inst* 65:559–569.

Ott MG, Townsend JC, Fishbeck WA, et al. (1978): Mortality among individuals occupationally exposed to benzene. *Arch Environ Health* 33:3–10.

Pearce NE, Checkoway H, and Shy CM (1986): Time-related factors as potential confounders and effect modifiers in studies based on an occupational cohort. *Scand J Work Environ Health* 12:97–107.

Peto R (1977): Epidemiology, multistage models, and short-term mutagenicity tests. In: Hiatt HH, Watson JD, Winster JA (eds). *Origins of Human Cancer,* Vol. 4. Cold Spring Harbor, NY: Cold Spring Harbor Laboratory, pp. 1403–1428.

Peto R, Roe FJC, Lee PM, et al. (1975): Cancer and aging in mice and men. *Br J Cancer* 32:411–426.

Rothman KJ (1976): Causes. *Am J Epidemiol* 104:587–592.

Rothman KJ (1981): Induction and latent periods. *Am J Epidemiol* 114:253–259.

Shavell S (1980): An analysis of causation and the scope of liability in the law of torts. *J Leg Stud* 9:499–507.

Thomas DC (1983): Statistical methods for analyzing effects of temporal patterns of exposure on cancer risks. *Scand J Work Environ Health* 9:353–366.

U.S. Environmental Protection Agency (1986): *Draft Criteria Document for Radon in Drinking Water.* Washington, DC: USEPA, Office of Drinking Water.

Walker AM (1984): Declining relative risks for lung cancer after cessation of asbestos exposure. *J Occup Med* 26:422–426.

White MC, Infante PF, and Chu KC (1982): A quantitative estimate of leukemia mortality associated with occupational exposure to benzene. *Risk Anal* 2:195–204.

Whittemore AS (1977): The age distribution of human cancer for carcinogenic exposure of varying intensity. *Am J Epidemiol* 106:418–432.

Whittemore A, and Keller JB (1978): Quantitative theories of carcinogenesis. *SIAM Rev* 20:1–30.

Index

The road into the city was crowded. They passed a row of shops displaying tyres and chrome car parts. 'The shops are still open,' Mahesh commented, squinting at his watch. It was almost eleven o'clock. They sped past lorries and bullock carts decorated with streamers and flowers. Pedestrians dashed between moving cars and buses.

At a traffic signal, a man on a bicycle with a small boy balanced on the handlebars whizzed by them. The bicycle was festooned with paper ribbons and noisy flappers on the wheel spokes, and the small boy was laughing excitedly. Some of the roadside restaurants had put up coloured lights, some of the larger establishments blasted music.

'Independence at midnight,' Motilal said, crossing his arms over his chest. 'Why can't the British conduct business at sensible hours?' He was excited about Independence, but he wasn't sure how the silk market would fare under an exclusively Indian government. He knew how things worked under the British. He imagined the new map of India. Lahore, Karachi, Peshawar, Islamabad . . . he had never been to any of these places when they were in India, and now they were in a foreign country – Pakistan. Freedom from British rule was a grand idea. But how would he feel tomorrow? Would he feel free? Would the image of the British officer who had thrown him off the beach be erased from his memory? Motilal let out a tired sigh and turned his head to the open window.

'Independence is not a business deal,' Mahesh said. 'Well, maybe it is,' he laughed lightly. 'It sounds glamorous, Independence at the stroke of midnight. The British do things with great ceremony, you have to admit.'

Motilal grunted and continued looking out of the window. He liked the confident way in which his son spoke. He would do well in America.

At Shivaji Park a convoy of police jeeps was blocking the road and the Vauxhall was forced to stop. Around them buses and lorries were also at a standstill. Loudspeakers hastily tied to lampposts and tree trunks were broadcasting a speech in Hindi. Men in dirty *lungis* chewing betel leaf and smoking beedis sat on their haunches on the footpath. Kerosene lamps from the handcarts of itinerant food vendors dotted the darkness.

Vincent opened his door. 'I'll go and see what's going on,' he said.

He returned in a few minutes. 'It's a rally. People are waiting till midnight. They've started a bonfire and there's a stage with a band. We'll have to take a side road.'

'Come on,' Motilal said to Vincent, tapping his hand on the seat.

Vincent swerved to the right, dodged a few pedestrians who were crossing at the intersection, and manoeuvred the car down an alley.

Pressed near the doorway of a seedy corner bar, two women in cheap saris, their arms burdened with bangles, their painted mouths plastered in smiles, waited for customers. Vincent tipped his cap at them. Motilal and Mahesh looked away.

When they reached the college the booth where the security guards sat was empty. Spotlights illuminated the stone portico in front, but the rest of the buildings, including the chapel spire, lay in darkness.

'Drive to the Dastoors' bungalow,' Motilal said. 'Pervez may know something.'

At the front stoop of Pervez's house, Motilal didn't bother to look for the doorbell. He beat on the door, calling over the sound of his fist on wood, 'Rustomji, open! Open the door! Pervez! Are you there?' The back of his kurta was drenched in sweat. Mahesh had never seen his father behave like this.

The porch lights came on and Pervez opened the door. His eyes grew wide and he fumbled with the buttons of his untucked shirt as he stepped back into the brightly lit hallway.

'Is Rohini here?'

'No.' Pervez felt in his pocket. The envelope he was supposed to deliver to Sagar Mahal was still there. He had promised to hand it in, but fearing the reaction it would incite, he'd gone straight home after the celebration at Gaylord. In any case, it was Independence eve – the letter could well wait until the next day. He had overlooked the fact that Rohini would not return home to Sagar Mahal that night and her parents would have no idea where she was.

'Have you seen Rohini?' Motilal stepped into the hall.

Pervez's hand shook as he gave the white envelope, which was no longer crisp, to Mahesh. 'It's in English,' he mumbled.

'From Rohini?'

'Uh . . . yes . . . no . . .' Pervez leaned against the wall, and tried to smile at Motilal.

Mahesh pried open the flap and unfolded the paper. His eyes narrowed in concentration.

> Please do not worry about Rohini. We have decided to
> marry at Zakaria Masjid today. This is what we both want.

We ask for your blessings, which we hope you will bestow upon us freely, for without your blessings both our lives will remain incomplete.

Hanif Wali Hussein.

The corners of his mouth twitched as he neared the end.

Motilal looked through the hallway. 'Where's Rustomji? And your mother?'

'They're both out of town. They've gone to Delhi to see . . .' Pervez stepped towards the drawing room. 'P-p-please come in. Please sit. Tea?'

Motilal glanced at Mahesh, whose face was slowly draining of colour. 'What is it?' The paper lay limp in Mahesh's hand. 'Here, let me see.' Motilal seized the letter and scanned the handwriting. Frustrated, he handed it back to Mahesh.

'She's married,' Mahesh blurted, waving the letter.

'What?'

'Rohini is married,' Mahesh said.

'What? How? Jagmohan . . .'

'No. Not Jagmohan. It's another fellow, Hanif. The letter is from him.'

'What? The Muslim? Rohini married him! How?' Motilal clenched his hands.

'You know him?' Mahesh asked.

'Of course not! I know about the letters,' Motilal puffed his cheeks, put his hands on his hips.

'What letters?'

'The letters that Saroj found. The Muslim letters!' Motilal began pacing.

A puzzled look spread on Mahesh's face.

'Never mind,' Motilal bellowed.

'They went to the mosque near Bhindi Bazaar,' Mahesh said, looking down at the letter. 'His name is Hanif.'

'Don't say his name to me!'

'But he seems modest,' Mahesh said cautiously. 'He's asked for your blessings.'

'My blessings to a Mussalman! Bah!'

Mahesh unfolded and folded the letter before sliding it into the envelope. He turned to Pervez. 'She married a Muslim?'

'Yes.'

Motilal looked angrily at Pervez. 'You knew about this?'

Pervez sank into a chair gripping the armrests. 'I tried to warn them. But—' A palpable silence filled the room. Pervez looked up at Motilal and said in the calmest voice he could muster: 'Please listen, Motilalji. Hanif is a good man. I've known him for some time. We're fast friends. Be reasonable, I know this is upsetting to you, but . . .'

'Why didn't you tell us earlier? For years I've known your father!' Motilal's eyes blazed. Perspiration dotted his forehead. 'You have no idea what this means.' Motilal stood over Pervez and leaned into his face. 'Do you know what this is going to do to us?' Motilal shouted. Pervez kept blinking. Turning to Mahesh, Motilal said, 'At least she's alive. Come on.'

The front door closed with a thud.

'I tried to warn them,' Pervez whispered to the silence.

Chapter 25

From the balcony of their room at the Peacock Hotel, Hanif and Rezana gazed out at the city and the sea beyond. The harbour lights sent long glittery ripples over the water. From the area around the Gateway came the boom of drums and trumpets. A struggling August moonlight picked out the ferries anchored near the docks and, farther out at sea, they could make out two big steamers.

'Rezana,' Hanif said, his eyes focused far away, at something on the water. He was hunched over, in a relaxed way, his elbows on the railing. The breeze passed over his shirt sleeves. 'Re-za-na,' he said again, slowly, delighting in each syllable. 'Do you know what your name means?'

She remained silent, self-conscious, and mesmerized by the way he said her name.

'It means "a beautiful bouquet of flowers",' he said.

Her gaze went to the white frangipani blossoms that came up on one side of the balcony.

He angled himself towards her. For the first time he noticed the dark brown birthmark near her left ear. He wanted to put his arms around her, press her to him, feel her body with his, but he suddenly grew anxious and turned away. He wanted to do everything the right way. But he had no clear idea of what that was. He stood quiet, although his mind raced. It would all happen in time, he kept telling himself. 'I wish we had the harmonium,' he said.

'The radio,' she said. 'The speech is tonight.' She went inside and switched on a lamp near the sofa. The lampshade cast a small pool of light while the rest of the room hung in semi-darkness. He followed her inside, leaving the balcony door open, and watched her twirling the knobs of the radio. 'Nehru's speech will come after the song,' she said, stepping back from the radio.

He watched as she undid her braid and shook her head, leaning back slightly, the long wavy hair falling abundantly behind her. He'd never seen her with her hair completely unbound like this. She was youthful, wholesome, and intensely beautiful, and even as his thoughts fumbled for restraint he felt a sense of abandon. The song ended. The departing Viceroy, Lord Mountbatten, introduced Jawaharlal Nehru as India's first prime minister. Rezana felt his fingers on her hair, moving the loose tendrils behind her ear, touching the earring, the small golden loops that she wore every day. She could hear herself breathing as she reached her hands to clasp his. The coloured glass bangles on her wrists clinked against each other. Nehru's voice sounded strong and clear; it was a good radio:

> Long years ago we made a tryst with destiny, and now the time comes when we shall redeem our pledge, not wholly or in full measure, but very substantially. At the stroke of the midnight hour, when the world sleeps, India will awake to life and freedom. A moment comes, which comes but rarely in history, when we step out from

> the old to the new, when an age ends, and when the soul
> of a nation, long suppressed, finds utterance.

'Rezana,' Hanif said. He couldn't help himself. His breath,
her name, remained suspended in the room. Her mouth was
closed, but her lips trembled.

> The past clings on to us still in some measure and we
> have to do much before we redeem the pledges we have
> so often taken. Yet the turning point is past, and history
> begins anew for us, the history, which we shall live, and
> act and others will write about.

Worry about the family she had left, the name she had given
up, this worry swirled within her. She touched a fingertip to
a mole on his face. He drew closer and ran his fingers
through her hair – tentative at first, then thrilling at the
denseness; growing more confident his hands plunged deeper
with fierce deftness.

> Freedom brings responsibilities and burdens . . . On this
> day our first thoughts go to the Father of our Nation,
> Mahatma Gandhi, who, embodying the old spirit of India,
> held aloft the torch of freedom and lighted up the darkness
> that surrounded us. We have often been unworthy
> followers of his and have strayed from his message . . .
> We shall never allow that torch of freedom to be blown
> out, however high the wind or stormy the tempest.

'The speech,' Rezana said awkwardly, and tried to pay
attention to the words. Lord Mountbatten would take down
the British flag; Nehru would hoist the Indian tricolour in
its place. She tried to imagine the scene, to focus on the
historic moment, to experience the euphoria. Nothing made

sense. She felt his breath on her face and his body close and insistent next to hers. 'Hanif,' she whispered.

> All of us, to whatever religion we may belong, are equally the children of India with equal rights, privileges and obligations.

Religion. She had traded her religion. She had given up her deities for Allah.

> We cannot encourage communalism or narrow-mindedness, for no nation can be great whose people are narrow in thought or in action.

A sultry breeze came in from the balcony and with it, the scent of frangipani. In the soft darkness of the room his hands went gently, quickly, to her neck, to her shoulders, to her waist. She didn't resist. She had become a sparkling drop of moonlight. The sari fell about her in a billowy heap. She groped with his shirt buttons. Her eyes focused on his chest, on the slight swell of muscle under the matted hair. His daring fingers went to the small hooks and clasps of the sari blouse and the drawstring of the petticoat. He fumbled with the knot, his fingers impatient at the loosening string. At the rickrack and frill of her undergarments, his gaze melted. This night, this incredible, amazing night. His hands moved over her skin. She felt a vein pulsing in her neck, under her ear as he led her down to the peacock coverlet.

> To the nations and peoples of the world we send greetings and pledge ourselves to cooperate with them in furthering peace, freedom and democracy. And to India, our much-loved motherland, the ancient, the eternal, we pay our

reverent homage and we bind ourselves afresh to her service.

The speech ended. In Delhi, on the ramparts of the Red Fort, Bismillah Khan raised the shehnai to his lips. The music rang out from the radio and filled the room of the Peacock Hotel. Outside, India approached a state of pandemonium with drums, firecrackers, shouting, dancing, and everywhere the smell of sweat and victory.

IV
PARTITION

Chapter 26

At Sagar Mahal the chandeliers in the main hall blazed all night; the servants were back and forth from the kitchen with tea. Harshaba wept and prayed. Motilal kept shaking his head in disbelief. Mahesh, Sumitra, Amrita, Shrikant and Prema talked among themselves – perhaps she was kidnapped. Yes, Muslims do things like that. How much money was he demanding? Was she beaten, violated? Did they really get married? Muslims can take four wives – does he have other wives? He made her convert in all probability. What kind, Shia or Sunni or Bora? *Muslim! Mussalman! Mohammaddan!* How old is he – eighteen, nineteen, twenty? Muslim houses smell of mutton. Even their clothes smell. What letters? She knew him from college. She knew the Muslim! He's a musician. Living in this house, she was having an affair, can you believe that? Our name is finished. Send a telegram to Dantali, ask Saroj to come at once. What about Ahmedabad? Somebody should tell Jagmohan. No, don't say anything yet.

Shrikant, who was quiet at first, shouted, 'It's a disgrace! We cannot tolerate this.' He said to his father, 'I will go to that Muslim house and drag him out myself.'

'And then what?' Mahesh said.

Shrikant ignored him. 'We should beat up the Muslim and have him thrown in jail. We should teach him a lesson.'

'Please,' Motilal said putting his hand on Shrikant's shoulder, 'be reasonable.'

Harshaba, on the sofa, didn't utter a word, but every once in a while a steely expression passed her face. Finally, she sat up and, in a low, composed tone instructed Sumitra and Amrita to pack Rohini's things. 'I want all of it out of this house,' she said, snapping her fingers. And to Mahesh, 'Go and deliver everything to her. But do *not* go inside the Muslim house. Do *not* drink their water.'

Sumitra and Amrita went to pack Rohini's things. Sumitra was sixteen, Amrita a year younger; both were slender with expressive eyes; and abundant wavy hair. Amrita, the more boisterous of the two, felt an odd sense of loss. But at the same time she realized there was purpose and meaning to what Rohini had done. It showed something. Hanif was probably tall and muscular with a thick moustache and a good face . . . Amrita had got used to the idea of Rohini and Jag. Now Rohini and Hanif? A musician. 'This Hanif, does he play classical music, or . . .'

'How should I know?' Sumitra frowned.

'He might be someone famous.'

'It doesn't matter,' Sumitra said. 'It's bad, what she did, running off with a Muslim. Come on, help me with this trunk.' Sumitra found it hard to believe that Rohini had pulled off such an act. The uproar in the household annoyed her, but the thought of her sister with a strange man also worried her. Rohini was much too impulsive. 'Just watch,' Sumitra said to Amrita, 'Within a month, she'll be back, regretting what she did.' The hinges creaked as she swung open the lid of the second trunk, releasing the pungent odour of naphthalene.

'Maybe he's a playback singer, in the movies. Maybe we've heard him and didn't know it,' Amrita said. 'We should look for his name. But maybe he doesn't play Indian music at all. Maybe he plays the piano and violin.' Amrita stood up, positioned her arms around an imaginary dance partner and started twirling around the room. 'Stop it,' Sumitra said, slamming the lid of the second trunk and clicking closed the latches.

౧౧

Hanif asked at the Hotel Peacock reception desk to use the phone, which Mr Kumar promptly placed before him, stepping back but remaining within earshot. Hanif dialled his home number and, cupping his hand around the mouthpiece, whispered the news to his mother. The earpiece squawked with her shock and anger. Hanif could only listen as she vented her fury – she would have liked to plan his wedding, she wanted to attend his wedding, she was his mother, had he forgotten that? When she asked the girl's name, Hanif said, 'Rohini.' There was silence. 'Rezana,' he said quickly. His mother drew a long breath. His father's voice came on the line and Hanif mumbled, 'I'll be home this afternoon with her.' Before his father could say anything, Hanif hung up.

Mr Kumar slid closer and took the telephone from Hanif. 'Everything okay, sir? The telephone . . .?'

'The best, the best. The best telephone in the world,' Hanif said as he ran outside. 'Let's go,' he said to Rezana, who was waiting on the steps by the front door.

'You told them?' she asked. 'What did they say?'

'Nothing really. They're waiting for us. Everything's fine,' he said. But she knew from his face that it was otherwise.

On the bus from Hotel Peacock to Bandra, the ticket collector grinned and refused Hanif's money. It was a free ride for Independence Day. There were parades everywhere. At Kala Ghoda, the famous junction named after Boehm's equestrian statue of King Edward VII, the crowds chanted '*Bharat Mata ki Jai*', and '*Long Live Mahatma Gandhi*.' Indian flags fluttered from rooftops and on makeshift flagpoles and in people's hands. Food wrappers and broken banners littered the roads, and the smell of spent firecrackers filled the air like incense.

When they arrived at Hanif's house, Rezana's heart was thudding. She'd imagined this moment a few times in the past couple of days, always with anxiety and foreboding. 'Do I look okay?' she asked, adjusting her sari.

Hanif smiled and nodded, ran a hand through his hair, then reached in his pocket for a handkerchief and wiped the back of his neck. A few twittering sparrows flew out of the banyan tree. 'The birds are singing to welcome you,' he said.

From the gate to the front door they walked up the path together, but at the steps she hung back adjusting her sari again.

The door opened before Hanif rang the bell.

'*Salaam Alaykum*,' Rezana said, bowing to Hanif's parents. She thought they offered the customary response, *Wa*

Alaykum As-Salaam, but she wasn't sure. She kept her eyes to the ground and she knew his parents were staring at her.

'Come in,' his father said, breaking an uncomfortable silence, and held the door open.

Hanif's father looked younger than Rezana had expected, certainly much younger than her own father. Tall and well built, he wore grey trousers and a white shirt. Her father never wore European clothes.

'Welcome,' his mother said, her voice polite but betraying no emotion. Dressed in *salwar-kameez* and *dupatta*, his mother was almost as tall as his father. 'Let's sit in the drawing room,' his mother said, as she led the way into the adjoining room. Her hair was twisted in a bun with the pins pushed neatly in. A perfume of gardenia or rose trailed behind her.

The drawing room was smaller than most of the bathrooms at Sagar Mahal. The open windows overlooked a tired garden with some grass and a few bushes along the wall. Hanif's parents sat in armchairs by the window. That left the settee. Rezana hesitated. It would be odd sitting so close to Hanif in front of his parents. But it would be even odder to remain standing. Smoothing out the back of her sari, she lowered herself onto the edge of the settee beside Hanif.

'I'll make tea,' his mother said, but made no move to rise.

Rezana fidgeted and looked at Hanif; should she offer to help? There didn't seem to be any servants. Did his mother do the cooking and cleaning? She wished she'd asked Hanif these details beforehand, and that Hanif had told her something about how his parents lived.

Hanif's father shifted in his chair, crossing and uncrossing his legs, leaning forward to adjust the cushion behind him, tossing it to the floor, folding his arms over his chest and studying the ceiling.

Rezana followed his gaze; his eyes avoided hers. The fan, set at a low speed, moved the air sluggishly; one of the blades was bent.

'What about your music?' Hanif's father asked, still looking at the ceiling.

Hanif frowned.

Outside, possibly from the neighbour's house, came the irregular staccato sound of someone expertly hammering. In the distance, the din of cars and buses on Carter Road.

'What does she know of the Koran?' his father asked.

Rezana glanced at him quickly. She had assumed that the Koran outlined different roles and obligations for men and women. But were there sections of the Koran that only women were supposed to read? Were certain pages barred to women?

Hanif sighed loudly and looked around the room. 'She will learn,' he said.

Rezana pulled a loose blue thread from her sari. She wondered how long they would sit there. The house smelled sour, like curdled milk. Her gaze slid uncertainly about the room. A porcelain vase was displayed on a bureau, and she was reminded of the porcelain Chinese statue in the divankhana at Sagar Mahal. The Chinese man was four feet tall with a long white beard, droopy earlobes, tiny black eyes, and a red mouth. When she was young her parents had said, 'Do not touch the Chinaman.' Yet, several times when no one was looking, she'd crept up to the Chinaman and touched the tip of her index finger to the statue. She wondered whether the porcelain vase on the bureau had been similarly forbidden to Hanif.

Hanif's mother stood up. 'Look, what's done is done. You both are married. Nikah is done. Is that correct?' She didn't wait for affirmation. 'Then you will live together as husband and wife.' Looking directly at Rezana, she smiled. It was an anxious but genuine smile. 'You will call me Ammi,' then gesturing towards Hanif's father, 'and he is Abbu. Okay?' Rezana nodded; she glanced at Abbu, the expression of shock was still there, but he was sitting more easily in the chair. Ammi continued, 'Good. That's settled. I'll show you Hanif's room. Where are your things?' Rezana gestured to her shoulder bag.

Ammi looked hesitantly at Abbu. 'We should invite people for dinner or do something to mark the occasion.' Turning again to Rezana, 'What about your family? Should we ask them to come? Oh, you must tell us about yourself. Hanif said you were in college together. You were reading English Literature, yes?' Again she smiled, this time more easily, more definitely. 'He likes literature,' she said, pointing at Hanif's father. 'Do you know cooking? You are Gujarati, no? He likes Gujarati *halva*.' Again she pointed at Hanif's father.

The tension in the room seeped away with every word. 'Don't worry, I'll teach you dishes of our style. Hanif likes chicken curry, also mutton biryani and *kheema*. Ah, Rezana, you are beautiful. My son has married a beautiful girl.'

The mention of her name startled Rezana. Ammi didn't even know her as Rohini, she realized. To the people she would meet from now on, she would be Rezana. And the way Ammi had said 'Rezana', so naturally and affectionately – that same wave of newness that had swept over her at the mosque came to her again, expect this time she felt light and easy; she was at the centre of an exciting new world. She smiled and looked down at the ruby ring on her finger.

'Yes, you must smile!' Ammi said. 'This is a happy occasion and . . .'

A car stopped outside the gate and they all looked to the window. Seeing the green Vauxhall, Rezana shot to her feet. 'It's someone from my house,' she said, her voice cracking.

'Let's see who it is, shall we?' Hanif said, striding towards the door. Rezana followed. Hanif couldn't imagine what exactly her family would do once they got the news, but he knew there would be consequences. He'd thought of a few things to say to her parents, and he would speak humbly and respectfully. He would first apologize for the rash way in which things had happened, then he would explain how committed he was to their daughter. He would say that he came from a good family – they were educated people and well respected in the community. Finally, he would tell them about his work at All India Radio, and that he was going to be a recording artist.

'Whoever has come from Rezana's house,' Ammi called behind him, 'invite them in. Have them sit. I'll make *sherbat*.' She said to Abbu, 'Bring extra chairs from the back room.'

Rezana looked down the road half-expecting to see a procession of cars and her mother emerging from one of them, yelling angrily.

It was Mahesh in the green Vauxhall. He and Vincent

carried the trunks up the path and laid them, one on top of the other, outside the door. Mahesh shook hands with Hanif, but he couldn't bring himself to look at his sister. He didn't agree with his parents' reaction and their unreasonable aphorisms about Muslims, but he couldn't commend Rohini either. Obviously she hadn't considered the repercussions.

'Please come inside,' Hanif said to Mahesh. 'Sit for a while . . .'

'No. I must go,' Mahesh replied hastily. With Harshaba's voice ringing in his ears – *Do not drink water in their house* – he headed down the path, towards the front gate, longing for a glass of water.

'Wait, Mahesh, please wait . . .' Rezana implored. She stared at his back as he walked down the path, his steps quick and definite. 'When are you leaving for America?' she called after him in a shaky voice.

'In ten days,' he replied as Vincent opened the car door for him.

'You'll come and see me before you go?'

Mahesh got in the back seat and stared straight in front.

Vincent raised his hand in a half-salute to Rezana before shutting the car door.

'He's going to America?' Hanif said.

Rezana nodded. 'He's leaving in ten days,' she said with a sigh.

'We should go to America. Maybe they need a playback singer for American pictures.' Hanif laughed. 'You can read American Literature. Maybe it's better than English Literature. We've certainly had enough of the British.'

If it's about literature we should go to France, she wanted

to say. She looked at the trunks, which were big and black with great brass latches. 'Okay, let's go to America,' she said. 'Why not? I'm already packed.'

Hanif laughed. The worst of what they could anticipate was over. What happened next would be, and Rezana practiced the word . . . *Inshallah* . . . as God wills it.

Chapter 27

Versova wasn't the kind of place that was on the way to anywhere, it was just somewhere on the outskirts of Bombay where people came to live. Andheri Station was four miles away, along a narrow road that cut across patches of quicksand, stretches of marshes, and fields dotted with palm trees. Apart from the fishermen, who lived in thatched huts and eked out a living from the shrimp and pomfret, or by smuggling gold across the Arabian Sea, there were fewer than fifty houses in Versova.

After Partition, Versova changed; it became a refuge for Hindu migrants from what was declared to be Muslim territory, West Pakistan. The pink mansion next to Sagar Mahal that belonged to the Maharaja of Kutch was sold to a high-ranking Congress Party commissioner who, instead of taking up residence and respecting the building's architectural integrity as neighbours expected, divided it into as many one- and two-room rental units as he could fit inside its walls. A new bus stop appeared near the dairy. More shops opened around the Ration Centre. There was talk of a municipal school on the vacant plot behind the public garden.

Mr Malkani, a Sindhi man with seven children, who fled from Karachi with his wife, bought the dilapidated sanatorium on the beach and converted it into a family house. They came to Sagar Mahal one evening to pay a neighbourly visit, Mr Malkani dressed in a light grey suit and a white bow tie, Mrs Malkani in a silk sari.

'Our life has completely changed,' Mr Malkani told Motilal and Harshaba. 'We had factories, acres of land, fruit trees, horse carriages, a big house, servants, everything . . . and now . . . well, at least we are still alive.'

While Mrs Malkani sat dabbing a handkerchief to her eyes, her husband told Motilal and Harshaba about the battle zone at the border. Fields covered with mutilated bodies, the earth charred beyond hope. Hindus and Sikhs crossing to India, Muslims to the newly created Pakistan. 'I'll never forget the stench of burning tyres and human flesh,' Mr Malkani said. 'Whole train cars were set on fire.' His eyes flecked with rage. 'People were stripped of everything they possessed, down to their gold teeth, and stabbed to death. We saw a group of girls being dragged away, screaming . . .' He clenched his jaw and swallowed. 'The journey was difficult for all of us, but especially for my eighty-three-year-old mother. We came to Amritsar by jeep with an army escort. We were lucky.' He paused after each sentence, as though in the telling he was reliving it. 'It's hard to forget such things. Memory is a curse sometimes.'

Motilal and Harshaba listened intently. That night in bed they were silent, both of them wondering if their daughter would go to Pakistan and fearing the calamities that might befall her at the border.

'She will require money,' Motilal said in the darkness.

Harshaba turned on her side. 'I'm tired. Let's sleep.'

Chapter 28

When Hanif returned home from work in the evenings, Rezana sat with him in the music room while he played the harmonium. Often he handed her the music book and they sang together. Some evenings they went to the seaside at Danda where they sat on the big rocks and watched the sun sink into the water. The small fishing boats would be careening towards shore and from time to time in the distance they could spot an oil tanker or a big steamer. On Sundays they spent the afternoon at the cinema; out of habit Rezana's eyes darted about the theater lobby when they entered and scanned the audience before the lights dimmed. Whenever Hanif brought home a gajra for her, she would open the banana leaf packet, sprinkle the flowers with water, and pin the string of white blossoms in her hair. At night she would place the flowers on his pillow and when he came to bed he would bury his face in the fragrance before reaching for her.

ന

Every morning Rezana awoke before the rest of the house to use the bathroom in the hallway. The white tiles with years of dirt in the cracks and the broken chain that she had to pull to flush the toilet bothered her. The clutter on the shelf below the mirror – combs, shaving items, toothpowder, and hairpins – bothered her even more. The dripping tap that left a rusty stain in the basin bothered her the most.

ꕥ

When Ammi asked Rezana to prepare the morning tea, Rezana nodded stiffly. The kitchen was surprisingly large with a white marble floor, a good window, and shelves lined with stainless steel canisters and cooking utensils. A small glass cupboard held the custard powder, saffron, almonds, and an assortment of other 'costly' ingredients.

'The milk is here,' Ammi said, lifting the lid off of a large pot. 'And sugar.' She shook the stainless steel canister and set it on the counter. 'The tea leaves are in that cupboard and, see in that bowl, I've already ground up the masala.' Ammi moved aside a few things cluttered around the stove. 'You have to pump the stove two or three times,' she said over her shoulder before leaving the kitchen. 'You know how?'

At Sagar Mahal, Rezana was never required to make anything. Except for the times she and her sisters snuck in to steal sweets, she never went into the kitchen. But she had a general idea of how to make tea. She surveyed the ingredients. Yesterday at the market with Ammi she was impressed by her mother-in-law's efficiency. Ammi knew exactly which vegetables were in season locally and which had come from somewhere else, and which bhaji-walla had the best lemons and chillies. She never haggled over price. When Rezana thought she had paid too much for a kilo of brinjals, Ammi said: 'We have been given more than we deserve. Why not give others more than they deserve?'

Rezana approached the kerosene stove, feeling resolute and in control. With only two pumps, she got it going. She put the milk and water to boil, as instructed, but misjudged her timing and added the tea leaves and masala too soon. As the mixture looked weak, she assumed she had got her measures wrong, and spooned in more tea. When she turned off the flame, she knew the colour of the tea was wrong. But, she reasoned, perhaps it would still taste okay. She poured the brew through the strainer into the cups set out on a tray; she splashed some and burned her wrist; she winced but did not let go on the pot. She used a kitchen towel to soak up the spilt mixture, and carried the tray to the dining room as elegantly as she could manage, wishing she hadn't filled the cups to the brim.

Abbu took up his cup first, slurped, and, looking like he wanted to spit on the floor, declared loudly, scornfully, 'Bitter!' He placed the cup on its saucer, returned both to the tray with a clatter, took up his newspaper and snapped the pages open. Ammi and Hanif didn't comment on the tea, but they left most of it unfinished in their cups.

Rezana carried the tray back to the kitchen, set it beside the sink and watched as the cooling milk formed a skin on the surface of each cup. Her eyes filled with tears. She reached for the small towel, damp and stained with tea, balled it up, and flung it across the room.

ରେ

Every evening as Ammi cooked, Rezana was expected to stay in the kitchen and help. She didn't mind cutting the vegetables, kneading the dough, or scouring the heavy pots. But the meat, the raw flesh sitting on the drain board, chicken or mutton or lamb, Rezana couldn't tell the difference, made her want to vomit. Pinkish brownish whitish . . . and red specks of . . . blood? She gagged.

Sometimes the chunks would be kept in a bowl to marinate for hours in a sauce. Rezana froze with horror the first time as Ammi picked up slippery globs of meat with her bare fingers and tossed them into the cooking pot. The stuff would sputter and snarl, and then the smell would start. Rezana felt her stomach heave and spiral upwards as she fled the kitchen.

At dinner, Hanif removed some meat from a bone and set it on Rezana's plate. 'Try it,' he said gently. Ammi and Abbu stopped eating and stared at her. She gaped at the brownish sliver on her plate. 'Come on, it's just a small bite,' Hanif said.

They were all looking at her. With her fingertips she picked up the meat, moved it towards her lips and placed it in her mouth. She couldn't breathe. Her heart began beating faster and faster. Her skin felt hot. The mass sat on her tongue. Nausea bubbled inside her. She looked at Hanif with imploring eyes that welled with tears. Oh, how she longed to be at Versova, away from these Muslims. By sheer will, she made her jaws move and her teeth pressed down on the lump, leathery and rubbery as it rolled about in her mouth. By the time she swallowed, tears were streaming down her face.

Ammi yelled at Hanif, 'Let her eat what she wants!' She rushed to Rezana's side and tried to put a comforting arm around her.

'*Tobah! Tobah!*' Abbu said to her, touching a hand lightly to one cheek, then the other. As Rezana dashed out of the dining room sobbing, he turned to Hanif and said coolly, 'Do we need such drama in the house?'

తి

The bedroom they shared was cramped with the signs of their conjugal existence: Hanif's single bed replaced by a double and pushed against the wall; her two black trunks lined up below the window; the wall hooks heavy with both their clothes. In his armoire, she rearranged a few of his things to make room for some of hers. On the writing table, in a new silver frame, was the photo Pervez had taken outside the mosque, the day of the marriage, black and white, and grossly out of focus. Hanif had his arm around her, his fingers resting lightly on her shoulder. It was difficult to tell whether they were smiling. When she looked at the photo the first time, she was reminded of Jag. She imagined his house in Ahmedabad with big windows overlooking the lawns, divans, crystal lamps, and his room with a huge bed . . . such sullied thoughts. Guilt welled in her throat and she vowed never to think of him again. But that very night, after her day of abject failure, lying next to Hanif, the image of Jag and his room in Ahmedabad invaded her mind.

తి

In the euphoria of being Hanif's wife, Rezana lost track of time, because the good days far outweighed the bad. Sometimes she went about in a daze, oblivious to whether it was morning or afternoon or evening. Her life had turned into a frenzied sequence of occurrences. One minute it was as though she were swept into a dream world, a scented vista or vision, where everything was ordered and perfect and full of promise. The next instant everything was on the brink of falling apart. There was nothing in between; no median state that claimed her time and synchronized her senses. She kept reminding herself that she had what she wanted most.

Outside, and all over the country, Nehru's government had declared a state of Emergency. The violence from the border was spreading to the cities and small towns of India. Hindus and Muslims were killing each other. The papers brought news of more riots and more rallies. 'It's good that we live in Bandra,' Abbu said. Bandra was the Christian area of Bombay and as such had not attracted sectarian attention. 'But stay indoors, we should not take chances.'

Each evening after dinner when they gathered around the radio to listen to the news, Rezana's sadness grew. 'What happened to Independence?' she asked Hanif. 'People are only speaking of Partition.'

ಜಾ

Rezana said to Ammi, who was peeling potatoes and humming softly to herself, 'The tap in the bathroom? I was thinking . . . uhhh . . .' They were in the kitchen preparing for Anwar-babu, Saira-begum, and a few other relatives who were coming for dinner. 'Ammi, I noticed that the tap in the bathroom has been leaking because it is old and there is some rust underneath, and even if we clean the rust, it will keep coming back if the tap keeps dripping water, so I was thinking we should get a new tap.' Rezana had not meant for it all to come out in such a rush of words.

Ammi stopped humming. She dropped the half-peeled potato and the knife on top of the mound of peelings. 'Finish the potatoes,' she said, before briskly washing her hands and leaving the kitchen.

Abbu had just returned from the office, and moments later, Rezana heard him in the drawing room. 'What? The tap is a problem? She wants a new tap? Who does she think she is, a high-class maharani? Send her back to Versova. Let her go to her father's house and use his golden taps. She's not fit for our house!'

The knife in Rezana's hand sliced into her thumb and she watched the blood rise to the surface.

'I told you,' Ammi said. 'I told you it was just a matter of time before she would start making demands, didn't I?'

Rezana left the potatoes and fled to her room.

When Hanif returned from work, Ammi met him in the foyer. 'Please,' he said, as he untied his shoes, 'give her some time to adjust. Something smells good. What are you cooking? I'm hungry.'

That evening when the guests arrived, Rezana's eyes were dim and puffy; the smile on her face as she carried the plates of samosas into the dining room was timorous and spiritless. During dinner, when she looked over at Ammi and Saira-begum chattering softly, she knew they were talking about her because neither would look at her.

Nothing was said about the tap. Rezana tried to avoid Ammi and Abbu as much as she could, and when she had no choice but to be around them during meals, she didn't have the courage to look at them directly. A week went by. Was her transgression forgotten? Each night, Hanif tried to reassure her, 'It's okay, don't worry. No, you have not fallen in their estimation.' But Rezana lay awake in the dark wondering if she should apologize to Ammi, whether that would be a noble thing to do – or should she put the whole matter out of her mind, as they seemed to have done?

It was in this state of uncertainty that Rezana heard Abbu come home and call to Ammi from the front door, 'Every day you remind me, now here it is.' He handed her a cardboard box from Bhogilal Bath Fittings, and said, 'Call the plumber tomorrow.'

ೲ

'Here, what do you think?' Abbu said, as he walked into the sitting room and handed Rezana a page cut from the *Weekly*. Abbu had never said anything directly to her before. A cursory nod was all he offered by way of acknowledgement.

Ammi, Hanif, and Rezana were in the sitting room eating the mango custard that Ammi had prepared for dessert after dinner. Rezana set her bowl on the table and unfolded the paper.

'What is it?' Hanif asked, looking over her shoulder. 'Ah, a poem. Why don't you read it to us?'

'Yes, let's hear you read,' Ammi said, adjusting herself in the armchair.

Rezana looked at Hanif and the paper in her hand. Read aloud? Here? In front of everyone? She would rather be subjected to endless hours of cutting vegetables in the kitchen. Abbu picked up his bowl of custard and settled into the armchair next to Ammi. Rezana glanced at Abbu, whose face gave nothing away. Hanif nudged her elbow in encouragement.

She took an uncertain breath and began, 'Partition, by W.H. Auden.'

> Unbiased at least he was when he arrived on his mission,
> Having never set eyes on the land he was called to partition
> Between two peoples fanatically at odds,
> With their different diets and incompatible gods.
> 'Time,' they had briefed him in London, 'is short. It's too late
> For mutual reconciliation or rational debate:
> The only solution now lies in separation.
> The Viceroy thinks, as you will see from his letter,
> That the less you are seen in his company the better,
> So we've arranged to provide you with other accommodation.
> We can give you four judges, two Moslem and two Hindu,
> To consult with, but the final decision must rest with you.'
>
> Shut up in a lonely mansion, with police night and day
> Patrolling the gardens to keep the assassins away,
> He got down to work, to the task of settling the fate
> Of millions. The maps at his disposal were out of date
> And the Census Returns almost certainly incorrect,

But there was no time to check them, no time to inspect
Contested areas. The weather was frightfully hot,
And a bout of dysentery kept him constantly on the trot,
But in seven weeks it was done, the frontiers decided,
A continent for better or worse divided.

The next day he sailed for England, where he could
    quickly forget
The case, as a good lawyer must. Return he would not,
Afraid, as he told his Club, that he might get shot.

Her voice slowed at the last line. She put the page in her lap and looked around the room.

'*Shabash!*' Abbu said. '*Subhan'allah!* How well you read!' He stood up and clapped.

Ammi smiled and nodded approval.

'Can you believe it?' Hanif said, 'A man with diarrhoea deciding the boundaries of nations!'

As she folded the paper and pressed her fingers over the crease, she knew Hanif was gazing proudly at her.

Abbu said, 'What do you think of the poem, Rezana?'

In her nervousness she had simply read the words, paid little attention to the meaning in the lines. 'I admire this poet,' she said quietly. 'He's English, but at least he shows how absurdly the borders have been drawn up.'

'Indeed, indeed,' Abbu said. 'A sub-continent divided with no regard for geography or history. And splitting Pakistan into east and west, with the entire landmass of India in the middle, what were they thinking? They're baboons, I tell you . . .'

ৡৠ

She liked her new name. Rezana. It sounded glamorous and seductive. Yet sometimes when Hanif accidentally called her Rohini, she didn't correct him.

Despite having given up the lifestyle to which she was accustomed – the mansion by the sea, the retinue of servants and cooks and gardeners and drivers – she never regretted her decision to marry Hanif.

Admittedly, sometimes he was impatient with her. 'You have to read this with feeling, with reverence,' he said when he heard her reading the Koran. 'This is the word of God, not one of your novels.' She wanted to say something back, but she held herself. In as much as she tried to imbibe the teachings of the Koran, and the sensibilities of a Muslim household, she realized she would never fully meet his expectations. But that, she rationalized, was her shortcoming, not his.

Indeed, she had no regrets, no misgivings whatsoever about Hanif and their life together. So why, then, when she looked at her silk saris in the two trunks that took up so much space in their tiny bedroom, and when she reached for the jade and lapis-studded hand mirror that her father had brought for her from Jaipur, did she feel so unhappy? Why did she try to listen each evening at sundown for the reassuring heaving and clanging of the iron gates and the chowkidar pulling the bolts through? Why did she look to the north whenever Hanif took her to the seashore and why did her eyes follow the line of sand towards Versova? Why did she long for the fragrance of sandalwood and the tinkling of prayer bells? And why, when she thought of Mahesh, Sumitra, and Amrita, did she feel so dejected and lonely? Why?

ಞ

Hanif admired the way Rezana appeared before his uncles and aunts and cousins, dressed in salwar kameez, as though it were the most natural thing for her. She had taken so readily to learning the Koran and going to the mosque each Friday. He was impressed by how easily she had developed a concern for his parents, making mental notes of even their minor likes and dislikes and adjusting her behaviour accordingly. How attuned she had become to his mother's whims – sugar in her tea only in the morning, no salt in her buttermilk, her allergy to lemon grass – and to his father's frugal-minded idiosyncrasies – fans at low speed only, one bucket of water for bathing, use the cheaper kerosene burner for cooking if possible, and not the gas. She joked with Hanif that the only reason he changed the tap was because she had pointed out to Ammi that every leaking drop was costing him money. After Rezana had read the Auden poem, his father had begun including her in discussions, asking her opinions, even praising the tea she prepared each morning.

Hanif liked the way she laid out his clothes every day. He noticed that she had replaced some of his old shirts with new ones and he wondered how much they had cost, and from where the money had come, though perhaps she had saved it from the money he gave her every week for 'incidentals'.

When they were going out one evening, he noticed her powdering her face. Although this delighted him, he teased, 'Do you think you're a film star or what?' She flipped her head back and swung her hips. The next moment she was in his arms and he was edging backwards and reaching to lock the bedroom door.

During the day at the radio station Hanif often thought about such intimate moments. The way she came into his arms with a slight teasing resistance, the way she touched his body, the way she let him touch her. And then he spent the rest of the day watching the clock until he could go home to his Rezana.

Yet, each night as she lay beside him, he sensed her sadness. Often he heard her crying softly. Once he sat up in bed. 'Listen, you have to stop this. Tomorrow is Sunday. We'll go to Versova and talk to your parents. You'll see, everything is okay.'

'No,' she sobbed. 'You don't understand my people. You don't understand my mother!'

Chapter 29

Loud knocking joined in with the sound of the persistent ringing of the doorbell. Rezana sat up in bed, annoyed, and shook Hanif's shoulder. It was the last night of Ramadan and the festivities had ended only a few hours earlier.

'What? What is it?' Hanif said, his eyes adjusting to the darkness. They heard Abbu and Ammi's bedroom door opening, and seconds later Abbu was shouting.

When Hanif and Rezana stumbled to the foyer, they found Ammi in her nightdress, an expression of panic on her face. 'Riots!' she screamed as she ran into the living room. Abbu stayed by the door, his shoulder to it, both hands fumbling to drive back the bolt.

Hanif and Rezana followed Ammi into the living room and edged to the window. In the light of the street lamp, they could see four men. One of them raised his arm and the long blade of a knife glinted in the darkness. Rezana gasped as Hanif pulled her back from the window.

'What do they want with us?' Rezana asked, her voice soft and urgent.

The men outside started shouting again, one of them seized the door handle and started pushing and kicking the door. The bolt shook but held.

'What should we do?' Abbu asked Hanif, reaching for the light switch, but Hanif stopped his hand from turning it on. Momentarily everything went quiet. In the hopeful silence Rezana heard the breeze shuffling through the trees.

'Open this door,' a voice outside commanded.

Hanif came into the foyer, put a hand on Abbu's shaking arm.

'Open this door.' Then more voices, chanting, 'Open up. Open up.'

In the living room Ammi collapsed onto the settee and Rezana went to her side. The reflection of fire danced in the living room window. Someone had lit a kerosene-soaked cloth tied to a pole.

'Open this door or your house goes up in flames!'

'Wait!' Hanif shouted and stepped in front of Abbu. He drew back the bolt slowly, and as the door fell open he put himself in the doorway. Although his heart pounded in terror, he stood firm and resolute, and bellowed as loudly as he could, 'What do you want?'

Four men in white kurtas crowded the door. Sweat glistened on their brows. One of them made to push Hanif aside, and seemed taken aback that he resisted. The man, thin but muscular, wore a white *topi*, the sides of his head were shaved bald. Hanif noticed a vein bulging around the man's neck.

'Is there a Hindu girl here?' the man asked, raising a stick and jabbing at Hanif's shoulder.

'No, we are Muslims here,' Hanif said.

'Hindus shouldn't live with Muslims,' the man said, jabbing again, harder, more painfully.

Abbu standing behind Hanif took a step forward. 'Is this about Hindus and Muslims?' he said. 'Have you no shame? Disturbing innocent families at this hour, and after Ramadan?'

Another man stepped forward, his hand balled in a fist, and punched Abbu in the stomach, driving the air out of him, and he fell gasping to the floor.

In the living room Ammi wailed as she saw Abbu fall. She tried to get up from the settee and rush to his side, but her legs refused to work. Rezana crouched next to Ammi and held her breath. They had come to kill *her*. She had the urge to run, but her body was numb. She looked towards the foyer for Hanif. He was pinned to the wall by two men. She saw a stick being raised in the air and coming down hard on Hanif's arm. 'Hanif!' she screamed.

The next instant there was a loud commotion outside. Some of their neighbours had gathered on the road in front of the house and the glare of flashlights came in through the windows and the open front door. A van, its horn blaring, stopped outside their gate.

'Police,' the bald man said.

The other man, the one who had punched Abbu, muttered, 'Who called the police? Let's get out of here.' Two of their gang members waiting outside threw their sticks down and took off running. The stick with the burning cloth fell on the grass, the fire flaring and cutting a streak in the ground. Someone picked up the stick and stifled its flame.

In the foyer, the man with the topi said, 'Let's finish the job. I'll kill her quick.'

'No. There's no time. We must leave now!'

Rezana looked up at the man with the topi. The voice

sounded familiar. She fixed her eyes on the man just as he turned and she got a glimpse of his profile, a crooked Bell's palsy jaw. *Shrikant?* Her breath came in heaving gasps. She shook her head. No, it could not be. It was just someone who looked like him.

The two men raced out and melded into the night. There was more shouting outside.

A policeman appeared at the door. 'Is anyone hurt?'

'No,' Hanif replied, rubbing his injured shoulder. Rezana had helped Ammi to Abbu's side and his breathing was more regular; he waved a hand at them to leave him be. 'I think we're okay.'

'We must write a report,' the policeman said, pulling out a small notebook and pencil from his pocket. 'God's grace you escaped. These thugs are striking all over Bombay.'

'Yes,' Hanif said to the policeman, then turned and looked for Rezana. '*Allah kI meherbani,*' he whispered – thank God she was okay.

'Did you recognize any of them?' the policeman asked.

'No,' said Hanif. 'They were not from around here.'

The policeman looked at Rezana for confirmation and she too shook her head.

ಞ

Pervez paced the drawing room in Hanif's house, hands in his pockets. He wore a dark brown jacket, and underneath it, his white shirt was crumpled and dirty. A large cardboard box sat by the front door. 'Please,' he whispered to Hanif. 'You have to help me.'

The room hung in shadows. Only the hall light was on. There had been a power outage earlier that day, and once in a while the bulb flickered off, sending everything into total darkness for several seconds.

Hanif, in faded white pajama and undershirt, went to the box and kneeling beside it lifted the flaps. 'Books,' he said, reciting titles: '*The Communist Manifesto, History of the Russian Revolution, The State and Revolution* . . .' Under the books lay dozens of pamphlets and a fat cloth-covered file. Hanif leafed through the file, shook his head and closed the box. 'What is all this?'

'Right now, don't worry about the box,' Pervez said, irritated with his friend. 'Get rid of it if you want. Where's Rohini?'

'Rezana,' Hanif corrected curtly, 'is sleeping. Everyone's sleeping.' He glanced at the clock in the hallway. It was five minutes past two in the morning. 'What do you need, Pervez?' Hanif went to the drawing room, sat on the settee.

Pervez slumped into a chair. 'All right, I'll tell you. There's this man, Sudhir, he's a friend of mine. He was arrested yesterday.'

'Why? What did he do?'

'Nothing! He didn't do anything. It's this new Indian government!'

'*Shush*, not so loud,' Hanif said. 'So they arrested him for no good reason?'

'We've been collecting guns and . . .'

'Guns? For what?'

'What do you think, Hanif? Sometimes you can be so . . . so . . . stupid.'

'Stupid?'

'Hanif. Just listen to me.' Pervez leapt to his feet.

'No, you listen to me,' Hanif said. 'We had an awful night here only two days ago. Do you know what happened? Do you care what happened?'

Pervez shook his head. He kept pacing as Hanif told him about the intruders.

'I'm sorry. I didn't know. I'm glad everyone's okay.' He took a deep breath. 'Please, Hanif. You have to help me. Sudhir's in jail. We used to work together for . . . for the Party. It's only a matter of time before the police come for me. If my parents find out . . . listen, just don't say anything, okay? The guns are at a warehouse in Mahim. I wanted to take the books there, but I can't now. Others are trying to get rid of the weapons. I should probably leave India.' He stopped pacing and stood before Hanif. 'I want to go to Pakistan.'

'Pakistan?' Hanif asked, bewildered.

'Yes.'

'I'm confused. What will you do there?'

'Some of the other members are going to Pakistan. We want to regroup and become stronger. We have money. Actually, the money is coming from Calcutta and some foreign countries. But anyway, we can reorganize ourselves in Pakistan and take up the cause again. It's the only way . . .'

'The only way? For what?' Hanif stood up slowly, put his hands on his hips. 'You're not Muslim. Why Pakistan?'

'Hanif, please. You said your uncle lives in Karachi. Can you contact him?'

'But the border . . .'

'I know the border.' Pervez took off his jacket, tossed it

over the chair. 'I'll be careful. Look, I'm doing this for . . . for our nation. I'm doing this to change the course of history. Don't you see?'

Hanif shook his head, sat down again and leaned back in the settee.

'Remember the Salt March? Remember Gandhiji's long walk from Ahmedabad to the sea at Dandi to make his own salt rather than pay the salt tax . . .'

Hanif stared at his friend and listened to his brave arguments. He had seen Gandhiji twice in his life – the first time at a rally at Shivaji Park, where he had gone with Pervez. There was a large crowd, and as Pervez elbowed his way to the front, Hanif was left standing towards the back, next to a pole holding two loudspeakers. He was struck by the way the crowd turned silent when Gandhiji took the microphone. He himself was hardly aware of anything else as he focused his gaze on the tiny figure on stage. With his head bent and shoulders hunched, Gandhiji spoke of the new Cabinet Mission that had just returned from talks in England; and he stressed the need for continued non-violence. Hanif would never forget Gandhiji's words, 'An eye for an eye will only make the whole world blind.' After the rally, Pervez had gripped Hanif's arm, 'Can you believe it? We actually saw him . . . don't ever forget this day.' The second time Hanif had seen Gandhiji was by chance, at Bombay Central station. Gandhiji was sitting on a bench, surrounded by people speaking in hushed tones. Hanif was crossing the train station and was about twenty feet away, and he stopped and stared. Gandhiji looked frail and thin; Hanif knew he had been fasting for weeks. He stood there for several minutes, craning his neck, trying to edge closer, until Gandhiji and his entourage made for a departure platform and vanished into the crowd.

Hanif looked up at Pervez and cleared his throat. 'You should go to Pakistan by steamer,' he said. 'My father knows a commissioner at the docks. I'll help you arrange the passage.' He heard Pervez take a deep breath and exhale slowly. Hanif stared at the floor, then put his head in his hands. Without looking up he said, 'Put the box under the settee. I'll sell the books with the old newspapers tomorrow.'

Chapter 30

It was late in the evening, long past the time of prayers, and although a servant had readied the puja utensils and fruits for the offering, Harshaba had not felt like praying. Her mind was preoccupied with earthly matters. Rohini had humiliated the family and she was worried that no one would marry her two younger daughters. 'We should perform the last rites,' she said to Motilal. 'We'll tell people that she's dead.'

Motilal stared at her. What demonic spirit had possessed her? What mother wished her child dead? And to perform the last rites on someone who hadn't even left this world . . .

Motilal tried to reason with his wife. 'Times are changing. We'll think of something to tell people. We'll say . . .'

'What? The truth? That she has run off with a Muslim?'

Motilal had to concede his wife was right; losing a daughter to Islam was as devastating as losing one to disease and he would have to accept that she was dead, or as good as dead. The pain inside him felt just as real. 'Who will do the ceremony?' he asked in a small voice. 'Who will explain to the pujari?'

A bewildered expression on Harshaba's face told him that he would have to do it.

'Let's wait,' he implored. 'I need time to think.'

'You can think all you want,' she said. 'This is the only thing we can do. We must think of our other daughters and look to their futures. Rohini has taken her life into her own hands, and it is no longer of our concern.'

Despite her measured outspokenness, Harshaba was tearing up inside. She had looked for another way, sending for Rohini and the Muslim and hosting a small reception at Sagar Mahal to acknowledge the marriage and give their blessings. But this wasn't about overlooking something like social status; he was a Muslim. The family name would be forever blackened and they would be cast out. Bombay would turn its back on them. Hashaba had come too far for that to happen.

She had grown up in a small village outside Ahmedabad, in a two-room house with three sisters, two brothers, parents, and grandmother. Her father worked in a foundry, making large metal parts for the railways. Harshaba's recollection of him was dim. He left early in the morning, returned late at night, ate solemnly, and then went out again. It was the image of her mother that clung in her mind. Her mother's skin, darkened from countless hours labouring in the fields behind their house, was the colour of moistened river rock, a glistening, brown hue. She wore a dozen bangles on each wrist, as well as toe rings, nose rings, and earrings, and she never took off any of the jewellery. She smelled always of the cooking fire, perspiration and coconut oil.

Harshaba could smell it now, as clearly as she could hear Motilal breathing next to her under the mosquito net. A slant of moonlight streamed into the room and she could see his arms folded over his chest. His eyes were open. She wanted him to reassure her and comfort her. Above all, she wanted him to recognize the sadness that was swelling within her and make it disappear, or, at least lessen it.

She couldn't bear the thought of Rohini lying in a shabby bed with a Muslim. Was she with child? Would Rohini do such things? Where? How? The uncertainty compounded her torment. The lewdness infuriated her.

Motilal could feel Harshaba shifting uneasily in the bed, pulling the white sheet to her chin, then a few minutes later, casting it aside. His head ached. She was right, he thought. There was nothing else they could do. Rohini had dishonoured them and it would be impossible to find good husbands for Sumitra and Amrita. People would talk. Maybe not directly to their face, but behind their backs, surely they would talk.

He made up his mind. They would erase their second daughter from their family, from their consciousness. They would move on with their lives. For an instant he felt an immense relief, and then an overwhelming surge of dread and guilt. He wanted the night to be over. But he feared also the coming of dawn.

Harshaba sat up in bed. The cicadas were hissing, ruling the night with their rhythm. She parted the mosquito net and eased herself out. The tiled floor felt cool. She stood at the window, her hair falling about her shoulders, a short, cheerless silhouette in the feeble moonlight. She heard Motilal murmur something. The breeze sifted through the curtains, bringing in the familiar damp, salty smell. For a long while she stood with her hands on the windowsill staring at the sea.

Then Harshaba walked out of the room, her legs commanded by some involute force. Through the dressing room, through the anteroom, down the stairs, she found herself on the verandah outside Rohini's room. She pushed at the door and the latch snapped against the wood as she let herself in. She groped her way through the shadowy sitting room. Finding the desk, she pulled out the chair, fumbled for the lamp switch and turned it on. Her eyes took in the contents on the desk – a sheaf of papers, an inkpot, a crumpled handkerchief, blotting paper, and pencils. Her gaze went to the bookshelf and lingered on a book on the top shelf that looked more worn and used than the rest. She wished she could read English.

She felt herself being pulled towards the bedroom where her daughters were sleeping, she hoped, soundly. The floor was covered with elongated patterns cast by the shadows of the window grilles, and she stepped into the design, interrupting the quiet geometry. Glancing at the two beds pushed against the far wall, she took in the sleeping forms of the two girls. She stood in the centre of room, not daring to direct her eyes to the left, towards the armoire, and to the other bed where the embroidered cover was tucked in tightly at the edges, and the mosquito net hung bunched above the bedposts. Clenching her fists she tried to fill her mind with images of happier times. But her thoughts were bleak. The harsh reality of what had happened struck her again, and she staggered out of the room.

Upstairs in her own bedroom, she held up the mosquito net and edged into bed. She turned on her side, her face away from her husband, the sheet in a messy heap at her feet. She heard him stirring and felt his hand on her shoulder; the tenderness of his touch stung as she closed her eyes.

ೲ

'I understand,' Shrikant said to Motilal. 'You want to preserve the upstanding name of our family. Staging her demise will put an end to the matter.'

Motilal, Shrikant, and Mahesh were at the dining table, Motilal in his usual position at the head, Shrikant to his right, and Mahesh to his left.

Mahesh said, 'Who thought of this? A mock cremation! It was my mother's idea, wasn't it?'

Motilal looked away.

'It's an excellent idea,' Shrikant said, glaring at Mahesh.

Mahesh glared back. 'It's ridiculous,' he said to Shrikant. Then to his father, 'Is it legal?'

Motilal remained quiet.

Shrikant stood up. He was done eating. 'Please excuse me,' he said to his father, 'I have some friends coming to see me this evening.' Stepping back he pushed the chair in with his hip. 'Don't worry about this . . . uh, Rohini matter,' he added to Motilal, while glancing severely at Mahesh. 'I'll make all the arrangements.'

Motilal nodded weakly.

Mahesh ate a few bites of rice and curd. 'Are you sure about this?' he said to his father.

'Yes,' Motilal said. He had barely eaten. He gestured to the servant to clear the table. 'Marrying a Mussalman? It's unthinkable!'

'What you want to do is even more unthinkable!'

'We don't have any choice,' Motilal said.

'Choice? It's not a question of choice,' Mahesh said, 'This is Rohini. She's your daughter. Just because she made a small mistake . . .'

'A small mistake. That's what you call this?'

Mahesh looked behind his father, at the framed painting on the dining room wall that depicted the battlefield at Kurukshetra – Arjuna, handsome and resolute surveying the armies amassed on two sides; and Krishna, his divine charioteer, proffering advice.

Mahesh got up; he could clearly see the anguish etched on his father's face. 'We've all made mistakes, haven't we?' There was bitterness and challenge in his voice.

Many years ago, as a boy in Ahmedabad, Mahesh had seen his father leaving the house late one night. Motilal, dressed in a silk coat and *pagdi* had left quietly through the side gate. Mahesh felt compelled to follow him, so he rode his Hercules bicycle, pedalling furiously to keep up behind Motilal's tonga. All the way down to Lal Darwaja, over the river to Gandhigram, down Netaji Road, past Mount Carmel Convent, and into Navrangpura. The tonga stopped outside a brightly lit bungalow. As Mahesh, sweating and out of breath, watched his father pay the *tonga-walla*, he could hear music and laughter from the bungalow's upper terrace. From his vantage point across the road, Mahesh saw a woman open the front door – he had an impression of her shimmering in the night – he heard her exclaim when she saw Motilal – there was no mistaking the seduction in her voice – then she took his elbow, led him inside and closed the door. Mahesh stood across the road for almost an hour, his thoughts tangled and messy. Then he got on his bicycle, and after one last sad look at the bungalow's lively terrace, pedalled home slowly in the dark. Many days later when he summoned the nerve to ask his father where he had gone in the night, Motilal replied much too hastily, 'Nowhere, I was here.' But the colour rising in his father's face told a different story. Mahesh knew, and Motilal knew too.

'A mock cremation!' Mahesh said now. 'What kind of tradition is this? Is it written in the Vedas?' his voice got louder and he tried to check himself. 'What Rohini has done is sad and shameful, I agree, but there's no need for such drastic action. She's already gone from this house.'

Motilal sighed. 'Rohini is dead to us, and let it be so to everyone else. She has left the Hindu world for the world of the Muslims and will never come back. We have done nothing wrong and will not have your sisters punished for her deeds. Our name, our reputation, must be protected . . .'

'Reputation!' Mahesh said harshly. 'We have traded all sorts of goods behind a façade of selling silk. We have crushed others for profit. Our money has come from Muslims, the British, even the Japanese, and let us not forget the Chinese – yes, father, I know all about that. How shamelessly our fathers profited from opium!'

Motilal rose, furious, 'Business and family are two separate issues.'

'Oh, please,' Mahesh raised his hand in the air, 'don't think I don't understand your pretensions. Your . . . your unsavoury affairs . . .'

Motilal coughed.

'Thank God I'm going to America,' Mahesh started marching out of the dining room. 'Soon, I'll be away from this nonsense!' he said over his shoulder.

Motilal sat quietly for a long time. He listened to the banter of servants in the kitchen. He didn't know what to think of his son's bravado. How could he explain to this young man the complex responsibilities of his station in life? And how could he tell him about the weight of the world that could be lifted, sometimes, in places other than home?

ראט

Three days later the bamboo stretcher was placed in the middle of the divankhana at Sagar Mahal. The women sniffled softly as they laid flowers on the body. The men, their faces withdrawn and defeated, hovered around the doorway.

Last night two servants had prepared the stretcher with pieces of wood swathed in white cloth in the form of a human corpse. It was an ersatz creation of a dead body with lopsided shoulders and a jagged, triangular head. Shrikant clicked his tongue and told Motilal that it looked horrible. After some inquiries in the fishing village, Shrikant returned with the body of a beggar woman. Her husband was reluctant, but Shrikant slipped him a fat envelope and said, 'She'll also get a good cremation.'

The servants dismantled the fake body and as they positioned the beggar woman on the stretcher and covered her with the white cloth, Mahesh entered the room. 'What . . .?' he whispered. 'Who is that? Where did you get . . .?'

'Don't worry,' Shrikant snapped, as Motilal looked away.

Now the pujari's chanting voice filled the divankhana. A stooped, white-haired man, he was summoned to Sagar Mahal for the dozens of major and minor pujas through the year. When Motilal explained the ceremony they wanted to perform, the pujari was dumbfounded. He'd never officiated at such a ceremony, he said, but he understood the rationale behind it. Harshaba said, 'We want all the rituals, no short-cuts, no one should say it wasn't a proper cremation.'

After the prayers, all the household staff members were summoned to pay their last respects. They lowered their eyes, whispered a prayer, and, enacting the rote gesture of mourning, touched fingertips to forehead.

Suddenly, disturbing the solemnity of the moment came Vincent's outburst: 'I don't believe this! What are you doing? She's not dead!'

The pujari stopped chanting. A collective gasp rose from the rest of the mourners followed by a strange hush. Motilal stared at the floor. Harshaba's face was rigid.

'Are you Hindus?' Vincent in his borrowed black suit gestured towards Motilal. 'Is this what your religion teaches?' He pointed at the stretcher. 'What kind of Hindus are you?' The servants queued behind Vincent murmured to each other. Vincent grabbed one of them by the shoulders. 'I'm telling you. I saw Rohini. Listen to me. I saw her with my own eyes.' He looked around the divankhana frantically. 'Where is . . .?' He pointed at Mahesh. 'Ask him. He saw her, too. I drove him there. We delivered all her things. Two big heavy trunks.'

Mahesh leaned his head against the wall and sighed. He

tried to catch his father's attention, but Motilal had closed his eyes and muttered, 'Rohini is dead.'

'This is evil!' Vincent was shouting now. 'Oh, you are evil people in this house.' He stood before the body lying on the floor, his face fierce, his defiant eyes assessing the other mourners. He bent down, his arms outstretched, as though ready to tear the shroud off and expose the body underneath.

The pujari cleared his throat, dismissed Vincent with the flick of his fingers, and resumed chanting: '*Om Shiva, Namo Shiva . . .*'

Vincent straightened himself, reached to his neck and from under his shirt took out his silver chain and, after putting his lips to the cross pendant, started: 'Hail Mary Mother of God . . . please help!'

'Be quiet!' Shrikant said as he pulled Vincent away and hurried him outside.

Vincent continued yelling, his hectoring voice louder than the pujari's chants. 'Oh most sacred heart of Jesus Christ . . . forgive these sinners . . . set them free by the power of Your mercy . . . we rejoice in your Kingdom . . .'

He's only the driver, someone whispered.

At the cremation grounds Motilal lit the pyre, placing the kindling on the corpse's head with a trembling hand.

A beggar woman received a wealthy funeral and her widowed husband had enough money to buy a new wife, drink, and live in luxury for a few years. But only a few people knew the truth and none had the guts to tell.

ೞ

That night, Harshaba drifted into a fitful sleep. She felt Sagar Mahal trembling. She awoke, realized she was dreaming, turned her head on the pillow, and closed her eyes. The dream resumed – it was late in the evening and the sky was streaked a riot of orange and red. The stretch of sea facing the house suddenly grew still, the water frozen in a wide strip. A violent wind started shaking the house. The wind seemed to have a wave-like rhythm, a succession of assaults. With military precision, it rumbled and rolled, as though under the orders of a furious commander, and brought with it a pounding rain. The thunder came in booms and bursts, as if the boulders on the beach had levitated to the sky and were blasting down as cannonballs.

Harshaba awoke and looked at the open window where there was only a gentle breeze. She lay in bed, too frightened to close her eyes, too frightened to breathe. On other nights Sagar Mahal, like any other old house, murmured, sighed, and creaked, harmless noises she'd grown used to. She got up and shut the window and, after glancing at Motilal's sleeping form, she lay down and closed her eyes.

The nightmare started again. All through the house, the windows and doors, defying their latches and stoppers, slammed open and close. Curtains ripped and chairs tipped over, almirahs crashed against the walls, pictures and portraits plunged to the floor, chandeliers swayed and jangled, pipes rattled and hissed, wires sparked and short-circuited. In the divankhana, the porcelain Chinaman wept uncontrollably.

When the first signs of dawn appeared at the window, Harshaba was drenched in sweat. She opened her eyes slowly and lifting her neck, surveyed the room. She saw Motilal opening the door to the verandah. She dropped her head back onto the pillow as the tears slipped towards her ears.

ಬಬ

Harshaba carried the guilt and sorrow of her daughter's death so well, no one knew the truth. But the reality of it haunted her. She took to wearing plain, saffron-coloured saris, and gradually turned the house over to the care of the servants, spending most of her day in prayer and meditation. For months at a time she lived at an ashram in Limdi, a small village in Gujarat. When Motilal got fed up with her being away and rebuked her for neglecting her family, she returned temporarily, but was soon gone again. Motilal acknowledged it made little difference whether she prayed at home or elsewhere; she had become oblivious to his presence.

Often she went away on pilgrimages to the Himalayas – to Kedarnath, Badrinath, Amarnath, or Gangotri. In her old age when she could no longer tolerate high altitudes, she travelled instead to Banaras and Haridwar, frequenting the ashrams along the Ganges River.

She never once uttered her dead daughter's name. But each day during her prayers, when the image of a familiar young girl, unbidden and unannounced, came into her thoughts, Harshaba sighed sadly and tried to ignore the lump that formed in her throat. Sometimes during these interruptions, when a solitary teardrop escaped down her fast-wrinkling face, she wiped it away with the edge of her sari.

Chapter 31

At the Shahs' house in Ahmedabad, it was early evening when the telegram arrived. Jag was dressing to play some badminton before dinner when he heard the commotion downstairs. His mother, running between the kitchen and the drawing room, her high-pitched voice fading then getting louder near the foyer; his father shouting for the servants, for Jag and his sisters. When Jag rushed downstairs his father thrust the telegram at him. Just then the doorbell rang. It was Saroj and Nalin sent as emissaries to convey the news.

Jag read and reread the telegram. 'Is this true?' he asked.

Saroj nodded. 'I'm sorry,' she said, 'she took ill. It was quite sudden . . .' She couldn't finish the thought. She felt the burden of Rohini's culpability on her back. She looked at Jag's parents but couldn't meet their eyes.

His father offered tea, but Saroj said they should go; it was a long drive to Dantali. At the door, she glanced at Jag. She would never forget the look on his face – a distant, vacuous expression imbued with regret. She lifted her hand a little, as though to touch his shoulder.

Jag wandered the luckless alleys of Ahmedabad, in the section behind Khajuri-ni-pol where the buildings butted against each other so tightly that not even the faintest breeze could penetrate. Except for a street sweeper, no one was about. A crescent moon hung high above the city and its light picked out a pack of rats raiding a heap of garbage in a corner.

His thoughts were in South Africa, on Katrien, the daughter of his Dutch business partner. He pictured her bluish-grey eyes, her light-brown hair, and her wholesome figure. She was studying Biology at a university in Johannesburg, researching cures for diseases that killed Africans in the bush. He remembered travelling with her family to the Cape on holiday and the afternoon he had spent with her on the beach at Hout Bay. It was June or July and a cold wind came off the ocean and tousled her hair and made her skirt flap around her legs. Gamely she took his hand and they ran towards the water, laughing and shrieking, the icy waves lapping their ankles. Later that evening, at the guesthouse, after her parents retired to their suite, he had taken her in his arms. Ultimately it was a deep sense of duty to his parents, combined with the notion that he was Indian and she European, that had prevented him from proposing to her.

He pictured Katrien trudging across the veld laden with medical supplies, drawing blood or injecting vaccines into bony black arms. Katrien, a small, determined figure in the fierce African landscape. The scene of his engagement ceremony a few months ago eclipsed the image of Katrien. He saw Rohini, adorned with jewels, beautiful in her silk sari, and his parents, happy and proud.

Now Rohini was dead. He spat at the darkness and yelled. Sweat glistened on his face. His lungs burned. From an open window someone shouted an obscenity and Jag volleyed back with a worse one. On the cobbled lane he came upon a cardboard box and began kicking it around, thoomp-thoomp, until the box fell apart. After drifting for a while, he found a seedy bar and ordered a glass and a bottle of whiskey, the best they had, and he drank to her death.

Chapter 32

Rezana waited, her pulse quickening whenever the phone in the sitting room rang, her heart lurching each afternoon the postman cycled up to the gate, and her eyes darting to the front windows when a car stopped outside the house, but there was no message, no news, no visitor from her family in Versova.

The night-time attack had left her terrified for weeks. She had heard it – 'I'll kill her quick' – and there was no question in her mind who they meant to kill, and why. The banging on the door, the menacing voices, the sticks and knifes – these had become the stuff of her nightmares, sleeping and awake. Abbu had filed police complaints and now there were triangular-patterned grilles on all the windows and a Nepali sentry – a trained Gurkha – who patrolled their road at night. None of the thugs were found, and the suspicion that one of them was Shrikant soon left her mind.

Gradually she gave up on hearing from Versova. Not because she stopped thinking about her family but because she decided to devote herself fully to her new life. What was needed, she realized, was a concerted effort to unlearn her past and embrace the traditions and rhythms of Hanif's house and his life.

Bandra was her home now, not Versova, and she had little by way of material reminders of her past. All that remained was her dignity, and that would be enough to sustain her while she forged a new identity. She believed that it could be done – from Hindu to Muslim, from Rohini to Rezana – she would reinvent herself.

She learned that her father-in-law spoke candidly about politics and in conversations with her, he criticized the freedom struggle. 'India behaved like a desperate cripple, made too many concessions to the British,' he said, clicking his tongue. 'Two separate parts of Pakistan, violence at the borders, problems in Kashmir, cronies and sycophants in Parliament, what a lovely mess we have struggled for. We all wanted Independence. But the British made sure it would cost us our unity; rather than hand back the jewel of its empire, they smashed it to pieces.' Rezana noticed, however, that he did not condemn the freedom fighters themselves. He had the highest regard for Nehru. 'Such a refined man, a first-class statesman,' he said. 'Except,' Abbu raised his index finger in the air, 'Nehru did not handle the Kashmir issue properly. Coercion is what made Hari Singh sign over Kashmir to India. Where was the diplomacy in that?' Nonetheless, he was pleased that Nehru was Prime Minister. He seemed less impressed with Gandhi, although on that January day, when Nathuram Godse – 'a madman, pure and simple' – fired the fatal bullet, Abbu mourned openly, and went to the mosque to pray for the nation.

Ammi rarely discussed politics but once in a while she worried about them staying in India. They had relatives in Karachi; it might be wise to immigrate. But Abbu puffed his chest and said he wasn't going to be driven out like that. Softening a little, he added, 'Don't worry, Bombay will not reject its Muslim population.'

Rezana had more mundane concerns and she set about learning the idiosyncrasies of the house – that the springs on one side of the settee in the sitting room creaked whenever someone sat down; that the music box with the dancing girls stowed in the glass cabinet worked only if the key was wound half way; and that the front door jammed when it rained. She discovered the crevices around the house where the ants lived and learned how to bait them with a pinch of chilli powder. She discovered that the drawer in the kitchen – the top one to the left of the sink where the big spoons were kept – had to be lifted and tilted back before being pushed in; and that the three-bulb light fixture hanging from the kitchen ceiling always flickered for a few seconds when it was switched on.

Rezana filed in her mind the times when the milkman came to the back door and the post was delivered, and which days the *pasti-walla* came to pick up old newspapers and the *dabbabatli-walla* to collect used boxes and bottles. Abdul, the old gardener who tended the desultory grass and unruly bushes, came and went by his own clock.

Ammi had taken Rezana soon after marriage to her tailor, an old man who worked in a small shed behind the mosque, and he made her some salwar-kameez sets. Rezana didn't mind the baggy pants and the long tunic – the ensemble was comfortable – but she had felt somewhat clumsy in the outfit. Now she went back to the tailor and, emptying a large bag of saris on the floor beside his sewing machine, asked him to stitch them into salwar sets. The old tailor admired the embroidery, the fine quality of the silk, and after many regretful sighs, agreed to cut them up.

Over the months she got used to the bathroom. She learned to be frugal with water when she bathed, but every day she marvelled at the shiny brass tap and the rust-free enamel. She arranged the objects on the shelf below the sink and, when they reverted to their usual state of disarray, she arranged them again. She got used to the cracked tiles, but already had the name of a mason should Abbu stop viewing renovations as 'needless expenditures'.

The patches of sloughed-off paint on the walls, the grimy corners in the hallway, the dark blotches of fingerprints around light switches and doorknobs, the gouges in the marble floor – all this, too, she tried to repair with a cleaning rag and elbow grease.

And there were things she simply learned to ignore.

When she was young she'd accepted the presence of beggars and slums as part of the natural order of things, separate and different from the world in which she lived. It was as though all the misfortune that might have come her way was absorbed elsewhere and she imagined 'elsewhere' as a remote reservoir in the Himalayas. Her childish bubble was soon busted and she started noticing poverty with new awareness. She noticed the women and children, their limbs maimed or diseased, sitting on the footpath in the bazaar with their begging bowls, the older children picking lice from the younger ones' hair. She noticed the hutment colonies at Danda, the open gutters breeding mosquitoes, men urinating against walls, and, when she and Hanif walked to the seashore in the evening, she noticed the cooking fires outside the huts and meagre meals being prepared in charred pots.

At night Rezana sometimes gazed into the flats in the building next door. It was a four-storey structure, hardly twenty feet away, and her eyes skipped over the lighted windows – a young boy sitting at a desk, a man in the balcony smoking a cigarette, a woman hanging out the washing – such random, ordinary images reminded her that her life was now closer to theirs, and although she didn't know any of the people in the flats, she felt somehow connected to them.

She learned to read the Koran. It was a slow process, but under the tutelage of Hanif's aunt, Farida-*fufi*, a bent old woman with a boisterous voice, Rezana tried to become a more devout Muslim.

Farida-fufi lived alone in a flat on Station Road, and two or three times a week she came to the house, one leg dragging as she walked. She took a liking to Rezana and, besides that, she said it was her duty and an honour, performing Allah's wish.

Ammi muttered and mumbled whenever Farida-fufi came over. According to her, the old woman just needed an excuse to come to their house, especially since each time she visited she stayed on for lunch and afternoon tea, sometimes even dinner.

Farida-fufi insisted on demonstrating the ablution rites before each lesson. 'First, declare your intention that the act is for the purpose of purity. Start by saying "*Bismillah*". Wash the hands up to the wrists thrice. Rinse out the mouth with water thrice. Sniff water into your nostrils thrice. Wash the whole face thrice with both hands, from the top of the forehead to the bottom of the chin and from ear to ear. Like this. Then wash the right arm thrice, right up to the elbow, and the same with the left. Wipe your whole head with a wet hand once. Wash your feet up to the ankles thrice, starting at the right foot. Try to keep this order in your mind. And remember, the *wudu* is valid until . . . you know the reasons?'

'Yes,' Rezana replied, recalling the reasons – using the toilet, sleeping with her husband, and so on – that invalidated the cleansing ritual.

This ritual accomplished, Rezana and Farida-fufi sat on the floor in the music room and took up the Koran. Farida-fufi was an exacting teacher. With her wattled chin trembling, her voice lilting but serious, her body rocking back and forth, she read a few passages aloud, after which, staring intently at Rezana, she provided a translation. When it was Rezana's turn she tried her best to imitate the older woman's inflections. If she forgot to rock back and forth while reading, she felt Farida-fufi's index finger nudging her shoulder.

For Rezana, reading the Arabic script was the biggest challenge. And not everything in the Koran was instantly clear to her in import. Once she asked Farida-fufi about the double meaning inherent in a long, complicated verse, but the old aunt's answer was a sharp, glassy stare and, after that, Rezana decided not to ask any questions. Sometimes Rezana was perplexed by the seeming contradictions in the text. In places it was written: 'Allah, the All Merciful, Full of Pity, Forgiving towards Mankind'; yet, in other places she read:

'Those who disbelieve, Allah taketh away their light and leave them in darkness. Those who disbelieve shall be tormented in Hell.' She tried to unite such opposites, marry each paradox, and occasionally, she succeeded.

When Rezana practiced reading the Koran on her own, she contemplated the structural complexity of the holy book. She liked the internal organization of the Koran, the verses containing the revelations grouped into one hundred and fourteen *suras*, arranged by length from shortest to longest. Farida-fufi said the shorter ones were revealed to the Prophet Muhammad at Mecca and the longer ones to him at Medina.

Every Friday she attended the mosque with Ammi. After some months she was reciting-kneeling-bending-touching forehead to floor, with the same ease and grace as the other women. During Ramadan, she ate before sunrise, abstaining from food and water until sunset. For Eid she learned to prepare *double ka meetha* with fried bread, cream, butter, and sugar. And she learned how long to let the vermicelli boil for the *sheer khorma*. The customary greeting 'Eid Mubarak' rolled off her tongue quickly and easily.

Yet Rezana hadn't forgotten about Diwali and Holi and Ganesh puja. In Bombay it was impossible to ignore these festivals. She often wondered if it was possible to totally disavow her old beliefs. Somewhere under the surface wasn't she a Hindu?

The question especially troubled her when she thought about death. The more she tried to put the whole subject out of her mind, the more intrusively it seemed to surface in her thoughts, especially the conflicting notions of life after death advocated by Hinduism and Islam. Karma and reincarnation were concepts instilled into her consciousness, yet her new life had little space for such views. In bed she tried to bring up the topic with Hanif. In answer, he pulled her closer to him and whispered,

> Don't speak to me of death,
> My world is complete, now
> Your breath renews an ocean.
> Tomorrow, whether we wake or not
> It is but a trifle thought.

Ultimately she deferred to Islamic prescripts. It was easier that way.

Within a year she trained herself to eat chicken biryani, mutton curry, *shammi-kebabs*, minced lamb, and . . . even beef. Minuscule helpings at first, placed tentatively in the mouth, and followed by several gulps of water. When she could eat the meat without flinching, without her stomach heaving, and, at times even with a sense of relish, she realized the transformation was complete. She had turned into a *pukka Mussalman*.

After that, she grew fond of the predictable rhythms of the household. No longer did she go about the house like a timid guest. No longer did she feel as though she would shrivel and perish like a plant in unsuitable soil. Rather, over the months, she exuded a quiet confidence in her status as wife and daughter-in-law.

A son was born in 1949. A daughter in 1950. Saleem and Sobia.

And then Hanif left for America.

V
AMERICA

Chapter 33

'A brave new voice for a brave new India' was how the record company said it wanted to promote Hanif's music. Bankim Chandra – 'Please, everyone calls me Banky' – was a fat garrulous man with a shock of black hair styled with a pouf, and his office at the record company was a wood-panelled room, cloudy with cigarette smoke, on the seventh floor of a building overlooking the bay. Banky had big plans for Hanif, but after listening to him for an hour Hanif grew restless and interjected, asking when they would get him into the studio so he could get down to work. Banky nodded and made a great show of calling in his secretary and checking his diary to see when the best sound technician was available. 'Things are always hectic around here . . . let me contact you when we have all the right people lined up,' Banky said, muttering something about making records being a more complicated process than the listener might think, and guiding Hanif towards the lift. Two weeks later, when Hanif inquired again, Banky asked Hanif to sit for a while, and as they drank tea, Banky repeated, 'Making records really is a complicated business!' Hanif listened to him for another hour, but managed to ascertain that the company didn't have the funds 'in the present climate' to launch a new artist.

'But I won the competition,' Hanif said. 'The prize was a recording contract, no?'

Banky took a cigarette from a handsome stone box on the table, lit it with a gold lighter, and drew on it slowly. Hanif stared at him as he tipped his head and exhaled smoke towards the ceiling. Something about Banky's silence told him that the record company's decision was final.

'I've been singing since I was a young boy,' Hanif said. 'I've trained under Iqbal Mehmood . . .'

'Things might get better next year,' Banky said, cutting him off and reaching for a monographed notepad. 'In the meantime, here,' he wrote on a page, folded it in two and handed it to Hanif. 'Here are the names of some people at other record labels. Tell them I sent you. If only we were in a position to take you on right now, but . . .' and Banky shrugged and smiled weakly, as if to say it was something beyond his control. 'I know you must be eager to get going.' Hanif found himself hustled to the lift and Banky's smiling, nodding face was slowly erased by the closing doors.

Hanif spent many hours in the same-looking outer offices lined with framed golden records drinking tepid tea and waiting to be seen by increasingly junior assistants. During one interview, a manager, who happened to be a fan of ghazals, asked him to sing on the spot, requesting certain songs and beaming in approval. Hanif was surprised, and irritated, to discover he had lost an entire morning entertaining the manager and his staff, but left thinking he had won the day. A week later he was rewarded with the same shrug and weak smile and cordial wishes for 'the best of luck' delivered by an assistant.

Hanif tried all the names on Banky's list, and more he had collected on his travels around the recording studios, but each successive call was met by an increasingly cool response, as if they had been half expecting him and were annoyed about having been forced into a position of saying 'no'.

'We do advertising jingles and a voice like yours deserves far better than we can offer,' said one manager. 'Advertising jingles?' Hanif said. He sighed and stepped towards a chair in the reception area furnished in better days and, before he even sat, was told they weren't signing any new artists.

He had devoted himself to music with a singleness of purpose, and the praise and accolades had led him to assume he was on the brink of greatness. But as the opportunities of turning himself into a professional slipped away, he lost confidence as a singer. He saw himself as a young, unsuccessful musician, ploughed under and forgotten, perhaps called upon every now and then to perform at a wedding or to entertain rowdy drinkers in seedy corner bars.

'Inshallah,' was all he could say at the end of the day when Rezana greeted him at the door with hopeful eyes – eyes that became instantly downcast on observing the disappointment on her husband's face, and clothes – the white shirt ironed crisp that morning – now, hanging off him like a sodden rag.

Abbu indulged his son's ambitions, but after three months he suggested he go to America for a degree in Business Administration. Studying abroad would require capital, but Abbu thought it would be a wise investment and would give his son a secure career. The degree would guarantee Hanif a high post in one of the new local and foreign-partnered financial companies opening all the time in Bombay and, after a while, Hanif might consider opening his own business. 'The social policies governing business are changing,' Abbu said to Hanif. 'India is moving forward in the industrial sector, and you have to take advantage of that.'

Ammi objected to her husband's decision. 'Music takes commitment,' she said, clearing bowls and plates at the end of dinner. 'He has devoted his life to it and he has such talent, and now you're asking him to throw away his dreams!' Rezana shared her sadness because they were her dreams too. She was confident the music business would pick up and Hanif would become the rising star of India he was destined to be. She even invoked Allah and said Hanif would not have been given such talent if it was not for some purpose. Abbu glared at her, and Rezana feared she might have transgressed some Koranic law she had yet to learn.

'Sometimes it has nothing to do with commitment or talent,' Abbu said. 'Sometimes it's a matter of meeting the right people, moving in the right circles.'

'What are you suggesting?' Ammi said, dropping the stack of dishes back on the table with a loud clatter. 'That we are nothing? That . . . we have no status? That we're not moving in the right circles?'

'I'm not suggesting anything,' Abbu said. 'Well . . . I am suggesting that he go to America.'

In their bedroom, Rezana begged Hanif to try the recording studios again. He had been promised a recording contract. 'Find a lawyer. It will be expensive, but you must demand what is rightfully yours,' she said. She had spent hours scanning the newspaper for schools and colleges that might need a music teacher. 'What about giving private lessons?' she asked.

Hanif shook his head. He was humiliated by the rejections. Going to America for two years seemed a good decision; besides, he was suddenly looking forward to the adventure. He had wanted Rezana and the children to accompany him, but in the end they had decided it would be best for him to go by himself. He would be more efficient that way. 'I'll come back from America and pick up my music,' he said to Rezana. 'Have faith!' But he was doubtful that the music industry in India would change – if they didn't want him now, why would they want him in two years' time, when lack of practice would have only diminished his artistry?

A cousin, Imtiaz, was at Syracuse University in New York and Abbu made inquiries and declared its business studies department to be 'excellent'.

'The children are still small,' Rezana argued, but knew that in the end Hanif was the one making the greater sacrifice by being wrenched apart from them. She brought out an old atlas and flipped to the map of the world, and measured the distance between Bombay and New York with her thumb. It was almost seven thumbs. She measured again, inching her thumb forward each time and checking it against the scale, trying to lessen the distance. On the map of New York State, she scanned the names: Albany, Rochester, Buffalo . . . Saratoga Springs, Syracuse . . .

Hanif boarded the Italian liner S. S. *Victoria* that took him to Naples. From there he transferred to another ship that took him to Southampton. From Southampton to London by train, and after a few days in London with the friend of an uncle whom he had never met but offered him rice and egg-curry for every meal and a thin mattress on the floor of his one-room flat to sleep on, Hanif took a flight to New York. He had never been on a ship or in an airplane and he tried to describe these new experiences in letters to Rezana, even as he felt a small tear in his heart. It was the beginning of a rift between them, but he believed they would withstand it. Of this, he was certain.

ಐಐ

To Rezana, the world suddenly seemed incomprehensible – Naples, Southampton, London, New York. These were at once imagined places she knew from her novels and real places she could see on the map to which people went to and come from and lived in.

The night that Hanif left, Rezana put the children to bed and locked herself in the music room. She uncovered the harmonium, and sat before it, turning the pages of his songbook. He could have been India's most sought after playback singer; he could have been a ghazal singer with dozens of records to his name. But instead he was off to America and she would not know who he was when he came back. He'd be a stranger to the wife and mother of his children. Tears streamed down her cheeks as she realized that the man she had married would never become a famous musician. She replaced the harmonium's cover, tugging at the cloth and causing a slight tear in the seam, and then sat with her hand on the instrument, staring at the moths flinging themselves at the ticking fluorescent light and listening to the pling-pling of their wings bouncing off the ceiling.

Chapter 34

At the Syracuse post office Hanif bought a dozen aerograms, sheets of thin, light blue paper on which he could write his letters. After pressing and folding into thirds, and running his tongue over the gummed edges, the sheets also served as envelopes. There was a pre-printed stamp on the corner, and a warning forbidding enclosures. Cheaper than airmail.

In the first aerogram to Rezana, Hanif wrote:

> The journey was comfortable, although I couldn't sleep much and arrived in America more tired than I've ever been in my life. I'm still tired and don't know how long it will take to recover. Perhaps it is the different air. The apartment has one bedroom, bathroom, and kitchen. There's a tub in the bathroom and hot water in the taps all the time. The stove in the kitchen is electric and I will start cooking the recipes that you wrote and sent with me after I go to the market on Saturday. Imtiaz and I get along well. He's quiet and studious.

Hanif didn't mention that his cousin Imtiaz had spent the last two nights at a friend's apartment in the same building, and that his friend happened to be a tall, red-haired American woman who smoked cigarettes and drank beer.

In another aerogram, Hanif told Rezana about the university campus – 'so big it takes half an hour to walk from one end to the other.' Everyone he passed said 'Hi!' even though he was sure he had never met them, so he just said 'Hi!' back to them and smiled. Sometimes he took longer routes to avoid them and he tried to stay away from what he dubbed as 'friendly areas'. The professors were passionate and learned, but they spoke much too fast and it was difficult for him to understand them. And the library – 'there must be millions of books, too many even for you to read'. He was getting top marks in all his classes and his professor wanted to recommend him for a summer clerkship with a financial firm in New York City. 'The work itself is not very interesting,' the professor said to Hanif, 'you might say it is very dull stuff indeed, but the pay is quite good, so you can have some fun, and the experience will be invaluable.' Hanif promptly agreed to the plan, if only to get away from the 'friendlies'.

Every time Hanif wrote, he said how much he missed her and the children. What he didn't tell her was that he missed the harmonium too and missed singing ghazals, and that sometimes lying awake at night, the distracted notes of a harmonium or the beat of tablas resounded in his head. He bought a Hallicrafters radio at Sears, but he couldn't afford the big antenna required for the short wave stations. In the evenings, after finishing a humble dinner, washing his plate and the ironclad frying pan, and laying them upside down on a towel to dry, he would switch on the radio and aimlessly turn the dial between the three AM stations – American football, American music, American news. He never heard

Talat Mehmood, Hemant Kumar, or Mohammed Rafi on the airwaves. As he listened to his professors expound the imperfections of the capital market, phrases of ghazals invaded his mind and his fingers played across the edge of the desk until someone looked at him oddly and he got embarrassed and stopped. He was a *kalakar*, an artiste, he believed; music was in his bones, in his blood. He should have stuck it out in Bombay. Sooner or later he would have got his break in the music industry. He felt a surge of anger towards his father for pushing him off to America, at himself for doubting his own talents. But a business career was logical and practical and he was doing it for Rezana and the children.

He made friends with two Americans, Frederick and Steven, who had fought in the war in Europe. They had a record player in their apartment and Hanif sat back and smiled as Frederick and Steven sang along to Frank Sinatra songs. After a while Hanif was singing, too:

> Night and day, you are the one
> Only you 'neath the moon or under the sun
> Whether near to me or far
> It's no matter, darling, where you are
> I think of you day and night . . .

'You're a natural,' Frederick said, thumping his back.

'What a fabulous voice,' Steven said. 'Like a professional. Did you sing much in India?'

'A little,' Hanif said.

On Saturdays, Hanif went to the movies with his two friends. He saw *Stalag 17* and *Roman Holiday*. It was a 'double feature', he wrote in his letter to Rezana, two movies for fifty-two cents. In another letter, he summarized the story of *An American in Paris* and the songs and dancing which reminded him of Hindi films. He told her about *The African Queen*: 'The actor, Humphrey Bogart, is like our Dilip Kumar.'

He wrote to Rezana about snow: 'It falls, not like the rains in mad, noisy, violent torrents, but silent and mysterious, a deluge of tender white petals dropping from the sky.' But he did not tell her how daylight ebbed a few hours after lunchtime and the evenings stretched dark and joyless into night. And he did not tell her about the cold-cold wind that cut him to the bones and numbed his soul.

ಎಲ

Rezana wrote to Hanif about the children. 'Saleem likes to make paper boats and float them in a bucket of water. He rarely talks,' she wrote, 'but he hums all the time, and whenever there's a film song on the radio, he stops whatever he is doing and sings along. Sobia walks without holding on to anything. She has learned new words, and she babbles incessantly.'

What Rezana didn't say in her letters, what she wanted to pen on those pastel blue pages and send across the six-thumb distance, but couldn't, was this: 'I feel abandoned. I am tired of singing lullabies to the babies, bathing and feeding them, and searching for the thermometer when they get sick. While you visit new places and meet new people, I sit here at the dinner table with your cheerless parents. I am disappointed that you gave up music. It is the mortar of our lives, what brought us together and keeps us together. What is left to impel our attachment, to fire our dreams?'

She didn't write this, could never say this, because . . . she was his wife. And a wife, she believed, should always support her husband's decisions.

Chapter 35

In New York City that summer, Hanif toured the Statue of Liberty, the Empire State Building, and Rockefeller Center. He wandered around Central Park. He ambled down Fifth Avenue, Madison and Lexington. He went to the office of Barclays Capital Investments, a large company with a range of government and corporate clients, early each morning and returned to the International Inn on Varick Street in time for dinner. The other residents at the Inn, young professionals or graduate students like himself, were mainly from Western Europe and Southeast Asia. One time, there was a delegation of Christian nuns from Ceylon.

The work was challenging. And it was dull. Hanif was assigned to the quantitative analytics division of the oil and gas sector where he worked with a team to propose pricing and risk taking. The internship required him to think in numbers and graphs, to solve problems using data; there was little scope for creativity.

All this he wrote to Rezana.

The money was good, and after paying for room and board he still had almost eight dollars left each week. He bought some souvenirs bearing the city's name – ballpoint pens, keychains, scarves, and ashtrays – to distribute to relatives in Bombay. At Woolworths he bought a red toy Ford for Saleem, a doll with curly blonde hair for Sobia, and a pink folding umbrella for Rezana. He considered a flowered dinner-set, but decided it would be too bulky to carry.

New York was a grander, taller, less complicated version of Bombay. Sometimes as he walked down Sixth Avenue to catch the bus to the financial district, he imagined palm trees and bougainvillea growing along the sidewalks, billboards advertising Hindi movies, and the kiosks at the corner selling paan, beedis, and *The Times of India*.

Strolling through Washington Square one pleasantly hot evening, he glanced at a hot dog vendor and superimposed the image of a bhelpuri-walla. He recalled how the bhelpuri-wallas in Bombay vied for customers by showering them with handfuls of puffed rice. Suddenly his eyes brimmed and he yearned for the city that smelled of green chillies, cilantro, dates, and tamarind, the city where he had left his wife and children, the city where he had left his music.

Soon he was packing to go back to Syracuse. Eight more months, he told himself, and home. It was in the last week of his New York 'holiday' that Hanif met someone from Bombay. The man was already seated at a table by the window when Hanif entered the dining room of the International Inn. Hanif couldn't help noticing him; he was the only other Indian in the room.

The hostess, Mrs Lily, a cheery, heavyset woman with short hair, said to Hanif, 'We have another Indian guest. I thought you might enjoy sitting together. I've already asked his permission.' From across the room, Hanif felt the man's eyes appraising him.

Hanif thought the man looked familiar – he had a distinguished face with a wide forehead and a small, straight nose, and was about the same age.

'Hello,' the man said, standing and extending his hand. 'Please,' he gestured towards the empty chair as though he owned the table. Dressed in a dark grey suit and red tie, hair neatly parted, he looked very stylish, almost flamboyant, more American than European. Rich, Hanif thought, at least compared to the few other Indians he'd seen in America. Hanif looked down at his own suit, poorly styled by comparison. In Bombay, his father had taken him to Wahid Rehman & Sons Tailoring, where an enthusiastic apprentice had helped them select the cloth, measured him for three suits and said they would be ready in three days, no fitting trial needed. When they returned to the shop the suits were hanging in the window, the coats and trousers on separate hangers. In the fitting room, Hanif turned this way and that in front of the mirror. It was the first time he had worn a suit. He was amazed at how dignified he looked and it finally occurred to him that going abroad was going to change him; for the better, he hoped. Inshallah.

The man at the table stared openly at Hanif, averting his gaze only as he sat down. Hanif watched the waiter pour water into his glass. Around their table, he heard the usual chatter of the other diners in foreign tongues. The smell of boiled potatoes and roast chicken and baked apples, American smells, permeated the room. He looked around the room at the blue striped wallpaper and matching blue drapery, the lighting deliberately dim during the day. Outside, it was still bright and hopeful. Potted red flowers on the windowsill. What time was it in Bombay now? A yellow taxi crawled down the street. A van followed. A woman in a white dress and a straw hat walked a big, fluffy dog. The dog, padding slowly and precisely, held its head smartly in the air.

The man cleared his throat. 'I'm Max,' he said.

'Max?' Hanif's eyebrows went up. He didn't know anyone called Max, which was a name he had only encountered before in movies and had always sounded mysterious to him, a contraction of Maximilian, which he had looked up and found to be Latin for 'greatest'. He appraised the man again. He was sure he had met him before.

'Mahesh, actually . . .'

Hanif's eyes shot open in shock. Of course! This man was his wife's brother. His brother-in-law! He was the same person who had come to deliver Rezana's clothes in the two black trunks. How many years ago? 'Your brother is here, in America, in New York, at the International Inn,' he would later write to Rezana. Hanif's shoulders tensed and he sat up straight. He stared at the two glasses of iced water, the flower in the vase, the carefully arranged forks and knives, the basket of bland bread rolls and the dish of butter.

'. . . but my friends call me Max.'

Hanif felt his leg twitching. Clenching his palm on his knee, he tried to steady the leg. He wanted to run from the table, escape to his room and never come down to the dining room again.

'I'm from Bombay,' Max continued. 'And you?' He picked a roll from the breadbasket and sliced it with his knife. He reached for the butter, took two squares, and then put the knife down on his side plate. Looking intently at Hanif, he said, 'I get the feeling we have met somewhere. But I don't know. I can't remember exactly. Somewhere in Bombay, perhaps at Willingdon Club, do you play squash, or . . .?' His voice trailed off and he shook his head. 'No. Never mind. It was probably someone else.'

Hanif noticed the hint of an American accent, the way Max flattened the 'a' vowel. It sounded almost put-on, especially since most of his words came out in typical Indian-English.

'W-w-we have m-m-met.' Hanif couldn't believe he was stammering, something he had not done since he was a child. He wasn't sure whether he wanted to hit Max or hug him. 'I'm Rezana's husband. Hanif.'

'Rezana?' Max's face drained of colour. 'Oh, God!' he mumbled. 'Of course. You're the Musl . . . Rohini's . . .' The disbelief, the incredulity, the memory of that day in Bandra outside Hanif's house some four years ago unravelled in the space between them.

Hanif felt like a criminal who had just given himself up. He ran an anxious hand through his hair. If Max didn't want him there, he would leave. He didn't care. Maybe he should leave anyway, before they said awkward, humiliating things to each other.

'Is she . . . Rohini . . . is she here?'

'No. She's at home . . . in Bombay. Rezana's in Bombay.'

'Re-*zana*?' Max said her name under his breath. 'How is she? It's been a long time.'

'She is very well, thank you,' Hanif said. He noticed that Max, like Rezana, tilted his chin upward when he spoke, and he had the same small, slightly curved mouth.

Max looked around the dining room as though searching for the waiter. Rezana. So she *had* become a Muslim. Did she know what they had done at Sagar Mahal? Did she know that they had cremated a beggar woman in her stead? Did this Hanif know? The whole thing had sickened him. It was his mother's doing, but his father had sanctioned it, and he pitied the man's weakness. He remembered leaving for America soon after that miserable day. With the fuss of the journey and, after that, his excitement at being in America, it had been easy to put the staged death of his sister out of his mind. Now, remembering that day rekindled his anger, his impatience – no hatred – for his half-brother, Shrikant. He looked in horror at Hanif and wanted to say: *Rohini's dead, or Rezana, or whatever you call her – she's dead.*

The sound of laughter from the next table distracted them. Hanif realized he had been staring at Mahesh, at Max, and a silence had fallen between them, neither knowing what next to say or do.

Max pushed the breadbasket and butter dish towards Hanif. 'Here, have some.' The gesture confused Hanif. Did this mean they were going to sit and dine together? He reached a hesitant hand to the bread. 'So, what brings you to New York?' Max asked. He wondered what his mother would say if she knew he was sitting with the infamous Muslim. *Don't drink the water at the Mussalman's house.* He reached for the glass on the table and, putting the glass to his lips, took a long sip.

Hanif placed a roll on his side plate. He had to go along with this dinner, he decided. It would be rude now not to. 'I'm working at Barclays for two months.'

'Barclays? The bank? I thought you were a musician?'

A waiter arrived at their table and set down their plates.

Hanif stared at his food, unsure of himself before his newfound brother-in-law. He wondered how long the pleasantries would last. Max seemed composed as he picked up his silverware and surveyed the food. He looked sophisticated and worldly in this dining room at the International Inn. Hanif wondered how he appeared to Max.

'I always imagine . . .,' Hanif said, still staring at the food, 'I always imagine it's cooked with masalas and fried in ghee. Then it tastes better.' He instantly regretted his words.

Max laughed. 'Yes. That's one way to survive in this country.' With his fork he started mixing the boiled peas with the potatoes on his plate, mashing them together into a paste, which he seasoned with salt and pepper and spread on the chicken.

Hanif's awkwardness faded and they talked, for almost an hour, laughing at the anomaly of their chance encounter, ignoring the messy history that connected them. Hanif gave him news of Rezana, and told him about the children. 'How wonderful,' Max beamed. 'But I cannot imagine her as a mother . . .'

Max was in New York City only for a few days. He'd finished his degree at a college in Ohio and was now considering Harvard for graduate studies. His father sent him an allowance of a hundred and twenty dollars every month. He hardly spent any of it and the money kept accumulating in the bank. He had tried to send it back, but the bank in Ohio couldn't convert dollars into rupees. So a few weeks ago he had bought a car, a black Chevy Sedan.

'Brand new,' he said. 'Model year 1952, with radio, heater, and white sidewall tyres.' Hanif had seen the magazine advertisement: *Brilliantly NEW for '52*. Max leaned confidentially forward. 'Fellows at my college are impressed when they see me driving this car. Before I bought it they pretended I didn't exist, their brains unable to cope with a brown face in a sea of white, I suppose. Even people who never talked to me before, now suddenly know my name. They even ask for rides. I don't mind, I'm happy to take them around.' Max had driven the Chevy to New York. 'On the Pennsylvania Turnpike,' he announced with authority in his semi-American accent, confident Hanif would be impressed that he had tackled the latest confusing manifestation of American innovation in transport – the freeway. Max didn't say he had got stuck in the centre lane for twenty minutes, unable to get to the correct off-ramp.

A waiter cleared their plates and served them dessert and coffee. Hanif stirred three teaspoons of sugar into his cup, added cream. Max drank his black, no sugar. Hanif immediately wished he hadn't added the sugar and cream. He thought Max would produce a pocketsize cigar case like Gene Kelly did in the movies. What if Max should offer him a cigar? He panicked as he rehearsed in his mind the proper way to smoke. They were the only guests left in the dining room. Mrs Lily came to tell them she was sorry they would have to leave in a few minutes, the dining room was closing, but she was happy to see them getting on.

Max described getting stopped by the police on the freeway. 'Twice, they pulled me over for no reason,' he said with irritation. 'The first time I have to admit I was scared. What if they thought I was a black man? Maybe they thought I had stolen the car. I told them immediately I was Indian, which confused them – so I had to add "from India", and they looked at me, skeptically, and double-checked my license and registration. When I gave them my passport, I think they understood I was a foreigner.'

Hanif's thoughts went to a diner in Syracuse where four men at an adjoining table had stared at him as though he had come from a gutter. Under their hostile gaze, he'd placed his order. No sooner had the waitress put his sandwich on the table, than the owner, a stocky man with a thick moustache, his belly bursting under his shirt, came around and asked him to leave. There was a wave of mumbling at the nearby tables before an eerie silence fell over the place. Not wanting to cause trouble, Hanif had got up and left.

Max leaned forward towards Hanif. 'The second policeman asked me how much the car cost and how I'd gotten the money.' His mouth slipped into a grin. 'You know what I said to him?'

Hanif shook his head.

'I said: My father is a Maharaja!' Max threw his head back and laughed. 'That policeman didn't know about Maharajas, he thought it meant "Mayor", but I explained that a Maharaja is a king, and I am a prince. You should have seen the look on his face.'

Hanif couldn't help but get caught up in the joke and marvelled at his companion's temerity, and envied his quick wits. 'He believed you?'

'Of course!' Max's eyes sparkled recklessly.

Hanif had a vision of Max dressed in a brocade *achkan*, a

fantastic silk turban, ropes of pearl necklaces, a diamond brooch. 'And then? What happened?' he asked, fascinated.

'The policeman bowed to me! He sputtered some apology, and he *bowed*! That's what happened. I swear. I waved to him, and drove off. No ticket, no nothing. Now, here I am. In New York.'

'Shabash! Well done,' Hanif said. He decided not to tell Max his diner story.

'From here I drive to Boston,' Max said. 'Why don't you come with me?'

'To Boston?'

'For three days, should be fun. Have you been there?'

Hanif was taken aback by the spontaneity of the invitation and the casual way in which Max had made the offer. As if it were no more than taking a picnic to Vihar Lake, and even that he remembered required days of advance planning. Boston. How far was that from New York? Hanif imagined himself in the black Chevy, sitting in the front with Max. How lucky Max was to own a car, he thought, and had the sudden thought to enroll in Chauhan's Motor Driving School as soon as he returned to Bombay. He had passed by the place many times, the Fiats parked in front with the driving school's name painted on the side doors and the red 'Learner' emblems on the back. He imagined himself cruising along Marine Drive, one elbow in the open window, up the slopes of Malabar Hill, down to Neapeansea Road, past the shops at Breach Candy. Ah, life. Yes, he must get a license, and a car. Suddenly he longed to drive off with Max. To do the things Max did, to be part of his world. But there was a full day of work at the office tomorrow. 'I'd like to go,' he said. 'But, the thing is . . .'

'It's settled then. We'll leave tomorrow and return by Sunday evening. No problem.'

'Sure, no problem.' The words stayed in Hanif's ears. He felt a sense of unease creeping into him again. Still, Max was willing to put the past aside. They could be friends, Hanif thought. Max wanted it. Now it was up to him. He flashed Max a smile. 'No problem at all,' he said.

ೞ

Max wanted to make an early start and the morning air was crisp and clear. It would get very hot later in the day, and Hanif was glad to get away. Max, in white linen trousers and a white shirt, a black cardigan thrown over his shoulders, its sleeves tied casually at the neck, chatted about the Chevy. He planned to ship it to India when he went home, he said.

Hanif was tired. When they had left the dining room last night, he had gone up to his room and packed from his suitcase a smaller bag for the trip. Then he'd written a letter to Rezana, not on the customary aerogram but on four sheets of letter paper. After sealing the envelope, he wondered if reading about her brother would upset her; she had made such strides in putting her family out of her mind. He slipped the envelope in a drawer; he would decide later whether to send it or not. When he finally went to bed, he couldn't sleep, so he got up and did something he hadn't done in more than a year – tried to write a song, a ghazal about two brothers. Humming the lines as he composed them, imagining the rhythm and the melody in his mind, all the while longing for his harmonium, he stayed up most of the night and then, for the first time in months, slept peacefully.

Now, sitting in the front seat with Max, watching through the wound down window the green pastures and dense woods and small towns of the American landscape, he wanted to talk about ghazals. Max probably fancied the opera and he possibly knew about Caruso. He wondered whether Max would be more, or less, impressed with him if he'd been a playback singer. He sat quietly, letting Max lead the conversation.

They passed a police car parked on the side of the road, behind some tall hedges. Max slowed the car. 'Yes, better go slow,' Hanif said, looking back at the police car. 'Don't worry; he's not coming after us.'

Max grinned. 'But I'm the son of a Maharaja. Actually, this time you can be the prince, and I am your trusted driver.' Casting a quick glance in the rearview mirror, he pressed the pedal and, as the car lurched to a higher speed, laughed loudly, 'We're both princes!'

Hanif turned around again, but there was a hill between them and the police car. 'Is it hard to learn . . . driving?' he asked, watching Max change gears.

'Not at all. It becomes natural after a while and you start understanding the car.' Max eased back on the accelerator and turned to Hanif. 'Want to try?'

Hanif smiled and shook his head, feeling a wave of affection for Max.

As they drove through Providence, Hanif asked, 'Where will we stay in Boston?'

'Eliza's place. Her parents have a big house.'

'Eliza?'

'Eliza Wiswall is . . . my girlfriend.' Max looked at the dashboard, pretending to check the fuel gauge, tapping the glass, but the needle didn't move from midway between half and full. For all his American accent and high-class ways, he seemed suddenly shy. Looking sideways at Hanif he added, 'We met in college. She took me to a baseball game against the Red Sox. The Boston team.'

'American girlfriend?'

'Fiancée, actually.' Max glanced at Hanif then fixed his eyes back to the road. 'Next year we're getting married. Or, the year after. Her family is planning the wedding. Church and all that.' He sensed the stunned look on Hanif's face and went on quickly, 'Baseball is a great game. Have you been? You must, at least once. Just for the experience, just to say you've seen a baseball game in America.' He cast a quick look at Hanif again. The distress on Hanif's face was clear, what he'd said about baseball hadn't registered. 'Cricket is better, of course. I'd much rather go to a cricket match . . .' Max launched into a long technical explanation of the differences between baseball and cricket, talking just to fill the silence.

Hanif could not fathom baseball's rules or its strategies. But he smiled anyway, recalling the Bud Abbot/Lew Costello skit, *Who's on First?* He had seen a rerun of the 1945 film *The Naughty Nineties*, as part of a double bill, and was puzzled at why the audience was close to tears with laughter. He wanted to tell Max that he had attended two baseball games and even a football match at Archbold Stadium in Syracuse. But all he could think about was Max and his American fiancée. She was probably the one who had given him the name 'Max'. Eliza and Max. Hanif wished he'd never agreed to this jaunt to Boston. He'd never been inside an American house, much less spent the night in one, and that, on top of Max's casual announcement, kept him in silent worry for a few moments. 'Do they know? In Bombay, I mean,' he finally asked.

'Of course not.' Max gripped the steering wheel tighter and sighed loudly. 'One of these days I'll write and tell them. Haven't figured out what to say. You know how it is. But they'll understand.'

'They'll understand,' Hanif repeated.

ॐ

Max presented Eliza's parents with a bottle of wine. From the way they thanked him and admired the label on the bottle, Hanif surmised it was an expensive gift. Eliza's mother, in a flowery dress and pearl necklace, was trim and athletic with short blonde hair. Her father, broad-shouldered and ruddy faced in a light blue suit, had a loud, hearty voice. Max had told Hanif he was an investment banker at Boston Trust, and Hanif had imagined a small, serious man. Eliza, in her too-tight blouse and big heels, was a youthful, flashy version of her mother. Max introduced Hanif as his brother-in-law, and that caused a flurry of excitement.

'I'm terribly happy to meet someone from your family,' Eliza said again and again.

Her effusiveness, as well as Max's introduction, filled Hanif with pride. He remembered the long letter he had written to Rezana that lay tucked in a drawer in his room at the International Inn in New York. He would send the letter, he decided; it would please Rezana to know he had met her brother. But he should be careful not to mention this American girlfriend in his future letters.

Eliza's house, in an area of Boston called Beacon Hill, was a two-storey structure with tall white columns in the front. Hanif was astonished at the clean furnishings – the art objects placed carefully on side tables, the well painted walls – the order and luxury that lived in each room. But he kept his astonishment to himself, and carried on as though he was used to it all. There was a maid and a butler, both in uniform, who moved quietly about the house. The maid brought a tray of lemonade while they lounged in the study, which was a wood-panelled room overlooking a swimming pool. When Hanif saw the others nod and gesture 'thank you' to the maid as she offered them a glass, he did the same. Max and he were shown to the guest wing – four bedrooms opening onto a small sitting room. Hanif's room, easily twice the size of his room at home, had a double bed, a bureau, a desk, and two armchairs by the window. A bouquet of fresh flowers and a small bowl of apples sat on the table between the chairs. Hanif stepped into the adjoining bathroom. His eyes went to a shelf on the wall; he had never seen a stack of towels quite like this before – at least a dozen, white and soft, and folded just so. Before dinner the butler knocked on Hanif's door and asked if he needed anything pressed or his shoes shined.

Dinner was served in a chandeliered dining room at a large table that glistened with silver and crystal. Eliza and her mother had cooked up a feast, with soup and casseroles and a flamed dessert. In Max's honour there were two different types of rice and a dish of vegetables with a heavy sprinkling of paprika. Eliza's father asked about Hanif's work at Barclays, and Hanif spoke self-consciously, thinking as they all listened to him, how much more they would admire him if he were a professional musician. Eliza's mother fussed over Max as though he really was a prince from India. Hanif noticed her angle the centerpiece of flowers so that the bigger blooms faced Max, and he noticed how she listened, leaning forward in her chair and putting her fork down, whenever he spoke. Was it because Max was taken to be equal to them in social stature, a foreigner who despite his foreignness exuded confidence and walked and talked like they did? Or, was it something else . . . Max had an innate charisma, Hanif decided, a natural sense of class and style.

Max's bottle of wine was opened at dinner and Hanif watched the others take delicate sips. Eliza's father gushed with praise at the year of the vintage, and Max beamed and nodded. Hanif had never tasted wine and when he lifted the glass to his lips he was surprised at the crisp bitterness that spread in his mouth. He couldn't decide whether he liked it or not, but halfway through the meal when the butler came to refill his glass, he said, 'Yes, please,' in the cool measured tone of a person who drank wine every day. He was well aware the Koran forbade intoxicating drinks, and sipping on the delicious wine and feeling its effects he could understand why. But it was simpler to drink than not drink.

The next day Eliza took Max and Hanif on a tour of the city. They set out in the morning in Max's car, Eliza in the middle of the broad front seat between them. She pointed out buildings and monuments and churches and parks. 'I can't wait to see Bombay,' she said to Max, who laughed. 'You'll be disappointed,' he said. 'It's not as nice as Boston.' 'It's nicer,' Hanif wanted to say, but kept quiet. They ate lunch at a glass-fronted restaurant near the harbour and she pointed out a place, Union Oyster House, where she said her father had proposed to her mother. As they strolled around Harvard Square, she slipped her arm through Max's, and Hanif, walking a step behind, was taken shocked. Max didn't seem to mind her arm at all; he even turned and whispered in her ear, then reached a hand to her blonde hair and moved it away from her face, letting his fingers linger at her neck. 'This is America,' Hanif told himself, trying to quell his uneasiness. He pretended to ignore their intimacy as he shuffled along behind them, but he couldn't help glancing furtively at her slender white arm entwined in Max's.

For Hanif, the three days in Boston went by quickly. He was just getting used to the lavish house and the generous hospitality of their American hosts when they were making their farewells and shouting 'Let's do this again soon.' On the drive back to New York, Max was quiet. Hanif knew that last night he and Eliza were alone in the main sitting room long after everyone else had gone up to bed. Had Max visited her room in the night? Hanif looked sideways at Max. He was driving with one hand at the top of the steering wheel, the other arm at rest in the open window. 'Are you really going to marry her?' Hanif asked.

Max straightened himself in the seat, put both hands on the wheel. 'She's in love with me,' he said, grinning gallantly and pushing the accelerator so that the car lurched faster and the sound of rushing air through open windows prevented further conversation.

Chapter 36

Rezana went about the days in a lighter mood, her mind filling with nervous anticipation. In two more weeks Hanif would be home. *The Great Caruso* was opening at Metro Cinema in Bombay on the same day Hanif was returning from America. Was it an omen? Rezana knew Caruso was Hanif's hero, and she knew they'd see the film. Perhaps there was still a chance that Hanif would take up music again as he had said he would.

The night before Hanif's arrival she brought out his harmonium, which had been relegated to a corner of the music room with a rolled up cane mat thrown on top. Moving the mat, she picked up the harmonium, her body bending with its weight, and placed it in the centre of the room.

Sitting cross-legged on the floor, she pulled off the cover. The harmonium hadn't been played in two years. She ran her fingers over the geometric design on the top before unlatching the bellows. The pleats crackled as they fanned open, releasing a faint odour of mildew. She played the scale: *Sa ... Re ... Ga ... Ma ... Pa ... Dha ... Ne ... Sa ...* Then backwards: *Sa ... Ne ... Dha ... Pa ... Ma ... Ga ... Re ... Sa.* It was badly out of tune, but she could still imagine a stage, velvet curtains, microphones, muted lights, and hundreds in the audience, the beat and the rhythm steeping the air. She imagined Hanif singing ghazal after ghazal, never tiring. She saw herself sitting in the front row, mesmerized like everyone else by his voice. She imagined the final ovation, the heady sound pushing everything else from her thoughts. She was a part of his world, a part of his music. She closed her eyes, abandoning herself to old memories and dreams.

Something welled in her throat. Disappointment? Regret? The sensation surprised her. This was not a time for discontentment. What was wrong with her? This was a happy occasion. Hanif would be home in less than twelve hours. Hadn't she been counting the months, the weeks, the days? Hadn't she channeled all her energy for the past two years into the moment of his return? Hanif's parents were waiting for him as well. Ammi talked about him every evening as she cooked dinner and worried about what he was eating, and Abbu talked about this and that business opportunity for his son. Saleem and Sobia had grown accustomed to his absence and mentioned his name in the abstract way that children speak of distant relatives; Rezana had been trying to rekindle memories of him for them.

Rezana had decided early on to accept his absence and occupied her days with a slew of domestic chores, the distraction of classes at the university and studying for her Master's degree. Yet never before had she held him more closely in her thoughts as she did in the months of his absence.

And now the wait was over. Tomorrow night he would sleep next to her again. Her skin tingled as she imagined him reaching for her in the dark. A wild tremor ran down her legs and she struggled to regain composure. She was happy, she told herself, as she squelched the messy, muddled thoughts that the harmonium had stirred. Of course she was happy. She clipped the latches of the air vents into place, reached for the cotton cover and stretched it over the harmonium. But instead of carrying the instrument back to its original corner, she left it in the middle of the room, in its rightful place.

ಜಞ

Early the next morning, Ammi, Abbu, the children, and Rezana met Hanif at Ballard Pier. The children gasped in awe at the great ship. As Hanif bent at the knees and swept them up in an embrace, they giggled and wrapped their small arms around his neck.

'Take us inside,' Sobia begged.

'Are you the captain of the ship?' Saleem asked.

Hanif laughed, 'I'm not the captain, I'm the happy-happy father of Saleem and Sobia! Come on, I'll show you the ship.'

In the evening, uncles, aunts, and cousins streamed into the house. The smell of an abundance of food was in every room. Neighbours who came to offer their congratulations were asked to stay and eat. Abbu stood at the front door brandishing Hanif's degree. In response to their 'Salaam Alaykum,' he said, 'See, Master of Business from Syracuse University in America.' He stressed 'A-mer-i-ca', saying the word in a slow, theatrical tone.

After the last guests had left, long after the children were put to bed and Hanif had got them settled with stories from America, Rezana fell into his arms. He held her tightly, pressing her to his chest. She hugged him back as fervently. Through the tears she choked, 'Two years, my beloved. It seemed like two lifetimes.' Gently he wiped away her tears. Then he, too, wept.

VI
CROSSINGS

Chapter 37

Motilal had heard of neither Harvard nor Boston, but soon understood from Mahesh's expansive description as he declared his intentions to pursue postgraduate studies there that it was a prestigious college where well-to-do American fathers sent their boys. He imagined his son in a domed library, sitting at a heavy mahogany table spread with books, his head bent in concentration. Motilal was impressed by the foreign flair his son had acquired after four years abroad. The way he walked and talked was different, and he exuded a hitherto unseen confidence.

'Perhaps I will visit America next year,' Motilal said.

Mahesh had hoped the distance and his father's general discomfort around all things 'foreign' would put him off such an idea, and he inwardly cringed at the thought of introducing his father, in his Nehru jacket and cotton dhoti, to Eliza and her garrulous parents; her glad-handing father and loud mother, and the shamelessness of American culture would be too much for his largely parochial sensibilities. His father would never accept Eliza, and Mahesh feared that his displeasure would manifest itself in the abrupt curtailment of funds into his account at First Federal of Ohio.

'You want to visit . . . America?' Mahesh stammered, and

even as panic pierced his heart, he beamed and nodded, 'Father, what a grand idea.'

ನಐ

'You're in Bombay?' Hanif asked, too loudly, into the telephone when Mahesh phoned. 'Can you come for dinner?' After their trip to Boston, when Hanif returned to Syracuse, he had received a letter from Max. Inside the fine white envelope were three photos – one of Hanif standing outside Eliza's house with her parents, another of Hanif outside a museum, and a photo that Eliza had snapped when they were leaving, of Hanif and Mahesh and the Chevy. On handsome white letter paper folded over the photos were four lines in a precise, careful hand, at odds with the breezy message:

Howdy Hanif,
It was a fun weekend, wasn't it? We should take another trip, drive out west to California.
                                                    Ciao, Max.

Hanif had displayed the photos on the windowsill above his desk, and after a few days mailed the last two to Rezana. He couldn't stop thinking about Max's letter. What was the meaning of 'ciao', and California . . . how many days drive was that? And imagining crossing India from one side to the other in a car, he wondered if it was possible, or safe. Hanif knew he could never go on such a long road trip, but his heart lurched at the thought. He was in a good mood for days. He repeated 'howdy' a few times, and then practiced saying, 'Howdy Max!' He had written back thanking him for the photos and his kind invitation and signed his letter: *Your brother-in-law, Hanif.*

Rezana was ecstatic when she heard Mahesh was coming to dinner. It was more than nine years since she had seen anyone from her family, though her memories remained vivid and, in spite of her attempts to forget, often came to her unbidden, so strong that she had to pause whatever she was doing and let them pass. She longed to hear news of her younger sisters, but then her thoughts would swing to her parents' humiliation and she longed to know if she had been forgiven, or simply forgotten. She had come to accept that her future would be as Allah willed it.

A dozen times she confirmed the day and the date of Mahesh's visit with Hanif. They argued about whether to call him Mahesh or Max. 'You'll see, he's not Mahesh anymore,' Hanif said. 'And he's requested kheema for dinner . . .'

'He eats *meat?*'

'He eats everything,' Hanif said. 'He's become a proper American.'

He did not tell her about Max's girlfriend; there was no point in creating drama, and he couldn't remember whether Max had asked him to keep it a secret.

Rezana rearranged the sitting room furniture, mended the sofa tassels and bought flowers for the dining table and new white-laced dinner napkins. In the kitchen with Ammi she tasted and re-tasted each dish, and thrust a spoonful into Hanif's mouth if he happened to wander in. The whistle of the pressure cooker, the clanging of pots and pans, the sizzling of oil – these sounds took over the house for the entire day. 'How much food are you making?' Hanif shook his head as he watched the chaos from the kitchen door. 'He's not a *kushti* wrestler.'

Saleem and Sobia fed off their mother's excitement and ran back and forth about the neighbourhood, announcing that their Mamu from Versova was coming to dinner, and Ma and Nani were cooking and cooking, and they had never met their Mamu before, but they hoped he would tell them Akbar-Birbal stories and bring them toys, but they were not to ask for anything, and they were to be quiet and sit nicely when he came, and Ma said someday they might go to his house in Versova, which was a big-big yellow house with gardens and fountains where golden fishes swam below the lotus flowers, and Ma said she used to live in the same yellow house when she was small, and she used to play badminton with Mamu on the beach and they skipped ropes at the edge of the water and sometimes Mamu would pull her hair which was long, even longer than it is now, and she would chase him into the waves.

Feeling left out of the final preparations and irritated by the women on the afternoon of Mahesh's visit, Abbu went for a haircut and shave, and took his time buying a new shirt, then hid behind his newspapers in the sitting room. The British were celebrating the coronation of Queen Elizabeth II, and New Zealand's Edmund Hillary and Nepal's Sherpa Tenzing Norgay had conquered the summit of Mount Everest, reaching twenty-nine thousand feet, and planted the British flag there. It was a proud day for the British Commonwealth, of which independent India remained a part. 'It's a glorious day for your brother to visit our house,' Abbu said to Rezana, holding up the newspaper so she could see the headlines and the photo.

Late in the afternoon, a courier arrived on bicycle with two boxes and a package wrapped in brown paper. 'Gifts from your brother,' Abbu called from the front door as he accepted the parcels. The children ran to the door, and were startled to be handed a box addressed to them, and they dropped to the floor right there and began prying it open. Rezana smiled at their happy faces as they held up picture books, American lollipops, and piggy banks already rattling with coins.

ಬಿ

Mahesh's taxi stopped at the gate, the door slammed, and the leather soles of his elegant shoes clip-clopped up the clean swept stone walkway. The street lamps were on and a light breeze mixed with drizzle filled the evening. He appeared at the front door, a svelte, smiling figure in dark blue trousers and a blue-and-white striped shirt. He bowed to Ammi and Abbu, and delivered the phrase he had practiced, 'Salaam Alaykum'. He embraced Hanif with one arm, Rezana with the other and, before turning his attention to the children, squeezed Rezana's shoulder, hoping in that gesture she would understand all that he could not say out loud.

'He's handsome,' Ammi whispered to Rezana as they followed the men into the sitting room. Rezana dabbed the edge of her *duppatta* to her damp eyes. Mahesh smelled of home, of washing soap and starch, of betel nut and rose. She missed that smell. The children hung back in the foyer, shy, peaking around a corner and giggling as they gazed at their Mamu.

Mahesh took in the humble furnishings of the sitting room and the content faces that now filled it, Rohini's especially; she looked very different from how he remembered her, not just the salwar kameez that fitted her so well but an air, an attitude, a happiness that went deeper than their meeting after so much time, something he didn't recognize. His little sister had grown up and become a woman and a mother and, there was no denying it, a Muslim. He looked at Hanif beside her on the settee and saw in his eyes the same undefinable joy; Mahesh nodded and smiled and sipped from the glass that had somehow materialized in his hand. Lemon sharbat. It tasted cool and sweet and he was glad that he had come.

'The gifts you sent ... too much,' Hanif said. 'You shouldn't have taken so much trouble.'

'It was no trouble. And it makes me happy to have a new niece and nephew to lavish with gifts.' His eyes drifted towards the window. 'It's a nice area, away from the main road, safe for the children to play outside.' He glanced at his sister and wondered if she had found it hard to adjust to this simpler life, and he wanted to ask Hanif how he'd convinced her to marry him, and where she had found the courage to leave home and family and faith and security to come here. He looked at her again, in awe.

'I've never been to Versova,' Abbu said. 'I know it's not that far, and there's a good beach and it's peaceful, no?'

Mahesh set his glass down on the side table. 'The name Versova derives from *vesava*, which means "place of rest". It was just a fishing village when the Muskat Arabs landed there in the early seventeenth century, killed off most of the inhabitants, and built a port. In about 1650, the Portuguese took the port and built a fort to guard their caravels that traded up and down the coast. The fort is still there on the hill, but the port has reverted to being a humble fishing village.' He looked around the room. They were all listening to him. 'You are right, Uncleji,' he said. 'Versova is very peaceful, and the beach is beautiful.'

Rezana had always been fascinated by the fort, an imposing stone structure with turrets that dominated everything in the shallow bay from its position on Mudh Island. On a full moon night, when the light glistened across the glassy water, the fort was mysterious and exotic. She'd been to the fort once with her cousins, but thought it dirty and dreary, crawling with lizards and infested with bats and she had to wash and wash to get rid of a stink that seemed to have penetrated the pores of her skin. She wanted to say there was nothing special about the fort, that it was mostly an illusion best viewed from afar, but Mahesh was a good storyteller and the children were gazing up at him with such delight she didn't want to spoil the moment.

'You've just returned from America?' Abbu asked.

'Yes. I'll be going back in a few weeks. But I wanted to come and see Rohini . . .'

'. . . Rezana . . .' Hanif corrected softly.

Mahesh glanced quickly at Rezana. 'It's been so many years, Rezana, Hanif . . . my apologies.' He suddenly wondered why he had come. Out of fondness for his sister? Certainly. And that he also liked Hanif? Of course. But it was more than that. Maybe what had really brought him here was a desire to be defiant, to turn his back on his parents and their hypocritical orthodoxy.

Rezana broke the awkward silence, clearing her throat and announcing, 'We ... we've prepared kheema for you. We hope it will be to your liking.'

On the phone, Mahesh had jokingly mentioned kheema to Hanif. He hadn't expected his request to be taken seriously. The conversation turned to food in America, and American habits, and Mahesh had many anecdotes to tell, and Hanif backed him up when the others laughed in disbelief, and they talked about President Truman and President Eisenhower and the dominance of the American economy, and the opportunities it offered. Mahesh spoke with confidence. Listening to him, Rezana felt proud of his knowledge, and a little grateful for his impeccable manners.

The children may have been bored by the talking, but they stayed close to Mahesh, sipping from their small stainless-steel cups of lemon sharbat, and whispering and giggling as they poked the ice with their fingers.

'Rezana,' Mahesh said, 'I must get used to your name. Re-za-na. I like the sound of it.' He raised his glass to her and the others joined in the informal toast.

She felt a wave of affection towards him. 'I hear *you've* changed your name, too, to Max.'

'Not officially. Just among friends. It's easier for Americans to pronounce.'

'Rezana completed her Master's in Literature,' Abbu said. 'She passed with honours.'

'Congratulations!' Mahesh said. 'I took a class in American Literature last year. Let me see, we read Fitzgerald, Faulkner, who else, Hemingway? Hemingworth?'

'Hemingway, Ernest Hemingway,' Rezana smiled, leaning forward in her seat. 'He has a strong hold over the American imagination. So independent and adventurous, but, ultimately, I think he is a self-obsessed, bigoted, drunk coward. Except for some of his short stories and one or two novels, there's no bite to his writing. They will probably put him on a high shelf, reserved for those they neither read nor criticize. He is of his time, nothing more.'

Mahesh was surprised at her eloquence. 'My goodness, such forthright and controversial views; what fun we'll have at dinner tables in America.' He rubbed his hands together, mischievously, and laughed, everyone joining in, including the children, though they had no idea what he was saying except they liked how he said it.

Saleem tugged Mahesh's trouser leg and asked if he knew any good stories. Mahesh looked down at his eager nephew and said he knew hundreds of them, and would tell some after dinner. 'What about magic tricks?' Saleem asked. 'For you, young master, of course,' said Mahesh and reached in his pocket for a handkerchief and a coin, covered the coin with the handkerchief, swirled his hands in the air, and made the coin disappear. Saleem jumped up and down. 'Where has it gone, Mamu?' he asked. And Mahesh reached behind his ear, flicked his wrist and produced the coin, as if drawing it from the startled Saleem's ear. Saleem rubbed his ear, looked at the coin, and rubbed his ear again. 'How did you do that, Mamu?' Mahesh ruffled Saleem's hair and said with a laugh, 'A magician never, ever, reveals his secrets.' He gave the boy the coin. Saleem accepted his Mamu's explanation and sat back down at his feet, turning the coin over and over in his fingers, and even tried to push the large coin into his tiny ear.

Abbu asked about the family business. 'Silk, I understand?'

'Trading, but silk yarn is a mainstay,' Mahesh replied.

Abbu said, 'It is an exotic business, silk. Tell me, if you can, what led your family to it.'

Mahesh paused for a moment, as though guarding a secret. Then suddenly, he relaxed; he was, after all, with family. 'Because of China,' he said. 'A long time ago our grandfather and his brothers were in the opium trade.'

'What?' Rezana sputtered and coughed. Hanif moved closer to pat her back, but with an incredulous look on his face, one shared by his parents.

'Yes, opium. During the nineteenth century, when the East India Company began shipping it to China, they were middlemen,' Mahesh said quietly.

'Opium? Wasn't that illegal?' Abbu asked.

'Yes . . .' said Mahesh calmly, '. . . and no. The Company directors in London publicly denounced the opium trade, but its British officers in India controlled a vast industry based on large-scale production. And it was very, very profitable. The fertile riverbed of the Ganges, the holy river of the Hindus, was perfect for growing poppies. The farmers, forbidden to grow anything else, harvested the opium, which was sold at auctions in Calcutta. My grandfather and his brothers, and then my father, were among the many Indian middlemen commissioned by the British to ship the opium into China – which really was illegal, so far as the Chinese were concerned – and shipments would sometimes be seized, which meant it was a risky business, but they were handsomely paid and the risk was well worth the rewards.'

They were all staring at him. Rezana had never heard the story before, but knew enough about the history of the British and the opium trade to hope her brother was joking. 'Are you sure we were involved in such a . . . such a despicable trade?'

Mahesh turned to Hanif and Abbu, 'You know of the Opium Wars?'

Abbu said, 'Of course.'

Hanif didn't, but he nodded anyway.

Mahesh wished he hadn't brought up the topic, but they were all looking at him, expectantly, and he saw no way of changing track after revealing such a shocking secret. 'In China, the effects of the opium trade were devastating. Millions of people became addicted to the drug. The Chinese Emperor tried to ban it, but it had penetrated even the palace walls, and several members of the royal family were hopeless addicts.

'Our surname used to be Dalal. The British gave the nickname, "China-walla", which our grandfather changed to "Chimanji",' Mahesh said. 'We took opium to China and brought back silk.'

'I had no idea,' said Rezana. 'How do you know all this?'

Mahesh laughed. 'I can't believe you didn't know.'

Rezana waited for him to continue, as did the others, but Mahesh took up his glass again, sniffed appreciatively at the lemon sharbat and drank down what was left.

'Are we ready for dinner?' Ammi asked after the silence had lingered too long, and went to the kitchen without waiting for an answer. Rezana followed, bringing the children with her. They wailed. They didn't want to eat in the kitchen; they wanted to eat with their Mamu.

In the sitting room, the men talked about business. Mahesh explained the new venture his father had started. It was called United Rayon, a large factory that manufactured a special yarn used for the production of lightweight silk. 'After the British left,' he explained, 'cloth from Manchester and Lancashire became hard to get, and the demand for textiles keeps growing. Mahatma Gandhi may have talked a lot about the virtues of the spinning wheel and homespun cotton, but India is on the path to industrialization.'

Abbu leaned towards Mahesh. 'Only last week I received a letter from my cousin-brother.' He looked at Hanif. 'You know, Anwar-babu.' Then, to Mahesh, he said, 'My cousin lives in Pakistan. He has a cloth mill outside Karachi and wants us to join in the business.'

'Do it,' Mahesh said, his voice sounding sincere and enthusiastic. 'Don't wait. Whether in India or Pakistan, from a business standpoint, I assure you the textile industry is going to hit the sky.'

Hanif was startled by Mahesh's temerity and feared his father might be offended, but Abbu was hanging on his every word, nodding.

Rezana called them for dinner. When Mahesh saw the spread of dishes on the table, his eyes widened. 'My goodness!' he said, with a low whistle.

It was stuffy and hot in the small dining room. A slight

breeze from the open windows brought in moths that whirled around the bulbs in the shell-shaped sconces. As Rezana served the food, Ammi asked Mahesh, directly, as was her wont, 'What about your marriage? Has anything been decided?'

Mahesh laughed. He felt gregarious and lighthearted, and longed to publicize his engagement to Eliza. He ran a hand through his hair in a nonchalant manner. 'Still time, still time. I have to finish my studies, Auntiji.'

During dinner Rezana mentioned Hanif's ghazals and his reposed ambition of becoming a playback singer.

'He told me about All India Radio,' Mahesh said, 'but ghazals, and a playback singer? Big-time stuff.' Arching his eyebrows and raising a hand in the air, palm turned upward like a classical singer, he exclaimed, '*Arre wah*, Hanif, I had no idea.' It occurred to Mahesh, especially from the tone in which Rezana had spoken about Hanif's music, the reverence, the enthusiasm in her voice, then the subtle disappointment when she described how he had put his music career aside, that it was music that had brought them together. She had fallen for his voice. What that meant, or what Mahesh was going to do with the information, he had no idea; but he felt triumphant, as though he'd calculated the answer to a difficult mathematics theorem.

'Will you sing a ghazal next time I come?' Mahesh asked. 'And next time, Rohini . . . I mean, Rezana . . . and Auntiji, don't prepare so much food. Just *chai* and some snacks. We'll have an evening of Hanif's ghazals. What do you say, Hanif?'

Hanif smiled, 'Inshallah, if I could only find the time to practice.' But already in his mind he was assembling a programme of the songs. He would bring out the harmonium tomorrow, perhaps he would even finish the ghazal he had started writing in America.

Rezana looked down and traced her fingers over the thin golden border of her kameez. Her mind swirled. Her brother would visit again, Hanif would return to his harmonium; perhaps they would go together to the Metro Cinema, to cricket matches at the stadium. Afterwards, they would stop at Cream Centre for cold *kesar* milk.

It was late by the time Mahesh left. The children were curled up asleep under blankets of *pashmina* scarves Ammi had laid across them on the settee.

Rezana and Ammi went to the kitchen and, as they cleaned up, they discussed the dishes Mahesh seemed to like best and what they should prepare next time. 'He's a fine man,' Ammi said. 'He will make someone a good husband.'

Her brother's wedding would be big, Rezana imagined. She saw herself arriving with Hanif and the children, all of them dressed in new clothes. They would bow to her parents, touch their feet, and ask for their blessings. The past would be ignored, buried, leaving only the joy of reconciliation. Her sisters would ask about her life, how she had passed the years, and she would talk about her studies and accomplishments. Saleem and Sobia would sit in their grandfather's lap, and he would smile, and proudly press them to his chest. Her mother would ask if she was happy, whether the in-laws were kind, and insist that she bring her husband and children to Versova every Sunday. Rezana turned to Ammi with shining eyes, 'I think my brother's wedding will be a grand affair.'

Chapter 38

'No!' Rezana wept to Hanif in their bedroom the next morning. 'A thousand times, no! We can't leave Bombay.' Sitting at the edge of the bed, she was in a blue salwar-kameez, hair uncombed and still wet from the bath.

Hanif stared at her for a moment, and returned to buttoning his shirt. 'It's for the best. You'll see.'

'I don't want to leave Bombay. What about my family?'

'What *about* your family?' Hanif repeated. '*This* is your family,' he gestured to the walls of their bedroom. 'Which tie should I wear? Come on, I'll be late for office. Please stop crying.' Crossing to the bed he tried to put a hand on her shoulder and pull her towards him, but she flinched and turned away. 'Think about Saleem and Sobia. Think about their future,' he said.

'Not Pakistan. I refuse,' she said through her tears. 'Delhi, Calcutta, Lucknow, anywhere, but not Pakistan.'

'Be reasonable. Karachi is on the seashore, not that different from Bombay.'

'Let them go; we can stay here.'

'There's nothing for any of us in Bombay.'

'There's Mahesh. I have to stay in Bombay for . . .'

'You mean Max!' Hanif laughed lightly. 'I told you, he's

the one who suggested we go to Pakistan.' Hanif picked a tie from his drawer, held it to his shirt.

'He wasn't being serious. My brother has always been like that, saying things to sound grand. You mustn't listen to him.'

'What he says makes sense. Anyway, your fine brother will be going back to America soon.'

Rezana stood up. 'Then let's go to America,' she said, surprised at herself.

'And what will we do in America?' Hanif began knotting his tie. 'It's expensive.' Yet even as he said that, he wondered, could they immigrate to America? He imagined the campus at Syracuse, the tall buildings in New York. 'It's one thing to go for studies, but to *live* there?' Hanif looked at Rezana and shook his head. 'It's cold, and it's much too quiet. *You* would not like it at all.' Hanif peered in the mirror and smoothed his hair with one hand.

Rezana stood beside Hanif, meeting his eyes in the mirror. 'I have no one in Pakistan,' she said evenly. 'I don't want to go.'

'Pervez is there, remember?' Hanif said. 'Rezana, don't be like this. We have to go. It's already decided. Abbu and I think it's best for the whole family.'

'We will be outsiders.'

'Don't bring up excuses,' he said. 'Think of it as a new beginning. Think of it as an adventure!'

'I've had too many new beginnings and too many adventures!' Rezana collapsed on the bed and began sobbing again. 'I can't do it. I don't have the strength.' She crossed her arms and buried her head in them, her wet hair falling over her shoulders.

Bending towards the bed and pulling her in an embrace, he whispered, 'You do have the strength, Rezana-*jaan*. Please, you're the strongest person I know.'

ಗಿ

The train slowed with a grating rumble. In the blue-grey darkness of the compartment, Rezana's eyes went first to the bedding rolls on the floor, to the sleeping forms of her children. Saleem had kicked off his blanket and she reached a hand to pull it back over him, then ran her fingers lightly over Sobia's hair. She glanced quickly at Ammi on the berth across from her. From the two upper berths she could hear Hanif and Abbu's irregular snores.

There was barely any room to move in their sleeper compartment. Every corner was jammed with their belongings – suitcases, duffel bags, boxes, and plastic baskets – every object a sad reminder of their departure from Bombay. Eleven pieces in all, Abbu counted frequently, expecting something to be stolen at any moment even though the compartment door was double locked. Larger trunks and corrugated boxes with their household things were in the train's luggage hold. Abbu pulled out the luggage receipt from his wallet every now and then and studied it carefully. Perhaps the piece of paper reassured him that their possessions were safe, or, was he looking at it in disbelief?

Ammi, usually cheerful and talkative, was quiet for most of the journey. She had brought along a book. Rezana had never seen her reading anything other than the newspaper before, and although Ammi kept the book open before her, she seldom turned the pages. Despite the abundance of food they'd packed for the journey and the snacks that Abbu bought from the vendors at each stop, Ammi hardly ate.

Hanif held the children on his lap and read them stories, or walked them up and down the corridor outside their compartment. Rezana sensed his anxiety from the way he hummed tunelessly to himself.

Abbu's cousin in Karachi had bought a second-hand car for them because the textile mill was several miles outside the city. 'We'll have to hire a driver,' Abbu said.

'Why?' Hanif looked up excitedly. 'I'll learn to drive. I could get a license.'

'We'll see,' Abbu said. 'It's not a bad idea, but we'll have enough to do . . .'

The train was gliding along sluggishly. Rezana lifted the curtain – outside it was still dark, a few dim lights barely visible through the morning fog. They must be nearing Karachi. The smell of coal and dew came in with the wind. It never smelled like this in Bombay.

How hastily Hanif and Abbu had made the decision to move to Pakistan. Within three weeks they'd sold the house in Bandra and packed all their belongings. She resented Mahesh for making this ridiculous suggestion to Hanif and Abbu. What did Mahesh know? Move to Pakistan and set up a cloth mill. Pakistan! Anger and bitterness swirled inside her, yet the image of Mahesh dining at their house brought her some joy. Perhaps he would visit them in Karachi . . . but even as she imagined this she knew he would never come.

She felt suddenly exhausted and longed for a bath. They

had been travelling for two nights and a day, changing trains in Baroda and again at Marwar Junction. She'd half-hoped that something would go wrong at the border; that the army guards would find something amiss with their papers and make them turn back. They waited for hours in a stifling hot carriage as the guards checked all the passengers' documents and rifled through everyone's luggage, the children fussing and wailing in unison. Nothing of consequence happened.

'We should be arriving soon,' Hanif said to Rezana from the upper berth. 'Wake them up.'

'I'm awake,' Abbu mumbled, raising his hands. 'Can you see anything outside?'

'I'm also awake,' Ammi said. 'I couldn't sleep at all.'

Rezana leaned towards the window and slid the curtain open. They were drifting past a high cement wall with barbed wire on top. At places there were big holes in the wall, as though someone had tried to tear it down. Turning from the window she looked around the compartment: Ammi getting the children ready, Abbu slipping a shirt over his singlet, Hanif climbing down from the top berth. Rezana adjusted the dupatta over her head, draped one end of it more securely over her shoulder, and exhaled softly.

The train was gliding less noisily now. A smart tapping on the door made all of them turn. 'Karachi in two minutes!' the ticket collector's voice announced.

ಬಬ

Anwar-babu and his wife Fatima-begum were waiting for them at the station. He was Abbu's cousin, older by five

years, and Rehana saw the resemblance immediately. Like
Abbu he was long-limbed and tall with a wide chest. He was
dressed in a beige salwar-kurta and black vest, grey hair
combed back and moustache precisely trimmed. Fatima-
begum was in a blue-black salwar-kameez with the dupatta
draped solemnly around her head and neck. They made a
stately pair, standing on the platform amid the general
commotion of the coolies and handcarts and scores of people
who had come to meet the train.

'Salaam Alaykum,' Anwar-babu said and waved, a smile
stretching on his face as he came striding towards them.
'Welcome to Karachi.'

'Wa Alaykum As-Salaam,' Abbu said, in a loud cheery
voice. 'What? No red carpet? No band to welcome us?' He
hugged his cousin, and their jovial banter gave Rezana
momentary reassurance.

Fatima-begum bowed to Abbu, then hugged Ammi and
Hanif. Rezana hung back with the children. 'Come,' Fatima-
begum said to Rezana, laughing and drawing her in with an
arm. 'Welcome, and what lovely children! How old are they?'

'Four and three,' Rezana said.

'Here, let me help you,' Fatima-begum took Saleem and
Sobia by the hand. 'The car is waiting outside. We'll go
ahead home. They'll bring the luggage in the taxi,' she gestured
with her chin to Anwar-babu, Abbu, and Hanif, who were
already surrounded by coolies.

In the car, Rezana sat in the back seat between Fatima-
begum and Ammi, holding Sobia on her lap; Saleem sat
next to the driver. Fatima-begum asked about the journey,
and Ammi leaned forward and chatted easily, her earlier

solemnity quickly disappearing. As the car honked its way out of the station and onto the main road, Rezana's eyes darted out the windows where the early sun sent wide shafts of light over the buildings and shuttered shops. She could still have been in Bombay. A few bicyclists and pedestrians, a sweeper woman bent over her task, a stray dog sleeping under a tree, its head on its paws. As Sobia squirmed on her lap, Rezana put her arms more firmly around her and kissed the top of her head. 'We'll be there soon,' she said, even though she had no idea how far the house was. The car sped down a tree-lined avenue, and Rezana focused her eyes outside again, looking for faults and flaws that might affirm the superiority of Bombay. It was only the first day and too soon to pass judgment, but she knew one thing clearly – she would never be happy in Pakistan.

The house was in a residential area of the city where landscaped medians divided the road and traffic circles were small parks with leafy trees and clean benches. The house, behind a low compound wall and fronted by a stretch of lawn, was a two-storey structure on a hill. A servant came running out and stood in the porch as their car swept up the driveway.

Fatima-begum led them inside. The sitting room, which was more than twice the size of their sitting room in Bombay, was furnished with carved colonial-style sofas, lamps with filigreed shades, and Kashmiri carpets. 'We'll eat after the men arrive,' she said, pointing to the dining room where under a colourful chandelier, the table was laid for breakfast. 'You probably want a bath first.'

'Yes,' Ammi and Rezana said in unison.

'Come,' she said, leading the way down a corridor.

Abbu and Ammi would have the guestroom downstairs, Hanif, Rezana, and the children the larger room upstairs. The house was not opulent, but quiet and tasteful, and Rezana felt her spirits lifting a little. They would be staying here for some time. On their behalf Anwar-babu had made an offer on a house at the Ministry of Housing and it would take four or five weeks for the offer to be approved and the title and papers to clear. It was a good house, in an affluent area, and the price was well within their means. Rezana had not given the issue much thought, but now she wanted their house to be as nice as this one.

Saleem and Sobia, excited by the bathtub, begged to fill it to the top. Rezana pulled them back; they were guests in this house she reminded them. But Fatima-begum said, 'Let's fill it!' She explained that both her daughters were married and lived near Dacca, in East Pakistan, and she rarely saw her grandchildren.

At breakfast, Hanif asked Anwar-babu when they could see the mill. 'Tomorrow,' Anwar-babu said, with a laugh. 'But it won't be just a tour. *Work* starts tomorrow, are you ready?'

'Of course,' Hanif said, and immediately thought about the white Fiat parked outside the gate in a clearing that Anwar-babu had pointed to when they arrived. 'And the car?' Hanif asked. 'I was thinking of enrolling in a driving school.'

'Driving school?' Anwar-babu clicked his tongue. 'I'll teach you,' he pointed to himself and laughed. 'In two weeks you'll have a license.'

'Really?' Hanif wore a wide grin. 'When I pass the driving test . . .'

'No need for test,' Anwar-babu laughed again. 'A few lessons from me, then two copies of your photo, and I'll handle the rest. If you wait in line to take the test you'll be an old man by the time they give you a license. Trust me, this is Pakistan.'

'Thank you . . .'

'For what?'

'For driving lessons . . . for your hospitality, for everything . . .'

'Please, Allah ki meherbani,' Anwar-babu said, raising his hand in the air. 'I am honoured that you all are here.'

ೞ

Pervez brought flowers for Rezana and a box of sweets for the children. In the foyer, Saleem and Sobia crouched excitedly to the floor, and tore off the wrapping. Saleem looked up at Pervez, 'You remind me of my Mahesh-mamu in Bombay.'

'You look well,' Hanif said to Pervez, hugging him.

Pervez had given up his communist dreams. 'I'm in the hotel line,' he told Hanif and Rezana as they led him into Anwar-babu's sitting room.

'Come, sit,' Hanif said, 'Tell us everything. We had such few letters from you . . .'

'I know,' Pervez said. 'I'm sorry. Letter writing is not my forte. Although, if you remember, I was good at letter *delivery*.' He grinned, Hanif laughed and Rezana rolled her eyes.

Pervez added, 'I got all your news quite regularly from your uncle. I wanted to telephone when they were born,' he pointed to Saleem and Sobia, who had followed the adults into the sitting room, their mouths stuffed with sweets, Sobia clutching the box with both hands, 'But the phones . . .'

'Yes, yes, I know,' Hanif said. 'We did get your telegrams. But what about the Communist Party?'

'Well,' Pervez said, scratching his head, 'I'll tell you, but first we must talk of happy things.'

When Rezana praised Pervez's stylish trousers and shirt with epaulets, he smiled and said he was engaged to a fashion designer who had studied in Paris. 'You will meet Parveen on Sunday,' he said. 'We're taking you out to dinner.'

'When is the wedding?' Hanif asked.

'In four months. On January the twenty-first.'

'Pervez and Parveen,' Rezana smiled. 'I'll have to get used to saying that.'

Chapter 39

It was a three-storey house behind Soldier Bazaar – past an open-air kebab stall lit up with strings of colourful lights at night, past the large compound of the St Paul's Grammar School – a sharp right after the wooden dairy shed, down a narrow road where old hefty branches of neem and eucalyptus trees arched over each other. The compound wall was blue like the house, and the wrought iron gate swung open on a long gravel drive.

In the sitting room there was a low round table, six easy chairs covered with cotton in a paisley pattern, and curio cabinets reflecting the windows. A long settee with steep slanted arms stood in the bay alcove, and in the semi-circular space behind it was a family of four wooden elephants on pedestals of advancing size. Overhead, fixed into carved white ceiling plates and spread at least twenty feet apart, were two fans, and, in the centre of the room hung a large white lamp.

The kitchen at the back of the house overlooked a courtyard and a garden beyond. Every cupboard was full with dishes, pots, and canisters. The door that led from the kitchen into a passageway and then out to a small building at the side was the servants' entrance.

A wide staircase climbed to the upper floors, to four bedrooms and bathrooms. There was polished wood furniture in the bedrooms, showpieces and lamps on corner tables, sheets on the beds and soap in the bathrooms, and, in the armoires, clothes of the previous owners – a Hindu family who had left suddenly during Partition.

'Isn't it strange,' Rezana said to Hanif, 'to benefit from someone else's misfortune?'

'Don't think about it,' he said, his eyes gleaming with satisfaction. 'Do you like it?'

She sighed deeply. 'It is beyond anything I ever imagined.'

∞

Rezana discovered that Karachi was not that different from Bombay. The buildings and roads, the trees and flowers, even the salty air had followed them there. She discovered the small bookshops in Urdu Bazaar, and the provision stores in Empress Market. Instead of Metro Cinema and Bandra Talkies they saw movies at the Palace and Rex Cinemas. The ships didn't dock at Ballard Pier but at Keamari Wharf. The banks and customhouses were not at Flora Fountain but on Bundar Road and Elphinstone Street. The promenade for strolls at sunset was not Marine Drive, but Lady Lloyd Pier at Clifton beach. Karachi proffered a collage of new names, but gradually Rezana found herself giving in to the new place.

She took up a lectureship, teaching twice a week at Karachi Women's College. A trustee of the college had offered her the position at a dinner party while they stood on the host's terrace, gazing at the gleaming Arabian Sea and discussing the history of the English novel. The Women's College was a prestigious institution and after the casual manner of the offer, not to mention the generous salary that came in crisp notes rubber-banded together at the end of the first month of teaching, Rezana understood that in Pakistan things happened easily if one knew the right people. Here people in power were held together by a common rhetoric that allowed them to glide through life with minimal effort. It was not a sudden realization, but rather something that she witnessed repeatedly in large and small instances, so that eventually it became less and less unusual.

If initially this new country had felt like a state of permanent exile to Rezana, it was now becoming familiar and comfortable. A three-story house, servants and gardeners, private tutors for the children, a car that Hanif drove to the mill and took them for holiday outings in . . . she knew that in India they could never have done so well.

ॐ

Stepping out of a fabric shop in a gully near Awami Markaz, Rezana was startled when an odd-shaped mass landed with a wet thump at her feet. She was alone. The taxi had dropped her at the corner, and she had walked down the cobbled alley to the shop. At ten o'clock in the morning, the shops had barely opened, but she had come early to avoid the brutal arid heat that seemed to smother Karachi at this time of year. She stepped back and looked down at her feet. And gasped. It was a writhing calf with its belly slit open, its guts

and blood spilling onto her sandalled toes. She stood, frozen
with shock for several moments, then turned to re-enter the
shop to ask for help. Buses, cars, and bicyclists moved along
the main road in the distance, but here around the shop it
was suddenly eerily deserted. A fat blue fly hovered near the
animal's eye, which was blinking absurdly. The calf's hind
legs were bound together with rope, the front legs splayed to
the side. It was only when a bearded man stuck his head out
from behind a corner and shouted an obscenity that Rezana
realized that the calf had been flung at her, that she was the
target of this humiliation. The next instant she was
screaming, clutching the parcel of fabric under her arm, and
dashing in the direction of the main road, her hands
overflowing with vomit as she tried to cover her mouth.
'*Haramzadi*, Hindu!' the man shouted behind her.

ನಾ

Hanif was in the annex office of the cloth mill, studying the
thick catalogue of the sanforizing machine that stood in the
main building, when two men in army uniform stormed in,
and shut the door behind them. After their initial hostility,
they were not impolite, and Hanif whose stomach was
knotted in fear, took a few slow breaths. Both men were
middle-aged, one of them had a puffy face with rosy cheeks
and a wide mouth, the other was muscular with broad
shoulders, his shirt stretched tight over his chest and upper-
arms.

They were paying a 'friendly' visit, they said, and after
they settled into the folding chairs across the desk, wanted

to know about the new machine, where it had come from, what it did, and how much it had cost. The broad-shouldered man picked up some letters and invoices from the desk, read them, and dropped them to the floor. He examined the boxed pen and pencil set on the desk, and then reached for the catalogue, which he fanned through. 'You know German?' he asked, almost in awe. Hanif shook his head and said there was English text on facing pages. The man glanced down, licking his finger and turning the pages slowly, before returning the catalogue ceremoniously to the desk.

When Hanif assured them that all the necessary import duties on the machine had been paid, all the licenses were in order, they both laughed. The rosy-cheeked man pulled out a chit from his shirt pocket and dangling it in front of Hanif's face, said, 'On the day you start the machine, keep this amount ready in cash. Understood?' When Hanif drew back and gasped, he added matter-of-factly, 'If you forget, we might raise the amount, or . . . we might have to take further action.'

The men stood up slowly. 'We'll go now, please excuse us,' the broad-shouldered man said. 'Our best wishes to your uncle. He's out this afternoon, the guard at the gate told us. We're sorry to have missed him, he's a fine man, always offers us tea. Perhaps he'll be here when we come next time.'

ॐ

'*Mohajir*. Immigrant.' At the mosque it was hurled as a harsh whispered insult at their backs, never to their faces. Rezana and Ammi turned to see a knot of women huddled on the floor in a corner. Evening prayers were over, but here in the upstairs antechamber of the women's wing, the women sometimes stayed behind to talk. It was a square room, about ten or twelve feet, with a latticed partition that overlooked the women's prayer hall below.

'Go back over the border, both of you,' a woman in a maroon *burqa* said. 'Go back to where you belong.'

'She's Hindu, isn't she?' another woman pointed a finger at Rezana. 'We don't want her at our mosque.' Her eyes were heavily lined with kajol and her face, which was youthful and attractive, bore a cold, mean expression.

Rezana clutched Ammi's arm. 'Please, Ammi,' she said. 'Let's go.' Rezana glanced at the huddle. There were five of them on the floor in a haphazard circle; the woman in maroon was sitting with one knee up, an elbow resting on it. She met Rezana's gaze defiantly, and then leaned into the circle and whispered to the others.

Ammi turned to the group, put an arm around Rezana. 'She is here, praying with us to Allah,' Ammi said. 'Have you no shame?'

The women on the floor stopped whispering, looked at each other and made some gestures with their hands. They stood up slowly; the woman in maroon was old, and had to be helped up. Two of them hung back, but the others moved purposefully towards Ammi and Rezana.

The woman in maroon, her hands clenched in fists and mouth set in a hard line, stood so close, Rezana could smell the rank odour of her perspiration. Rezana thought she might strike Ammi and she looked frantically to the door and pictured the staircase that led out of the building.

'Go now,' the younger woman said, stepping forward with a hand on her hip. 'For your own good.'

'No,' Ammi said, stamping her foot, her grip on Rezana's shoulder tightening.

Rezana looked sideways at Ammi, her heart hammering loudly, and the next instant she found herself turning to the women. She said: 'We will go when we're ready.' Her voice was shaking but she kept on. 'I took the vow at a mosque in Bombay, and since then I have studied the Koran daily. My children's names are Saleem and Sobia; they are still small but I teach them about the life of the Prophet. Next year, Inshallah, my husband and I will go on Hajj.'

There was a long silence.

'I see,' the younger woman said, and took a small step back, her hand dropping from her hip.

'One more thing,' Rezana said. 'Yes, we have come across the border from India, but we are all equal in Allah's eyes, are we not?'

The woman in maroon stared at Rezana. 'No need to lecture us,' she muttered as she turned away. She nudged the younger woman and Rezana watched them whisper to each other as they shuffled towards the door.

∞

Rezana and Hanif's lives were changed in a single evening, and they would later puzzle about the path they took that led them to that moment. Almost as soon as they arrived in Pakistan, they were introduced to Anwar-babu and Fatima-begum's large circle of friends and also to Fatima-begum's relatives who lived in Karachi, and every Sunday they received a *dawat* to attend a party or picnic, play cards or watch cricket at the gymkhana.

At a businessman's house where thirty people were invited to a dinner party, someone mentioned ghazals, and Anwar-babu said, 'You should hear my nephew sing!' The host produced a harmonium from some room of the house, and announced to his guests that it was time for a little entertainment. The servants came in to move the coffee table from the centre, and brought in more chairs from the dining room.

Hanif tried a few notes. The instrument was old, some of the white keys had yellowed and were chipped, but after a few adjustments the harmonium could still hold a tune if he didn't demand too much from it.

His pitch was a bit shaky. It had been a long time since he'd rehearsed. But the applause was warm and sincere, and following the first ghazal his impromptu audience asked for more. Soon there were requests from every corner of the room, and as Hanif's voice loosened up, and he played the opening notes of a requested song, they cheered happily, and swayed to the music.

Rezana felt a hand touch her elbow. 'Do you sing, too?' asked the businessman's wife, Hooriyah-begum, an elegant middle-aged woman with a thoughtful face. Rezana drew a quick breath. 'Oh, no. I used to . . . but it has been a long time,' she stammered.

Hooriyah-begum touched her elbow again, a little more definitely. 'Please,' she said, gesturing with her other hand around the room, 'You are among friends.'

Hanif rose from the floor and held out his hand as Rezana approached, his face bright and excited from singing. 'Rezana?' he said, and for a moment she thought that all the wonder and beauty that existed in the world had gone into the way he said her name. As they both bent to the floor he shifted the harmonium to make room for her beside him. She looked at him and nodded, and there was no need to ask or discuss which song they would sing. Looking around the sitting room that had turned into a small performance hall, he announced the song: *Jeena hé Téré Muskurahat ké Leeyea*, I Want to Live Only for Your Smile. 'It was our first song together,' Hanif said, and as 'ahs' and 'ohs' swept around the audience, his fingers took to the keyboard. Over the opening notes, he added shyly, 'We were in college then.'

After that evening, at subsequent dinner parties sitting rooms were rearranged beforehand, the furniture pushed to the sides and a harmonium positioned on a handsome carpet in the centre of the room, and soon it was understood within the elite circles of Karachi society that Hanif was a talented singer and his lovely wife, Rezana, who sometimes sang with him, had a remarkable voice, too.

Chapter 40

A year or so after arriving in Karachi, Hanif and Rezana received a letter from Mahesh. He hadn't gone to America after all. He included a card-size photo of himself and his new wife, Nandita, taken during their wedding reception at the Wellingdon Club in Bombay.

Hanif was bewildered. Who was this Nandita ... what happened to Eliza? The image of Eliza and Max walking arm in arm in Boston had stayed with Hanif and, over time he'd come to believe that Max would marry Eliza because Max was bold and determined and always got what he wanted. Now studying the wedding photo, the flower-garlanded groom with his hands clasped in front, the bride decked in red and gold finery standing to his left, Hanif felt demoralized. He was disappointed in Mahesh, who he realized did not have the guts to stay in Max's shoes. Hanif sighed loudly, and as he pushed the photo back into the envelope, he had the feeling that all the heroism and brio had slipped out of the world.

Rezana was shocked at Mahesh's letter. While she had imagined a splendid reunion with her family on the occasion of Mahesh's wedding, they had carried on without her. In one stroke her link with the past had snapped.

In October 1965, Rezana received a telegram from Mahesh. Motilal had died of a cardiac arrest. Immediately Rezana started packing. Her mother, her brothers and sisters, surely they needed her. She would go to them and as they grieved together all the bitterness would evaporate. But with the war between India and Pakistan just over, the Indian government refused the entry permit. Rezana grew frantic and angry. Haunted as though by a tenacious ghost, she longed for Bombay. She felt the pull of an entire city, an entire country. 'I hate Pakistan,' she said to Hanif, who was busy telephoning friends, trying to find someone who might know a high-ranking official in the Indian government.

In 1968 there was another telegram from Mahesh. Harshaba died suddenly, of no apparent cause. Again the Indian government declined the travel permits. But this time Rezana endured the news with resignation. She told Saleem and Sobia who were both teenagers in high school that her mother had died, but there was no reason to cancel their upcoming family vacation that they had been looking forward to for some time.

In the months after her mother's passing, Rezana received a letter from Saroj. It was a short impersonal note, penned hurriedly, conveying snippets of news about herself.

Opening Saroj's letter brought unwelcome memories of the day she had struck her face. For years, Rezana could think of her only with hostility. Yet now, in Saroj's written words there was nothing but friendship and, strangely, even a hint of remorse. *If you choose not to write back, I'll understand . . .* Rezana considered the letter a peace offering and sat down to write a reply immediately. How would it be, to see Saroj again?

ಬಬ

Rezana started following the news of India and Pakistan's turbulent relationship more closely. She prayed for the issue of Kashmir to be resolved. At the slightest lull in the news, she believed the animosity would soon end and the borders would be thrown open.

Three years later, in 1971, there was another war, this time over the independence of East Pakistan, when Dacca, tired of the resource exploitation by and the political hegemony of West Pakistan, declared Bangladesh a separate Muslim state and Islamabad sent in the armed forces to reinforce its control. Pro-Independence leaders and sympathizers were slaughtered. India sided with Bangladesh. In Karachi, they stayed locked inside their three-storey house. They covered the windows with black paper, and when the black paper ran out they used brown paper bags and pages of old magazines. Air-raid sirens screamed incessantly. At night the sky lit up with anti-aircraft fire. Mobs shouted in the alleyways. Each night in the darkness they feared for their lives; at dawn, if the lines were working, they phoned their friends around the city.

Terrified, too, for her family in Bombay, Rezana prayed the Pakistani fighter pilots would miss their targets, for the Muslim army to back down against India's superior forces. She kept the radio on all the time. Every hour she waited for the news that Pakistan had surrendered. She read all the newspapers. A US warship was deployed in the Indian Ocean, its missiles aimed at Pakistan? Or India? It was difficult to tell. Commentators said the Cold War had got hot as the US, the Soviet Union, and China postured on the sidelines.

After the war, Pakistan was shrouded in disillusionment and uncertainty. Images of the saddened, trounced General Yahya Khan dominated the papers for a few days, finally replaced by photos of the new president, Zulfikar Ali Bhutto, who spoke of democracy, a better Constitution, and a modified parliamentary system. He outlined a plan to negotiate the return of the ninety-three thousand prisoners of war and a peaceful settlement with India. He promised to build a new Pakistan.

Rezana wanted to believe him. She worried about the children's future. Saleem was studying to become a barrister, getting ready to sit for his first-year exams, and Sobia who had grown into a tall, self-assured woman wanted to attend medical college.

Chapter 41

A group of businessmen who had hosted Hanif and Rezana in their homes sponsored Hanif for a concert in the two-tiered auditorium of the National Arts College of Karachi. The day after the sold-out event there was a long, favourable review in the Arts and Events pages of the *Sunday Times*.

Within weeks his voice was being carried on the airwaves of Radio Pakistan. At ten minutes past nine, after the news bulletin, the host of *Melody Night* introduced Hanif Wali Hussein as 'the singer who lays bare his soul, and touches ours'. At home, even before the start of the news bulletin, Rezana turned the radio volume to high. Ammi, Abbu, Saleem, and Sobia were all in the sitting room with her; the two servants stood grinning in the doorway.

In the months following the radio broadcast, Hanif gave performances in Lahore, Peshawar, and Islamabad. His voice took on a subtle humility, an altogether different mellowness that seduced even the most casual listener. He wrote seven new ghazals, each infused with haunting pathos, and with the debut of a record album called *Yaadein*, one side featuring ghazals by Ghalib and Zafar, the other his own compositions, he became Pakistan's most revered artist, a household name.

Rezana, immersed in running the house and teaching at the college, had not stopped yearning for what they had left behind. She visited India often in dreams and daydreams. She vowed to return to Bombay for the next Diwali, for Holi, after Ramadan, after Eid, after the next monsoon. The years slipped by.

ಬಿಬಿ

In India, riots raged against Indira Gandhi's divisive rule and policies. Forced sterilization to control population growth, violation of election laws, mass bulldozing of slums. The list of grievances was long. To preserve her precarious position as Prime Minister, she declared a state of Emergency. With India under military rule, Rezana lost hope of visiting Bombay.

But in 1977 when Mrs Gandhi was finally voted out, there was talk of a cultural exchange between the two nations and Hanif's name came up as the best musician to represent Pakistan. When the Culture Committee approached Hanif, he said he was honoured, but he could not go without his wife. He could not give a performance without her, he said, she was his muse, and they always sang a duet midway through the show.

While Hanif practiced gloriously for his return to India, Rezana kept her enthusiasm in check. Too many times her hopes had been crushed . . . something was sure to get in the way again. Besides, did she really want to go back? How would it feel to have all the years of despair suddenly rush into a full stop? Would the happiness be too much to bear? Battling a hodge-podge of emotions she was struck with an astonishing realization – that Karachi had become home.

But . . . *Bombay!*

VII

HOMECOMING

Chapter 42

Rezana watched Hanif, who was clicking the ballpoint pen beside her on the Air India flight as he read the immigration documents. He wrote 'Pakistan' in the space beside 'Citizen of . . .', and copied their passport numbers on the forms.

It had been a while since she'd had to wrestle with that muddied question of national identity. Born in Hindu India, long-time resident of Muslim Pakistan, Rezana had thought herself hardened by time, and sentiment, about her allegiance. Yes, India was the land of her birth. But Pakistan . . . Pakistan was the place where roses grew in lustrous reds and pinks, where the call of the muezzin at dawn rang pure and soulful, where they owned a beautiful house, in which they had raised and educated their children, and where Hanif's voice had become famous. She belonged to Pakistan. It was a strange feeling arising out of years of struggle and sadness.

'Purpose of visit . . .?' Hanif muttered.

Rezana turned to the window and looked out at the ocean below them, reflecting back through wisps of cloud the sunlight and blue sky around them. 'Music,' she said. 'Put "music". That is the purpose of our visit, isn't it?'

'You think the airport-wallas will understand? Something more, I think. How about . . .'

'You can't write a ghazal there,' she laughed. 'Look at the space on the form and put whatever fits.'

Hanif had no problem standing before thousands of people and singing and making music, but the thought of an immigration officer terrified him. 'Invited by Indian govt. for music programme', he wrote, the last word spilling out of the allotted space. His foot felt for his briefcase, which contained the letter of invitation. Their passports had visas for Bombay and Delhi, which suited their plans, though he was puzzled by the restrictions. His harmonium, cleaned and tuned for the trip, was in the luggage hold and he could only hope its wooden crate would survive airport handling.

The chance to perform in Bombay elated Hanif. It scared him, too, returning as a star to the city that had rejected him and his music. But one glance at Rezana, who looked peacefully out of the cabin window, reassured him. It had been a long journey, not least getting from Karachi to Dubai to pick up a flight the next day to Bombay. India was not disposed to allow direct flights with its neighbour. Rezana had dressed for the trip in a sari, and as she'd stood before the mirror adjusting the pleats, Hanif was reminded of their college days. That first time he'd seen her – the pink sari, the long hair, the chuum-chuum of her anklets – that image had never left his mind. And drinking tea at Café Royal, seeing movies at Metro, strolling along Apollo Bunder, Marine Drive, and the gardens behind the High Court . . . he could will those memories into animation and watch them unfold in his thoughts as radiant dioramas featuring their younger selves. He noticed now the lines and creases around her eyes and cheeks, the slight droop of the lips, but still . . . still the beauty hadn't left her face.

'Finally, back to Bombay,' Hanif said, rubbing his hands together. 'How do you feel?'

'Things must have changed, it won't be the same Bombay,' she said nonchalantly. Inwardly, though, she believed everything had held, that it would all be just as she had left it, that the years wouldn't dare swindle her of this homecoming.

She clenched and unclenched her fingers. Excitement, anger, joy, and disbelief . . . the emotions churned inside her. Mahesh would be at the airport to meet them. She wondered how much he'd changed, and whether there was anything left of 'Max'. The night he'd come for dinner to their house in Bandra was the last time she'd seen him. She distinctly remembered that evening, how he had amazed them all by his intelligence and confidence, and how his visit had prompted Abbu and Hanif to pack up the family and move to Pakistan.

The city began to fill the cabin window. Terraces of apartment buildings, clusters of palm trees, power lines, ribbons of roads, miniature cars and lorries . . . under a bright blue evening sky.

Her heart quickened as she stepped behind Hanif down the rickety metal stairs that rolled up to the plane. They followed the other passengers towards the terminal, the hot wind whisking around them bringing whiffs of jet fuel and burning tar. The evening sky was still a bright blue. She scanned the front of the terminal. People were waving from a terrace where an Indian flag on a flagpole hung from the railing. She squinted at the crowd, but it was difficult to make out individual faces.

They waited in queues to pass through security checks

and passport control. Their papers were in order and she felt relieved as they walked through the wide passageway where brightly coloured advertisements exhorted tourists to the Elephanta Caves, Gateway of India, Kohinoor Silk Centre. Hanif pointed to a picture of a hotel with a swimming pool and said, 'Sun-n-Sand Hotel. Must be new. It looks nice, doesn't it?'

Rezana didn't hear him. They had just emerged into the Arrivals lounge and her mouth was open in shock. She spotted Mahesh at once – a well-dressed, well-built figure, waving enthusiastically at her. Next to him, a striking lady in a bright yellow sari, who Rezana guessed was Nandita, his wife. And with them, standing in welcome, was *everyone* from her family. Saroj and Nalin, Sumitra and Amrita, two men who she surmised were their husbands, children of various ages, and several aunts, uncles, and cousins. Momentarily her eyes stopped on Saroj.

The next instant she was among them, enveloped by their arms and smiles and tears. Giddy with excitement, feeling like a toy top, she was spinning and whirling from one person to the next. She wanted the universe to stop, to allow her a moment to memorize their faces, to file in her mind the glory of this welcome for which she'd hoped and waited so many years. *This* was the unbounded joy of the world. Her eyes grew teary and she gave in to the purity and sanctity of crying. Someone placed a flower garland around her neck. Everyone was talking at once – '. . . this is my husband . . .', '. . . meet my wife . . .', '. . . this is my son . . .', '. . . my daughter . . .' – Rezana didn't know which way to turn. Her brothers and sisters, familiar and strange at the same time; nieces and nephews she'd never met; aunts, uncles, and cousins she'd forgotten about. She couldn't speak, the past twenty-five years suddenly congealed into a lump in her throat.

She looked for Hanif. He'd hung back at first, but now, he, too, wore a marigold garland around his neck and was pulled into the circle of happy commotion.

They stood around in the airport lounge, talking and exclaiming. Finally, someone said it was time to go home, and they piled into the procession of cars and headed for Versova. Mahesh drove Hanif and Rezana in his Fiat.

Hanif got in the front and watched Mahesh close Rezana's door and then get in the driver's seat. Mahesh in his mid-fifties had lost the litheness of his youth, but in his trousers and bush shirt, sunglasses, and hair styled in a wave, he still had the swagger that Hanif remembered from their days in America.

From the airport the narrow rutted road took them past an industrial complex before suddenly putting them on a wide, tree-lined strip. 'This is the new airport highway,' Mahesh said, as he changed gears. 'But you'll see, every two minutes there are traffic signals. This is what's holding up India.

'The farmers are doing well, but the crops they grow can't get to the markets in a timely fashion because the roads are horrible. Our factories produce surplus, but we can't get the stuff to our ports, which don't work anyway because they retain a coolie mentality in a containerized world. Look there,' Manesh tapped Hanif's elbow and pointed to some workmen with shovels on the opposite side of the road.

'Those are men from the telephone exchange laying new cables. Tomorrow there will be men from the electric company digging the same hole . . . But the phone and electricity lines won't be going to your house or business unless you've paid the right "fee". Do you know what I mean?'

Hanif clicked his tongue. 'Pakistan's the same, even worse. We end up paying for things we don't want. Politicians are everywhere, with their hand out, interfering. The solution—'

'Solution?' Mahesh laughed again.

Rezana rolled down the window and felt the warm, heavy air rushing past the car. It smelled just like Karachi, the complex mix of scents, some sweet, but underscored by a cloying note of rot and decay. They drove past a busy hutment colony, and a shabby and almost deserted hotel, and the Parle Bottling Company, trucks spanning two-decades of models pulling in and out. After a few kilometres they left the stop-go airport highway and entered a road lined with tenement blocks where clothes were drying on balconies barely wide enough for a flowerpot. Small shops at street level spilled their wares onto the footpath. Big billboards promoted Hindi films – *Khoon Pasina*, *Anurodh*, *Amar Akbar Anthony*. A poster advertised Saridon analgesic tablets. Lamp-posts were festooned with small triangular symbols promoting birth control and family planning.

'. . . That black Chevy was a first class car,' Mahesh said. 'Do you remember how we drove from New York to Boston? Good fun, wasn't it?' Glancing quickly at Rezana in the rear-view mirror, he added, 'You should have seen Hanif's face during that trip. He was so scared.'

'I wasn't scared,' Hanif said. 'I was . . .'

'You were *scared* . . . admit it. Eliza and her world scared you. I thought you'd jump out of your skin when she tried to shake your hand. And her father and mother . . . they are an odd couple, I agree.' The car stopped at a railway crossing, where bells rang and lights flashed; a man stood next to the boom barrier, which he began to raise once the track was clear. He was slow, and the abrupt clamour of car horns made Rezana cover her ears.

'Who is Eliza?' Rezana asked.

'You don't know about Eliza?' Mahesh said.

'No.'

'You kept my secret, Hanif. Thank you. You're a good man. Who's Eliza? She is married now to a politician husband, a senator, and has four children. Nandita has met her, and they get along well. We're all good friends now.'

'But who is Eliza?' Rezana said.

'Eliza Wiswall,' Mahesh said. 'It's a long story. I used to be Max in those days . . .'

Hanif wondered if Mahesh regretted not marrying Eliza. From the expression on his face Hanif surmised that he might still be in love with her. What had happened? Perhaps it had ended when Mahesh told his parents. Clearly, he had opted for the more straightforward path. Hanif looked directly at him, and Mahesh, aware of this scrutiny, sighed heavily and kept looking in front.

'That's new,' Mahesh said, pointing to a square, modern-looking building, the Oscar Ambar Theater. 'Nandita likes Hindi movies, but I only like American films . . .'

Rezana recognized the bus depot, and the road leading up to it that was congested with taxis, rickshaws, double-decker buses, and traffic-dodging pedestrians. She searched for more familiar landmarks and there was the Nadco General Store, its front now enclosed with glass and sporting a modern neon sign, and Ahura Bakery, where her father had ordered an enormous, round cake for her tenth birthday, with chocolate icing and rings of white sugar roses. Her mother was angry, because the cake contained eggs and good Hindus didn't eat eggs, but she looked happy when she ate a big slice of it anyway and said it was good.

After the main bazaar, they drove past Ramji Mandir, the whitewashed temple that housed statues of Rama and Sita. She'd forgotten about the temple, but now recalled coconut offerings and sandalwood incense and conch shells and was surprised when she realized she had unconsciously joined her hands and bowed her head . . .

Past Navrang Cinema, past the road that led to Bhavan's College, past Dena Bank . . . Rezana kept looking for telltale signs of the old Bombay. But the city of her memories seemed to be eluding her, escaping around every bend just as she thought she had her bearings. On the long stretch of road to Versova, she felt even more disorientated. She waited for the marshland and quicksand, and the water buffaloes that lazed in the murky water, and the stick thin boys who tended them. But the marshland and quicksand and water buffaloes were gone, replaced by tracts of housing stretching endlessly on either side.

'All reclaimed land . . .' said Mahesh, watching her reaction in the mirror. He pointed to a row of expensive apartment buildings, each with its own little compound that contained either a swimming pool or well-tended garden, and each with its own guards. 'Bombay is growing, you see.'

To Rezana, Bombay seemed to have shrunk, the crowds, the shops, the buildings, everything, bearing down on her, stifling her. The roads didn't look as wide as she remembered. And the sky wasn't the clear blue of her memories, but seemed to be brushed by a gauzy haze. Versova was smaller than she remembered. She closed her eyes, and tried to ignore the constant honking of horns and the jostling traffic along what had once been such a solitary road. Mahesh and Hanif were talking and laughing. She felt the car slow to a halt on crunching gravel and heard the creak of big iron gates opening, but she kept her eyes closed. She concentrated on the sound of more crunching gravel, and waited for the tyres to lock and slide to a stop.

'Here we are,' said Mahesh, shutting off the engine with a final, throaty rev. 'Welcome, Hanif, to Sagar Mahal. And with your permission, my friend ... for the sake of convenience ... welcome to you, too, Rohini. Here you are Rohini, not Rezana. There are simply too many people who know you as you were, and it will take time for them to know who you are now ... so, if I may beg you this indulgence ...?'

Hanif smiled and, seeing the amusement on Rezana's face at her brother's eloquent request, told Mahesh that they were only here for five days and did not want to waste time with confusion. He knew her people would never call her Rezana, but they'd work it out, so there was no point making a thing of it. 'Maybe I should change my name to Hasmukh ... or Harshad?'

Rezana leapt out of the car and in one breath took it all in – the fountains, the palms, the jasmines, the terraces, and the house, which was still the same pastel yellow. Behind the house, she could see the endless sea. There was no horizon that evening, only a blur where sea and sky came together. The setting sun was leaving a lustrous glow in the sky.

She looked down as she walked towards the porch. The asphalt had split and weeds had sprouted through. For a few minutes they were caught up in the commotion of everyone returning from the airport, children darting here and there, and their luggage being unloaded from the car and sent to their room.

'Was Shrikant-bhai at the airport?' Rezana asked Mahesh. 'I didn't see him.'

'No,' Mahesh said. 'He couldn't come.'

As she and Hanif were shown to the guest room on the second floor, Rezana gripped the banister. The wood felt smooth and strong. The windows with the patterned glass panes, the tall carved doors, the mosaic tile on the floors, the cut-glass chandeliers . . . all this she remembered. The furniture – a sofa, a table by the wall, a lamp in the corner – there was much she recognized. But somehow everything looked different. The word 'neglect', or some connotation of it, came to her mind. She looked around more deliberately. The floor mosaic was chipped and gouged in places, the chandeliers dim and dusty. The sofa that once had bright floral upholstery was now covered in orange vinyl. The mirror on the dressing table was cloudy around the corners; the window grills crusty with rust. She noticed the sloughed-off paint on the walls, a two-year-old calendar that no one had bothered to remove, and an electrical wire from a light switch exposed and stapled to the wall.

What Rezana didn't know was that the family fortunes

were dwindling. Just before Motilal died, his silk business had suffered a major setback. Polyester had appeared on the scene and was fast becoming the new rage. Motilal refused to invest in different machinery and looms. 'Artificial fabric! Bah! Never!' he said to his business associates. In the proxy fight for his silk mills he lost the majority share.

Rezana turned to Hanif now, to judge his reaction. He'd never asked about the house and between them the opulence of Sagar Mahal had been taken for granted. She felt embarrassed, and braced herself for the disappointment on Hanif's face. But Hanif, busy unpacking his harmonium, didn't seem concerned with the decor.

They went down to the divankhana where everyone had gathered before dinner. There were trays of cold drinks and platters of fried snacks. Rezana wanted a hot cup of tea, but felt awkward about asking one of the servants. She sat on the sofa next to Saroj, Sumitra and Amrita in chairs across from them.

Rezana's eyes went to the porcelain statue of the Chinese man on the side table, to his long flowing beard, red lips, and thin black moustache. He had withstood the passage of years; no rambunctious child had knocked him over. Had the statue been brought back on an opium ship by her grandfather? Should she now loathe this revered childhood object? Did her sisters know the family history? She stared at the statue, the family talisman, the silent accomplice in the workings of their lives.

Amrita said, 'You come after more than twenty years and we get to see you for five days!' Still the fair, rosy skin, Rezana noticed, the same warmth in her voice.

Rezana glanced at Amrita's diamond earrings and necklace. Obviously Amrita had married into a wealthy family. Rezana said, 'I know, five days is a short time. Next year, we'll plan it differently.'

'Your husband is quite famous,' Saroj said.

Rezana glanced at Saroj. What was that in her tone – a trace of sarcasm or jealousy? But Saroj smiled, and Rezana knew, even as the searing image of being hit by her sister flooded her thoughts, that Saroj had put the bitterness behind her. Saroj looked old, her hair completely grey, the years marked in the many lines on her puffy face.

'You must tell us about Pakistan,' Sumitra said. 'We heard you eat mutton. Do you actually cook it?'

Rezana nodded resignedly. What could she tell them about Pakistan? That sometimes they were treated as second-class citizens because they were immigrants from across the border? That a bearded man had thrown a writhing calf at her feet and shouted an obscenity? Could she tell her sisters about the time she and Hanif had witnessed bomb blasts at the cricket stadium? Hanif had gripped her hand and they had charged out of one of the back gates, but the next day they learned that the stadium had turned into an execution ground and dozens of people were killed, not from bombs but from police gunfire. Could she tell her sisters about how their cloth mill had been looted and Hanif, Abbu, and Anwar-babu had been held at gunpoint? No . . . she would tell her sisters only about the beautiful parks in Karachi, the tranquil grounds at Mazar-E-Jinnah, the American-made bridges and tree-lined roads, the fancy markets and shops on Tariq Road, the *biryani-wallas* in Bohri Bazaar. She would tell them about the ancient archeological sites of Mohenjo-daro and Harappa, and the verdant resorts of Murree, Quetta, Gilgit, and Swat.

'Have you brought photos of the children?'

Rezana nodded. 'I'll bring out the album tomorrow. By the way, I haven't seen Shrikant-bhai, where is he?'

Saroj, Amrita, and Sumitra looked at each other. No one answered.

Saroj said, 'Next time you must visit me in Dantali. But if you bring Hanif-bhai with you to Dantali,' she cleared her throat. 'In our house—'

Rezana smiled awkwardly at her. 'Don't worry, we can always meet here. You like coming to Bombay, don't you?' There was an affinity between the four sisters that had held despite their estrangement. But Rezana sensed they were keeping something from her, something that the three of them had shared and was now camouflaged by the passage of years.

Indeed, there were some things no one wanted to discuss. These contentious subjects were best left buried deep below the bedrock of the house. For instance, no one could tell Rohini that, a few months after she'd eloped with Hanif, Jag's parents asked for Amrita's hand in marriage for their son. On the wedding night, however, Jag disappeared. The rumour was he had started drinking copiously, and, the next day rushed off to South Africa and never returned. It was difficult to say what Amrita felt; she was sixteen at the time, and with her naturally cheerful disposition was good at concealing her emotions. Eventually, she married a man from Surat and everyone forgot about her very short marriage to Jag.

And no one wanted to discuss the whole matter of their father, Motilal, and his two concubines, Chandrika and Mridula, both young and exquisitely beautiful. He'd installed them in houses in Ahmedabad, within a kilometre of each other, and provided them with money to live comfortably. Chandrika had borne him a son and a daughter, and Mridula, two sons. When Motilal passed away the two women and their children appeared in Bombay, and while everyone was shocked, Harshaba let them sit among the other mourners in their white saris, and endured the tears they both shed for her husband. But now, Harshaba too had died. Chandrika and Mridula never visited Bombay again, and nobody talked about them anymore.

Finally, there was the matter of the fake funeral. A daughter of the house had done the unthinkable – she had married a Muslim. Unable to bear the shame, her parents told the world she had died.

All this was hidden under the bedrock and what reason was there to bring up such stories now, during this happy reunion?

Amrita said, 'That's right. Any excuse and Saroj is here in Bombay.' She laughed lightly. 'Even if Rohini comes to Dantali, what will she do there, Saroj? Go with you to the village library that has four books on the shelves? Rohini, did you know, Saroj is now president of the Dantali library?'

Saroj glared at Amrita and said, 'We have almost twenty thousand books! It's actually quite peaceful in Dantali. It's a good life there.'

Rezana stood up to look for Hanif. She walked to the far side of the divankhana, past the big marble pillars. From here, beyond the front verandahs, she could see the outlines of the fountain, the lotus pond, and the bougainvillea creeping over the compound wall. The ebbing evening light threw shadows here and there. Soon the insects would start their droning. For a moment she felt as though she had never left, that nothing had changed. She tried to will herself into an alternate reality in which she was nineteen again, and Sagar Mahal was glorious and familiar. She wanted to go outside, sit on the bench alone, and fill herself with the salty evening.

She noticed Saroj coming behind her, and stopped as she reached for the light switch. The glow from the chandelier came down softly and, as it did, it brought up a large oil portrait of Harshaba and Motilal. Harshaba sitting upright in a chair, her sari covering her hair, a slight smile on her lips; and Motilal in a dhoti and long coat, a turban wrapped smartly around his head. He stood behind her, his hand resting self-consciously on the chair. In muted shades of brown and maroon, it was a carefully done portrait exuding a certain intimacy, as though the artist had adopted the role of a biographer – Harshaba's pugnacious chin, her too-serious disposition, her fierce gaze; and Motilal's distinctive forehead, his perfect nose, his regal demeanor – it was all there, extracted and made into art.

Rezana gasped and stood motionless before the portrait. She hadn't seen her parents since 1947, when she was nineteen. And now here they were before her, older versions of her father and mother, created with brush strokes, immortalized in paint. For years she had tried to imagine their faces and hold on to some memory of their physical forms. She looked again at the portrait and felt oddly relieved.

She had the urge to pray. The words 'Allah-O-Akbar' started in her mind, but instead of the prayer came a childhood memory – the bright, hot morning when her father was arriving from Ahmedabad and she had accompanied her mother to the station. With their platform tickets in hand they walked past the benches marked 'European Ladies', to the ones marked 'Indian Ladies', and before the train pulled in they spent a few minutes eating peanuts that Harshaba purchased from a kiosk. As a young girl she had hardly gone anywhere alone with her mother and a routine trip to the station had seemed unusual to her even then. After the peanuts she was thirsty but knew better than to ask for a glass of lemon water from the cart. She'd never forgotten the image of her father stepping off the train, how confident and stately he looked, and the easy smile that came to his face when he saw them.

Rezana gazed at the portrait again, more critically. Harshaba and Motilal appeared mythical, at once larger than life, but also absurd caricatures of what she remembered as their real selves. She tried to imagine her mother singing the morning prayers, her father joining in at the last verse, but the sounds of their voices eluded her. Had they forgiven her? Had they come to understand that what she had done was not out of malice towards them? Everything is predetermined, her mother believed, we live out the pains and pleasures of our past lives. In her mother's eyes now she might see the flicker of forgiveness she had long coveted. Surely it resided, howsoever minutely, in the hazy shading of her painted irises. But Rezana didn't dare look closer. She sniffled and reaching for the handkerchief tucked into her sari at the waist dabbed her eyes and nose.

Saroj put her arm around Rezana, held her for a moment, then tried to lead her away. Saroj regretted finding those love letters in the armoire, carefully hidden behind Rohini's clothes. If only she had left them there and kept quiet. Every time Saroj visited Bombay, from the minute the train pulled into the station, she would scan the crowds. She assumed each slender figure of medium height, with a long thick plait of hair down her back, was Rohini. She would focus intently on such figures, excitement bubbling inside her, and when it turned out to be someone else, the excitement fizzled, until she spotted another slender, medium height figure with long hair. In this bubbling-fizzling state she passed her days in Bombay before returning to Dantali.

Once the curiosity to visit Rohini's house in Bandra became unbearable. She decided to go in the afternoon; they would drink tea together and she would tell Rohini she was sorry about everything. She would find Rohini cheerful and content in her new life – and this, Saroj imagined, would absolve the guilt she wore around her neck like an amulet.

Saroj took a bus to Bandra station and walked all the way to Carter Road. On the way, she kept practicing the phrases – Salaam Alaykum, Khuda Hafiz. For hours she roamed up and down the footpaths, but, ultimately, she didn't dare look for the side road past Bandra Talkies where she knew Rohini lived. She returned to Versova late that evening, the sound of her mother's warning – *no one will talk about Rohini, we have nothing to do with her, we will not mention her name in this house* – ringing in her ears. After that, Saroj recognized the problem with herself – the ability to face danger and adversity without qualm was missing in her constitution. Now, with her arm around Rohini, she tried to understand the extent of her sister's courage and resilience. Saroj's fingers tightened around her sister's shoulders, the pressure conveying what she felt for her – admiration, affection, and envy.

Hanif stood away from the sofa and walked towards them. He had known this would be an emotional visit for his wife. He remembered the times she cried at night as they lay in bed, and how her gulps and sniffles would pierce his heart. Once he'd jokingly told her to stop crying because he was tired of wringing out handkerchiefs, and even in the darkness he had sensed her smiling through the tears. He thought that his own family had made up for the loss of her old home, but now, seeing her here, among her own people, he felt humbled. He had worked hard to provide her with a comfortable life, but he realized now that more than money and material luxuries, it was something much deeper, an intangible connection to home and family that defined who she was. His eyes searched her face for a long moment. He wondered whether she still considered herself a part of them. Or had the years apart forced her to subdue and relinquish those feelings of attachment? He thought about the Rezana with whom he'd discussed music, the Rezana who was usually deliberate and enthusiastic and tireless. The Rezana now standing near him seemed withered and weakened and there was nothing he could say to lighten her mood.

Saroj directed Rezana's attention to the opposite end of the room. Here, on the wall, flanked by two cut-glass lamps with dusty silk-fringed shades, hung a large framed sepia photo – about forty people, men standing in the back row, their wives in front of them, the children kneeling or sitting cross-legged on the ground. Motilal and his brother were in the centre, their wives and daughters on either side, and, behind everyone, the house as the backdrop.

Saroj beckoned Hanif to come closer. 'Look, this is Rohini. She must have been twelve or thirteen years old.'

Hanif smiled broadly, arched his eyebrows, and gazed at the photo, taking in the whole family before focusing on the figure Saroj pointed to. He looked back and forth between Rezana and the photo. 'Yes, yes, the resemblance is there. I see it,' he announced. 'What a face it was, even then!' he added teasingly.

Rezana had forgotten about the photo, but now squinting as she tried to identify the others, she recalled the day when everyone had come to the house early in the morning. A thick fog had rolled in from the beach, so the photographer had waited an hour or two, and when the light was right, it had taken a long time to organize everyone in their correct positions. She was amazed that the photo was still here in the same frame on the same wall.

It suddenly occurred to Saroj that Harshaba had not fully succeeded in expunging Rohini from the family, though she had gone to great lengths. Rohini's clothes were packed and sent out of the house. After the cremation the ashes from the effigy were scattered in the Ganges. The jewellery in Rohini's trousseau was sent to the jeweller with instructions to melt and recast and reset everything. How carefully her mother had attempted to erase Rohini's existence. Was the photo an oversight? Saroj imagined her mother in the photographer's shop, instructing him to open the frame and blot out Rohini's image. Perhaps the photographer had convinced Harshaba it was impossible. Or perhaps Harshaba purposely wanted to preserve a tiny memory of her daughter.

Saroj said, 'Tomorrow evening, we've planned a party in your honour. The Kapoors will be coming, and several others.'

'Dr Kapoor?' Rezana asked.

'He passed away a few years ago,' Saroj said. 'His son and his family still live in Versova, although not in the same house. Actually, the house isn't even there. They've built a tall apartment building on the property.'

'Versova has changed,' Rezana said sadly.

Mahesh joined them. 'Why don't we have a ghazal night tomorrow?' He looked at Hanif enthusiastically. 'What do you say?'

'Where?' Rezana asked. 'Here?'

'Of course,' Mahesh said. 'A private performance, here, in Sagar Mahal! Hanif, think of it as a dress rehearsal for your show.'

'Yes! It's a great idea,' Rezana said.

Mahesh said. 'Why don't we invite your friend from college? Pervez? Does he still live in Bombay?'

'Pervez is in Karachi,' Hanif said. 'He's been there since Partition.'

'What's he doing in Karachi?'

'Well, he's married and has a family. He runs a big hotel now.' Hanif told them of Pervez's involvement with the Communist Party – the underground meetings, the weapons, and his part in organizing riots around Bombay.

'So, what happened? Was he arrested?' Mahesh said.

'No. My father and I took him to the dockyard where my

uncle was an officer, and Pervez boarded a ship bound for Oman. From Oman, he made his way to Karachi by bus and on foot – imagine! On the way he came down with typhoid and almost died. In Karachi our relatives took care of him. After some months he wanted to immigrate to the Soviet Union, but he was turned back at the border. My uncle finally got him a job and he ended up settling in Karachi.'

'What about his communist activities?' Mahesh said.

'Nothing. He joined a small communist cell in Karachi, but nothing happened. He had some grandiose notion of organizing the peasants in a mass uprising – like in China. But people were scared in Pakistan. One never knew which hit list one was on, and when the government was watching. Not to mention the mullahs. By the time we got to Pakistan in '56, Pervez had given up all that. And today, if you see him today,' Hanif gestured with his hands, making a large circle in the air, 'you would never imagine the man used to be a communist. He lives in a fancy house in Clifton, servants, cars, everything. Always, the finest European suits. His wife is a dress designer; she studied in Paris and speaks fluent French. And you should see the big parties at his house. Where he gets the Scotch, no one knows. Friends in the American embassy, probably.'

Mahesh folded his arms over his chest. 'If I come to Karachi, I would like to meet Pervez,' he said, amused.

Rezana said to Hanif, 'I want to show you my room, come.' She led him out to the verandah and then down a hallway.

Mahesh's son, Bimal, appeared at the door. Twenty years old, he was tall and lean, in blue jeans, and a black t-shirt.

Rezana knew he was studying to be an architect. 'Come in, come in, no need to knock,' Bimal said. The sound of rock music set at low volume came from a stereo behind him. Before closing the door, he called a servant and gave instructions for drinks and ice.

The mosquitoes, the heat and dust, and the general dilapidation of the house were nowhere to be found in Bimal's room. An air conditioner hummed quietly, the off-white walls matched the off-white sofa. Showpieces – a brass Nataraj, an ivory elephant, and a few abstract sculptures – were placed carefully in the built-in cabinetry that held the stereo. Recessed lights from the ceiling shone down, illuminating the space smartly, but quietly. The smell of aftershave or perfume trailed the air.

A girl stood near the stereo looking through the records. She turned as they entered. 'This is Tejal,' Bimal said. 'We're in college together.' With his foot he pushed aside the high-heeled sandals she'd taken off and left by the door.

Tejal shook hands with them. In jeans and kurta and big silver earrings she wore her long hair loose, the front strands falling around her face. With her bangles jingling on her wrist, she flipped the hair back in a smooth, seductive gesture. Rezana smiled to herself. When she was in college she could never have dreamed of having a male friend in this room. Even letters from a male friend had caused such trouble . . .

The servant entered carrying a tray with four glasses and a jug of iced lemon squash. Bimal moved aside the vase of flowers on the table to make room for the tray. Rezana and Hanif sat in the armchairs; Bimal and Tejal, not the slightest bit self-conscious, sat together on the small sofa across from them.

Rezana's eyes wandered around the room that was nothing like the space she remembered. She could hardly believe the transformation. Briefly she felt resentful, but told herself that at least Bimal had taken the trouble to update a small part of the house.

Bimal noticed her studying the room. 'Well, what do you think?'

'It's tasteful and modern,' Rezana said. 'You will be a good architect.'

Through the open doorway, her eyes wandered to the bedroom. She immediately recognized the armoire, though it had been refinished in a lighter stain, and recalled the letters wrapped in silken *rumals* sequestered among petticoats and saris.

Hanif said jokingly, 'What? The room wasn't like this when you lived here?'

'No, not at all.' Rezana focused on the corner, near the window, and she pointed to it. 'My desk was there. And there was bookcase next to it.'

'Ah, yes, let me show you,' Bimal said, walking towards the built-in cabinetry. He threw open one of the cabinets below the stereo. 'I've kept the books. I thought they would be collector's items one day.'

Rezana stood up slowly and stepped to the cabinet, bending to look at the books. She gasped softly as she ran her fingers over the tired spines. Picking out a book she fanned through the pages. She didn't notice the tattered front cover, or the discoloured paper inside. Glancing at Bimal with grateful eyes, she pulled out another book. 'You can take them,' Bimal said, 'I'll have them packed up for you.'

The door opened. Saroj and Amrita stood in the doorway. 'Dinner will be ready soon,' Saroj said.

Tejal smiled at Rezana. 'Over dinner you can tell me how you and Hanif-uncle met and how you both got married.' Tejal raised a hand to her forehead, flipped her hair back. 'I've heard it's quite a story.'

'Over dinner? That won't be enough time,' Hanif laughed. 'Be prepared to stay up all night, Tejal. It's a long story, almost as long as the Ramayana.'

Rezana felt Amrita's hand on her elbow. Amrita said, 'Let's take a stroll in the back garden before dinner.'

In the corridor, they ran into Shrikant and his wife, Prema.

'I've been looking for you,' Rezana attempted to bow as a gesture of respect, but he moved aside.

Shrikant and Prema didn't say a word and waited for Rezana to pass in the corridor.

'What's happened? Don't you recognize me?' Rezana asked.

There was a long pause. Shrikant, in a white kurta over beige trousers, a small arc of white hair on his balding head, had grown thin and stooped. He wore black-framed spectacles and his white moustache dropped around his small mouth into a tufty white beard on his chin. Prema, in an orange sari, her neck and arms decked with gold jewellery, a big orange bindi on her forehead, and orange lipstick, looked glamourous next to him.

'Okay, let's go,' Amrita finally mumbled and took Rezana's hand to lead her out.

Shrikant clicked his tongue. 'I know who you are,' he said, coolly. 'You used to be part of this family until you ran off with a Mussalman. Do you have any idea of what we went through? Without a backward glance you carried out your selfish plan. What good did it do you?' Shrikant glared at Rezana. 'Ha, I hear he's some third-rate harmonium player with a thick voice. Good, you deserve each other. Muslims like you should stay on the other side of the border! Everyone here may be happy to see you but I don't care. I cannot accept you as my sister.' He took a step back, and then raising his voice, added, 'Let me tell you something else.' His jaw slipped into an awkward angle, 'As far as I'm concerned, you're dead.'

Rezana was stunned. She glanced towards the dining room for Hanif, then at Prema, who seemed taken aback by her husband's outburst. Amrita tightened her grip on Rezana's arm, 'Come on, come on, let's go,' she said, pulling her away.

One night, many years ago, along with three of his cronies Shrikant had attacked her house in Bandra. He had in mind minor harassment – throwing stones on the windows, shouting insults – he had never meant to enter the house – but on the way there, in the taxi, one of his friends produced a knife and sticks and a small can of kerosene. 'We'll teach those Muslim pigs a lesson,' the friend laughed, and, as the others in the taxi cheered and whooped, Shrikant found himself drawn into the bravado of the little mob. But the plan fell through – perhaps the taxi driver went to the police station after he dropped the foursome at the corner of Carter Road – and when the police arrived on the scene, Shrikant ran all the way to Bandra station without stopping or looking back for his friends.

After that, unlike Mahesh who had roundly argued with

Motilal and Harshaba about performing the mock cremation, Shrikant supported his parents' decision. As the dutiful eldest son, he went to Haridwar for the final prayers, and immersed the urn of ashes into the Ganges.

'Don't pay any attention to him,' Amrita whispered to Rezana. 'He's become Member of Parliament, so he thinks too much of himself. Just forget about him.'

But Rezana couldn't stop thinking about Shrikant. His words, and the hateful expression on his face stayed in her thoughts as she quickened her steps to keep up with Amrita.

The lulling rhythm of the waves came to them before they reached the compound wall. Tinted in darkness, the air was thick with the smell of spray, drying fish, and, every once in a while, a sudden tang of burning garbage. Their saris billowed with the breeze as they stood at the wall and gazed out, their silhouettes diminutive against the sky and the sea. There was a half moon that night and its glow came down on the water in a slow, lazy streak. Along the coastline to the south, the bright busy lights from apartment buildings and the television tower at Worli interrupted the darkness, but to the north, towards the fishing village and the Portuguese fort on the hill, the night hung calm and complacent. It was as though modernity and progress stretched on one side, tradition and history on the other, and their house, the grand Sagar Mahal, stood stranded in the middle.

'It's always beautiful here, isn't it?' Amrita said. 'My husband and I live at Marine Drive, and we have an excellent view from our flat, but this . . . this is something else.' She threw her arms towards the scene. 'What about your house in Pakistan? Do you live by the sea shore?'

Rezana shook her head and rested a hand on Amrita's arm, and Amrita understood from the gesture that her sister didn't want to talk. They stayed by the wall for several moments, staring at the sea in silence. Rezana wondered what she should have said to Shrikant. *Whatever you feel about me, about Muslims, I'll always think of you as my brother –* she wished she could have said that. She understood the shame and anguish she had brought upon her people, but surely, now, thirty years after Partition, she could be forgiven. Perhaps during her next visit to Bombay, Shrikant would be different, but she knew this was unlikely even as she imagined it . . .

Tomorrow Hanif would sing in the grand hall and his ghazals could turn the minds of enemies. She closed her eyes and as a wearied peace settled in her head, she lifted her chin to the breeze and to the softly heaving sea.

Acknowledgements

Creating a novel is mostly done in isolation. But this book would not exist were it not for the kindness and brilliance of many people.

Renuka Chatterjee, Dharini Bhaskar, and the team at Westland. Thank you for your interest in this novel and imposing on it your exacting standards.

Rita Juster. If it weren't for you, I would never have written fiction.

Nancy Allen. Thank you for your careful comments on every chapter.

Victor Rangel-Ribeiro. Thanks for showing me the 'germ' of my story.

Writing group friends – Jane Saginaw, Kaleta Doolin, Lauren Embrey, Trea Yip, Julie Hersh, Donna Wilhelm, Sudeshna Baksi-Lahiri, Linda Weinberg, and Eden Elieff. Thank you for sharing your talent and love for stories.

My gratitude to the teachers and students at the Iowa Summer Writers' Workshop, and the Bread Loaf Writers' Conference. Jan Pendleton – thanks for telling me to develop the music of the novel.

Hedgebrook Writer's Retreat. Thank you for the gift of quiet days of writing, and most of all, thank you for helping me believe in myself as a writer.

Larry and Claudia Allums. Your encouragement and assurance fuelled my confidence. And, members of the Dallas Institute Book Group, you won't believe how often I felt as though I were writing for each of you.

Marly Rusoff. Thank you for your enthusiasm, for reading numerous drafts and offering invaluable critique.

Toby Tompkins and Deborah Artman. Thanks for nurturing the manuscript during its early stages.

Tim Cribb. Your wisdom, judgment, and intrepid editing have made this a better book.

Niti and Saurin Patel. Thanks for intelligent as well as banal discussions. Had we but world enough, and time . . .

Satchit Srinivasan. Your friendship has been a steady wind in my sails.

Harish. Thanks for constantly reminding me of who I am. Where would I be without your affection?

Jai, Kirun, Sarath, and Monica. You have influenced me more than you know. It is an honour to be your mother.

Raghu. From the beginning, how astutely you critiqued the manuscript . . . every page bears your trace. And, one more thing: In this lifetime there is nothing better than being your wife; but you gave me space and time and dignity to be a writer as well. Thank you.